Basic Medical Statistics

Basic Medical Statistics

ANITA K. BAHN, Sc.D., M.D.

Associate Professor of Biostatistics,
Department of Community and Preventive Medicine,
Medical College of Pennsylvania, Philadelphia, Pennsylvania;
Department of Medicine, Washington Hospital Center, Washington, D. C.

Grune & Stratton

New York and London

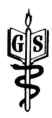

Library of Congress Cataloging in Publication Data
Bahn, Anita K.
    Basic medical statistics.

    Includes bibliographical references.
    1. Medical statistics. I. Title. [DNLM:
1. Biometry. 2. Statistics. HA 29 B151b 1972]
RA409.B34   519.5′02′461   72-6822
ISBN 0-8089-0782-4

Grune & Stratton, Inc.
111 Fifth Avenue
New York, New York 10003

Library of Congress Catalog Card Number 72-6822
International Standard Book Number 0-8089-0782-4
Printed in the United States of America

Preface

Statistics need not be awesome! As I have emphasized in my lectures to physicians, medical students, nurses, social workers, and scientists, a few basic concepts underlie all statistical reasoning. If these few concepts are thoroughly understood and the proper framework laid, the different statistical formulas can be appreciated as but variations on the same theme applied to different situations.

My "obsession" in writing this text was to gradually and logically develop a holistic view of what statistics is all about, to "guarantee" that the least quantitatively inclined reader could attain sufficient statistical comprehension to follow the research aspects of current medical literature and conduct simple statistical tests.

To achieve these ends, the text provides a semiprogrammed type of self-learning and testing experience. In each chapter, the "lecture" is followed by (1) exercises, both the true-and-false type and numerical problems with step-by-step solutions and discussions, (2) a summary of the chapter, and (3) glossaries of new terms and of symbols. Cumulative reviews interspersed at critical points as the story unfolds aid the reader in synthesizing the material. Chapter 16 provides a synopsis of all the statistical methods presented. The last chapter (Chapter 17) offers a potpourri of exercises with solutions as a final "test" of comprehension. The many examples drawn from both classical and current literature in medicine and the health sciences confront the reader with the practicality of what he is studying.

The first twelve chapters of this book were serialized in *The Woman Physician* (now the *Journal of the American Medical Women's Association*), beginning with the September 1969 issue. The enthusiastic response from the journal's readers has been most gratifying. The many requests from these readers for the entire set of twelve articles and the successful use of this text in mimeographed form by a number of schools of medicine and allied health in this country and abroad have prompted the updating of these articles and their publication, with five concluding chapters, as this book.

The content and illustrative examples of this text reflect the author's view that statistics is best taught initially "in one piece" to further understanding of the cohesiveness of basic principles and to demonstrate their application to all of medicine — the basic sciences of genetics, pharmacology, microbiology, physiology, anatomy, and clinical medicine — as well as their traditional role as tool in epidemiology and public health. Further discussion of epidemiologic concepts and methods may be found in a forthcoming book by Judith S. Mausner and Anita K. Bahn entitled *Epidemiology and Preventive Medicine,* as well as in other works on this subject.

ACKNOWLEDGMENTS

This material is dedicated to two truly eminent women: Margaret Merrell, Sc.D., an outstanding teacher of biostatistics, whose lectures at the Johns Hopkins University School of Hygiene and Public Health served as the model for much of this material; and Katherine Boucot Sturgis, M.D., who foresaw that continued self-education of medical students and physicians requires training in biostatistics.

The training program in epidemiology and biostatistics which led to the writing of this book was supported under grants PHT6-76 and 5 DO4 AH 00676.

Permission for use of illustrative material was generously granted by Dr. Merrell, by John Fertig, Ph.D., of Columbia University School of Public Health and Administrative Medicine, by Colin White, M.B., of Yale University School of Medicine, by Peter Armitage, Ph.D., of the London School of Hygiene and Tropical Medicine, and by others as indicated in the text.

I want to express my appreciation to the class of 1971 of the Medical College of Pennsylvania for stimulating the preparation of these written lectures and to the class of 1972 for "testing" the original draft. I also wish to thank my colleagues Hyman Menduke, Ph.D., Judith Mausner, M.D., M.P.H., Mrs. Lucy Goldman, M.Sc., Mrs. Gladys Nigro, B.S., and Carol Currier, M.D., for invaluable suggestions and criticism.

I am grateful to the Publications Committee of the *Journal of the American Medical Women's Association (The Woman Physician)* for suggesting the initial series of articles on which this text is based and for permission to reproduce the first twelve chapters of this book, and I am indebted to Dorothy Macy, Jr., M.D., Associate Editor of that journal for invaluable editorial advice in the early preparation of this manuscript.

I also wish to acknowledge the helpful criticism of the final manuscript by Joseph Ciminera, Ph.D., of Merck, Sharp & Dohme. I am particularly indebted for advice and suggestions to Nathan Mantel, M.A., National Cancer Institute, National Institutes of Health, Department of Health, Education and Welfare, and the University of Pittsburgh School of Public Health.

I am indebted to the Literary Executor of the late Sir Ronald A. Fisher, F.R.S., to Dr. Frank Yates, F.R.S., and to Oliver and Boyd Ltd., Edinburgh, for permission to reprint Tables III, V, and XXXIII from their book *Statistical Tables for Biological, Agricultural and Medical Research,* sixth edition, 1963.

Finally, I wish to thank Mrs. Eleanor Burne and Mrs. Virginia Jensen for their invaluable typing and secretarial assistance.

ANITA K. BAHN, Sc.D., M.D.

Contents

1

Introduction

Role of Statistics: Important Differences Versus Significant Differences • Qualitative Versus Quantitative Data • Populations and Samples • Bias; Precision and Accuracy • Use of Controls (Retrospective and Prospective Studies)

ROLE OF STATISTICS

How can statistics help the physician? Let us take an example: Suppose Treatment A is tried on one sample of patients and Treatment B on another comparable group of patients. A difference in outcome is observed. There are two questions that the physician must pose: first, Is this difference large enough to be important? This decision, the statistician cannot help with since it is based on clinical judgment. If the answer is, "Yes, the difference is *large* enough to be of interest," a second question should follow: Is it a *real* difference? Equivalent ways of stating the second question are: Could the difference be explained by *chance alone*? Is the difference *statistically significant*?

The second decision is one in which statistical reasoning can aid by use of a few concepts which revolve around the central theme: the evaluation of the factor of chance. Such evaluation is often done intuitively by the physician when he says: "This outcome is based on too few cases for us to be certain," or "Treatment A does appear to be better than Treatment B." In the following chapters, we will develop a formal procedure by which the physician can make

decisions of this type in the face of uncertainty, with a predetermined error risk.

QUALITATIVE VS. QUANTITATIVE DATA

Another general concept is that data can be classified into two major types: *qualitative and quantitative*. Qualitative data relate to attributes or categories into which persons or things can be classified, such as sex, race, immune status —items one can enumerate or count, or record as "yes" or "no", binomial or multinomial data. Such data give rise to *discrete* or *discontinuous* distributions (there can be 3 survivals, but not $3\frac{1}{2}$). In contrast, quantitative data result from measurement. Typically, we are concerned with a *continuous* variable such as height, weight, enzyme output.[1] For example, there are an infinite number of possible points along a continuum of height: our calibrating instrument determines how finely we can distinguish these points.

In these chapters, qualitative data will be discussed first and then quantitative data. It will

[1] Certain discrete variables such as number of teeth also may be considered as "quantitative".

become apparent, however, that there are many similarities.

POPULATIONS AND SAMPLES

A *population* is the entire group about which information is desired (a synonym is *universe*). The population may consist of a breed of mice, or children in a community or one school. Within the population there is *biological variation* so that one cannot predict with certainty the outcome of a procedure or the physiologic response of an individual.

Suppose we wish to study a physiologic response in a particular population. The population is called *homogeneous* if no further subdivision is necessary for appropriate analysis. It is *heterogeneous* if it can be subdivided on the basis of some characteristic (such as age or sex) into subgroups that differ significantly among themselves, with respect to that response.

If it were feasible or economical to study an entire population, or if there were no biological variability, there would be little need for most of the statistical methods that will be described. Usually, however, one must depend on only a portion of the population, or *sample,* about which information is actually obtained. If the sample is properly drawn, it is possible to make inferences from it to the entire population, with a known level of "confidence". A leading presidential candidate in the 1968 election discounted the results of public opinion polls solely "because they involve only about 3,000 people across the country." The candidate was way off base on purely statistical grounds.

With appropriate procedures inference can be made from small samples to population values. *Random sampling* is a procedure for selecting a sample which gives every item in the population a known opportunity *(probability)* of being selected. If each item has the *same* opportunity of selection, then it is called *simple* random sampling. Examples of this are drawing a name from a lottery, or selecting a case number by use of a table of random numbers. Table I-1 lists some random numbers and illustrates their use. More complex sampling procedures may involve *stratifying* a population on the basis of some characteristic such as income, or geography *(chunk sampling)* and then randomly sampling within each group at either equal or different rates. Samples such as nationwide public opinion polls use a combination of methods for efficiency.

BIAS; PRECISION AND ACCURACY

One of the most important dangers in sampling, questionnaire construction, or any other statistical procedure, is *bias*. Bias may be defined as a systematic difference between a population or true value and the corresponding value derived from samples taken from that population (bias does not necessarily involve *prejudice*, which is a state of mind of an individual that leads to a desire for a particular outcome). Bias can occur where the entire population one wishes to make inference to is not included in the sampling frame (i.e., part of the population has a *zero* probability of being selected). A well known example is the *Literary Digest* survey for the 1936 presidential election which purported to sample the total voting population, yet excluded persons without telephones (note that it was not the *number* of persons sampled that led to biased results). Sometimes a study is biased because one is not measuring the specific item one had intended (e.g., surveying a voting attitude when one is really interested in surveying a voting behavior). Thus it is important to delineate carefully the objective of the study and what is to be measured.

Another major source of systematic error is *nonresponse*. Nonrespondents may differ from respondents with respect to the characteristic studied — data from a health examination survey where there is a high rate of nonparticipation may be considerably biased because of self-selection of participants on the basis of their health. Another type of bias occurs when incorrect information is obtained from the respondent, consciously or unconsciously, or because questions are poorly phrased. Bias may also result from improper methods of tabulating or analyzing data. I hope that the reader will become aware of the common methodological pitfalls that lead to bias.

Two other terms frequently used are *precision* and *accuracy*. Precision refers to variation among repeated measurements of the same object, such as the consistency between first and second measurements of an observer's counts.

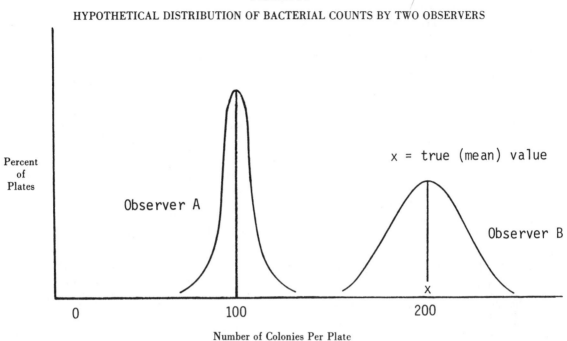

FIGURE 1-1

HYPOTHETICAL DISTRIBUTION OF BACTERIAL COUNTS BY TWO OBSERVERS

Percent of Plates

Observer A

x = true (mean) value

Observer B

x

0   100   200

Number of Colonies Per Plate

Accuracy, on the other hand, refers to the closeness with which measured values agree with "true" values. In Figure 1-1 it can be seen that Observer A is more consistent in his bacterial counts than is Observer B (Observer A's counts tend to agree with each other and show less variability), and yet A's counts are always under-estimates (perhaps because he fails to count the colonies on the edge of the Petri dish). Observer B tends to be less consistent, but is more accurate (his counts are closer to the true value).

USE OF CONTROLS

Before concluding this general overview of statistical methods, below is a still-too-common type of fallacy, quoted from a recent newspaper article:

"HEART ATTACK SURVEY FINDS DANGER IS TO LAZY MAN . . .

A statistical jolt has been dealt to the widely held idea that . . . ambitious and hard-driving males are more prone to heart attacks than more relaxed ones . . . Drs. . . . investigated all the persons under 50 in a community of 1 million population who died of heart attacks within one year. There

were 133 of them, 122 men and 11 women. Their statistics indicated quite the opposite. A statistical preponderance of the <u>122</u> youngish heart attack males presented a 'picture of indolence,' they reported. This picture was highlighted by physical inactivity and habitual peace of mind. '<u>Sixty-six</u> per cent customarily occupied themselves, for the most part, with television, reading and visiting when not at work,' . . . <u>Twenty-seven per cent</u> were slightly more ambitious and were generally busy with such activities as house repair, light carpentry, and gardening during the evenings and on weekends. <u>Eight per cent</u> performed heavy carpentry, cement work and other arduous labor on their own time . . ."

Would you agree with the authors' interpretation? What other data do you need to arrive at the conclusion that indolence leads to heart attack? Does not one need comparable data on the percentages "indolent", "slightly more ambitious", and "heavy worker" among those who <u>did not</u> suffer a heart attack (i.e., a *control group*)? Perhaps the majority of males under 50 today engage in little physical activity, and the proportion of lazy persons is even higher among the noncardiac cases. Thus either a comparison must be made of cardiac and noncardiac cases by level of physical activity (a *retrospective* or *case-control* study), or the relative risks of a heart attack must be determined by following a large population of "exercisers" and "non-exercisers" (a *prospective* study).

The topic of controls brings us full circle to one of our first questions: Is an observed difference between two treatment groups statistically significant? In answering this question, use is made of a type of "control" — the probability distribution of chance differences under the assumption that no true difference exists (the *null hypothesis*). Against this probability distribution our observed outcome is evaluated. If it is very unlikely that such an outcome could occur if the null hypothesis were true, then the hypothesis is rejected and the alternative hypothesis, that a true difference exists, is accepted.

In the next chapter, we shall discuss how probability distributions are generated and their use in significance tests.

PROBLEMS AND SOLUTIONS

A note to the Reader —

The exercises at the end of each chapter are an integral part of the presentation. The reader is urged to "dig" into these exercises since only through application of statistical principles and logic to real problems in medicine can one test and reinforce understanding of concepts. At the very least every problem should be read and the answer reviewed. Omit computations not needed for checking or for appreciation of the reasonableness of the answer. The *principle* is more important than the arithmetic.

PROBLEM 1-1

Suppose you were interested in estimating the immunization status with respect to polio myelitis of children aged 6 and 7 in a large city. The following proposals for selecting the sample were offered:

(a) Children found upon inquiry at every tenth house in the city

(b) Children drawn by lot from public school records of 6 and 7 year olds

(c) Family contacts to chicken pox

---

*To help you with your computations, a table of squares, square roots, and reciprocals is shown in the Appendix (Table E, p. 246).

(d) Family contacts to diphtheria cases

Discuss briefly your views with regard to each of these suggestions.

ANSWER 1-1

(a) Children found upon inquiry at every tenth house in the city: this method will result in the most "representative"[1] sample of the methods proposed but it is the most time-consuming and costly. It may involve listing of all houses to draw a sample, call backs, transportation, enumerator expense, as well as visits to houses without 6 and 7 year old children.

(b) Children drawn by lot from public school records of 6 and 7 year olds: the sample cannot be representative of all children, primarily because it will exclude children attending private and parochial schools. In some cities, this group may be relatively large. If the survey is extended to these children, the sample representation would be adequate even though a small number not attending school due to physical or mental handicaps are excluded. This method would be much more practical than a house survey. It would probably be necessary, however, to obtain the information from the parents of the sample children by questionnaire.

(c) Family contacts to chicken pox cases: the chief difficulty with this method is selection due to differential reporting of chicken pox. Cases are not likely to be reported unless there is a physician; reported cases, therefore, may be correlated with medical care and immunization. Also, "only" children rarely would be included.

(d) Family contacts to diphtheria cases: this proposal is much worse than (c). Major problems are (1) the very small number of diphtheria cases today and (2) the almost certain inverse relation between the occurrence of diphtheria and polio immunization. This would lead to a gross underestimate of the true proportion immunized.

PROBLEM 1-2

Explain the *fallacy* in logic of the following statement:

"Each year, more men are seriously injured or killed in the United States in manufacturing

---

[1]This type of sampling, called *systematic*, could lead to bias if every tenth house is a corner house with a higher-income family.

	Industry	
	A	B
Number of industrial fatalities per year	100	50
Average number employed in the industry	10,000	1,000
Rate or *risk* of an industrial fatality per year	$\dfrac{100}{10,000} = .01$	$\dfrac{50}{1,000} = .05$

This illustrates the common fallacy of the lack of a *denominator*. A denominator is needed to form an appropriate *rate* in order to evaluate risk.

---

plants than in mines. Hence, we must discount claims by officials of mining unions that mining is more hazardous than is manufacturing in general."

ANSWER 1-2

Two groups cannot be compared as to *risk* of an event, such as accident, simply by comparing the number of events. In the hypothetical example above, industry B has the higher risk of industrial fatality (.05 compared with .01) but since many more persons are employed in A, the number of industrial fatalities is higher in A.

PROBLEM 1-3

A simple random sample is always a good representative of the population.
True or *False?*

ANSWER 1-3

False. On the *average* a simple random sample will provide an unbiased estimate of the characteristics of the population, and, therefore, will be representative of it. However, any one sample may have values that are not typical.

PROBLEM 1-4

Explain the *fallacy* in logic of the following statement:

"In a recent study of several hundred men, none of whom had been exposed to gunfire or what we normally consider intense industrial noise (all had been sewing machine operators in the garment trade for 30 years or more), more than 90 per cent had a very marked hearing loss at the higher test frequencies and more than two thirds had a noticeable hearing loss at the speech frequencies. The effect of heavy industrial noise on hearing is well known; on the basis of this recent information, it is evident that prolonged exposure to noise even as mild as the whirring of sewing machines has a deleterious effect on hearing."

ANSWER 1-4

This statement illustrates the fallacy of the lack of a "control" or normal group for comparison. It is possible that the same degree of hearing loss occurs as a "natural" part of the aging process and can be just as readily demonstrated in occupational groups exposed to even less noise than sewing machine operators.

TABLE I-1

USE OF A TABLE OF RANDOM NUMBERS

Problem: Given a population of 90 cases, to select a random sample of 20 cases.

Procedure: 1. Arbitrarily assign a number to each case from 01 to 90.

2. On the table of random numbers, arbitrarily pick a 2-digit column.

3. With closed eyes, select a random start in that column.

4. Beginning with the starting number, continue to sequentially select every 2-digit number in that column (and in the next 2-digit column, if necessary) until 20 cases have been selected.

5. In the event a random number not included in the sequence 01 to 90 occurs (e.g., 98), skip that number and proceed to the next random number listed.

6. Similarly, if a random number already used occurs again, disregard it and continue to the next random number listed.

7. To assure that a number is not picked twice, keep some record in numerical sequence of numbers selected.

Example: In the tenth 2-digit column, a blindfold random start is made with the number 61. The 20 numbers used to select the sample are shown by check mark. Numbers not used lie outside the sequence 01 to 90, or are repeats, and are crossed through.

(In this example we have moved down a column but we could have chosen to move in some other direction).

25	19	64	82	84	62	74	29	92	24
23	02	41	46	04	44	31	52	43	07
55	85	66	96	28	28	30	62	58	83
68	45	19	69	59	35	14	82	56	80
69	31	46	29	85	18	88	26	95	54
37	31	61	28	98	94	61	47	03	10
66	42	19	24	94	13	13	38	69	96
33	65	78	12	35	91	59	11	38	44
76	32	06	19	35	22	95	30	19	29
43	33	42	02	59	20	39	84	95	61 ✓
28	31	93	43	94	87	73	19	38	47 ✓
97	19	21	63	34	69	33	17	03	02 ✓
82	80	37	14	20	56	39	59	89	63 ✓
03	68	03	13	60	64	13	09	37	11 ✓
65	16	58	11	01	98	78	80	63	23 ✓
24	65	58	57	04	18	62	85	28	24 ✓
02	72	64	07	75	85	66	48	38	73 ✓
79	16	78	63	99	43	61	00	66	42 ✓
04	75	14	93	39	68	52	16	83	34 ✓
40	64	64	57	60	97	00	12	91	33 ✓
06	27	07	34	26	01	52	48	69	57 ✓
62	40	03	87	10	96	88	22	46	04̶
00	98	48	18	97	91	51	63	27	00̶
50	64	19	18	91	98	55	83	46	09 ✓
38	54	52	25	78	01	98	00	89	85 ✓
46	86	80	97	78	65	12	64	64	70 ✓
90	72	92	93	10	09	12	81	93	00̶
66	21	41	77	60	99	35	72	61	22 ✓
87	05	46	52	76	89	96	34	22	37 ✓
46	90	61	03	06	89	85	33	22	80 ✓
11	88	53	06	09	81	83	33	98	29 ✓
11	05	92	06	97	68	82	34	08	83 ✓
33	94	24	20	28	62	42	07	12	63
24	89	74	75	61	61	02	73	36	85
15	19	74	67	23	61	38	93	73	68
05	64	12	70	88	80	58	35	06	88
57	49	36	44	06	74	93	55	39	26
77	82	96	96	97	60	42	17	18	48
24	10	70	06	51	59	62	37	95	42
50	00	07	78	23	49	54	36	85	14

PROBLEM 1-5

Use the Table of Random Numbers (Table I-1 — preceding page) to select a random sample of 10 cases from the attached list. Determine the proportion who are male in your sample.

(1) Why may your sample differ from the true proportion?

(2) Why in general would you expect a better estimate if the size of the sample (n) were larger?

PROBLEM 1-5

LIST OF CASES AND SEX

CASE NO.—SEX		CASE NO.—SEX		CASE NO.—SEX		CASE NO.—SEX		CASE NO.—SEX	
01	M	11	M	21	M	31	F	41	M
02	M	12	F	22	M	32	F	42	F
03	F	13	M	23	F	33	M	43	M
04	M	14	F	24	M	34	F	44	M
05	F	15	M	25	M	35	M	45	F
06	M	16	F	26	F	36	M	46	M
07	M	17	F	27	M	37	F	47	M
08	F	18	M	28	F	38	M	48	F
09	M	19	F	29	M	39	F	49	F
10	M	20	M	30	M	40	M	50	M

Total No. of cases 50

No. of males 30

Proportion male .60

ANSWER 1-5

(1) The sample proportion may differ from the true proportion because of chance variation (sampling error).

(2) In general, the sample is more likely to be a good representative of the population as the sample size increases because there is greater likelihood of selecting elements from all parts of the distribution.

PROBLEM 1-6

Is the following statement justified?

"In 1920, 10 per cent of the deaths in a certain age group were due to cancer. In 1940, such cancers accounted for 15 per cent of the deaths in the same age group, therefore, the risk of dying from cancer has increased."

ANSWER 1-6

No. The percentages above reflect only proportionate mortality figures. It is possible that the number of deaths from cancer decreased in the 20 year period but that there was an even greater decrease in deaths from other causes. It is essential to compare probabilities of death or death rates in order to make such statements:

$$\text{Death rate} = \frac{\text{Number of deaths during year}}{\text{Number in population exposed to risk of dying}}$$

PROBLEM 1-7

Non-response in a health survey can be properly handled by assuming that non-respondents do not differ from respondents with respect to the characteristics studied. *True* or *False*?

ANSWER 1-7

False. Respondents and non-respondents are "self-selected" groups and, therefore, are likely to differ from each other. Data on the demographic and other characteristics of each group (e.g. age, sex, color, economic status) may provide some insight into factors accounting for non-response. However, the health of the individual may determine his participation in the survey. Non-participants may be too sick to participate or on the other hand may be healthy and, therefore, uninterested in participation. For this reason, it is necessary to obtain a high response rate to avoid bias in the data collected.

PROBLEM 1-8

In a simple random sample every element in the universe has an equal chance of being chosen. *True* or *False*? If *false* state the reason.

ANSWER 1-8

True. In a simple random sample, every element has an <u>equal</u> probability of being selected.

PROBLEM 1-9

In designing a survey, it is sufficient to consider only the sampling design. The construction of the questionnaire is less important since just as many people will overstate a fact as will understate it. *True* or *False*?

ANSWER 1-9

False. A proper sampling design (i.e., protocol for selecting the sample) is not sufficient to obtain the true information. The sampling design and questionnaire complement each other.

A good sampling design will:

(a) provide an estimate of the *sampling error* in the survey (i.e. error due to chance in the sampling process);

(b) assure that certain *non-sampling errors* are eliminated — such as erroneous exclusion from the sampling frame of a group about which reference is to be made.

However, other types of *non-sampling errors* can easily arise. For example, a question can be so phrased that the data obtained will consistently underestimate the true value, that is, result in a systematic error or *bias*. Therefore a well-constructed questionnaire is important also.

PROBLEM 1-10

We wish to assess the effect on the teeth of 5 to 6 year old children of regular use of a toothpaste containing a new ingredient, Q. The children who are to take part have their teeth examined at the beginning of the experiment and are given a dental health score, the D. M. F. index. Each child is instructed in the correct use of the toothpaste and provided with sufficient paste for 12 months' use. Some children receive the new toothpaste containing Q, and others a control paste without Q. After 12 months each child is re-examined and a new value for the D. M. F. index obtained.

Discuss the steps you would advise to ensure a meaningful trial of Q, considering in particular the choice of control toothpaste and assignment of pastes to children. It is possible that children with bad teeth to begin with may respond somewhat differently to Q than those with good teeth.

ANSWER 1-10

In a controlled experiment we attempt to (1) select two groups which will be as similar as possible in all characteristics except that under investigation, (2) exclude as far as possible opportunity for personal preference or other bias in the evaluation of the results. It is recommended, therefore, that:

(a) Groups be formed corresponding to different states of dental health (i.e. low, medium, and high initial D. M. F. score) and test and control pastes be assigned at random to children within these groups.

(b) Control toothpaste be identical in color, taste, smell, and container with the paste containing Q. The parent and child as well as the dentist assessing the final D. M. F. score be unaware which paste has been used.

SUMMARY OF CHAPTER 1

In summary, we have introduced the concepts of:

—statistical significance
—qualitative vs. quantitative data
—random sampling from populations
—precision and accuracy

Also we have noted some major fallacies in reports of medical research:

—lack of a control group
—lack of a denominator
—self-selection of respondents
—clinical trials which are not rigorously designed to minimize bias

CUMULATIVE GLOSSARY I: TERMS

CHAPTER I

Population (Universe)	The entire group about which information is desired.
Sample	That portion of a population about which information is actually obtained.
Bias	A systematic difference between a population value and the corresponding value derived from samples taken from that population. Bias does not necessarily involve prejudice.
Homogeneous Population	No further subdivision of population is necessary for appropriate analysis.
Heterogeneous Population	Population can be subdivided on the basis of a characteristic other than the one under consideration into subgroups that differ significantly among themselves with respect to the item being measured.
Qualitative Data	Data based on the categorization and enumeration of individuals according to some characteristic which they either have or do not have, such as living or dead. Such data are always discrete.
Quantitative Data	Data obtained by measurement, e.g., height or weight. Typically such data are continuous, although they may be discrete.
Continuous Data	Data representing an infinite number of possible points along a continuum.
Discrete Data	Discontinuous data.
Inference	Estimation of population values (parameters) from sample data.
Random Sampling	A method of selecting a sample which gives every element in the population a known opportunity (probability) of being selected for the sample.

Simple Random Sampling	Every element has *equal* probability of selection.
Null Hypothesis	Assumption that no true difference exists, i.e. that the difference is zero.
Significance Test.	A test of the null hypothesis. If the null hypothesis is *rejected* the specified alternative hypothesis is *accepted*.
Control Group	Comparison group for evaluating the effect of an experimental procedure.
Chance	The happening of events, the way in which things occur.
Precision	Consistency of repeated measurements of the same thing.
Accuracy (Validity)	Closeness with which a measured value agrees with the "true" value.
Prospective Study	A study in which a group classified by presence or absence of a factor is *followed* to determine association of the factor with the frequency of occurrence of some subsequent event e.g., the risk of developing a disease.
Retrospective (Case Control study)	A study in which cases and controls (non-cases) are compared as to presence or absence of an *antecedent* factor to determine its association with the risk of developing a disease.
Rate	$$\frac{\text{Number of events (cases) in a period of time}}{\text{Population exposed to the risk of this event}}$$
Sampling Error	Error due to chance in the sampling process resulting in some difference between the sample outcome and the complete count carried out in the same manner.
Non-Sampling (Systematic) Error	Error due to other than chance in conducting a statistical investigation, e.g., bias due to faulty measurement, interviewing method, the design of the questionnaire, interpretation, etc. These errors may be present in a complete count as well as in a sample.

2

Probability;
Binomial Probability Distributions

Probability: Measurement, Limits and Rules • Binomial
Probability Distributions — Tree Diagram • Binomial Probability
Distributions — Binomial Formula

Previously we stated that in evaluating an experiment, the physician must decide whether Treatment A is really different from Treatment B in terms of survival rate. To make this decision, he goes through a negative type of reasoning. "Let us assume there is no true difference *(null hypothesis)*. How often would a difference of this magnitude (or greater) occur just by *chance (sampling* variation)?"

If, under the null hypothesis, such an event occurs very frequently by chance, then he cannot rule out chance as a likely explanation. Although a true difference may exist, there is insufficient evidence of it. On the other hand, if, under the null hypothesis, such an outcome is very unlikely to occur by chance, then he will reject this hypothesis and make the decision that a true difference exists. The risk of error in these decisions will be discussed later along with the formal procedure for decision making.

To determine whether a particular outcome is very likely or unlikely by "chance alone," we need to determine either (1) experimentally, or (2) theoretically, how often all possible outcomes occur in a sampling situation. The result is a *probability distribution* on which we can locate our sample outcome, the observed proportion ($\hat{p}$). We can use the experimental approach by tossing ten coins one million times and graphing the results. Figure 2-1 is a frequency distribution indicating how often, in a million trials of ten tosses, there are 0 heads and 10 tails, one head and nine tails, two heads and eight tails, etc. Similarly, one could over and over again draw cards from a deck, toss dice, or select beads of different colors from a jar.

Alternatively, identical results can be obtained on a theoretical basis through application of the laws of probability and some elementary algebra. We will define and illustrate these laws of probability and from them develop probability distributions.

PROBABILITY:
MEASUREMENT, LIMITS AND RULES

The *probability* of an event is the proportion of all possible events that are of the specified type. There are six possible outcomes of one toss of a die, each of which is equally likely if the die is not loaded. The probability that the number 5 will turn up represents its proportion among all possible outcomes. Since there is only one way in which 5 can turn up, the probability is 1/6:

$$\text{Prob. (5)} = \frac{\text{the number of equally likely ways in which a five can occur}}{\text{total number of equally likely outcomes of a die}} = 1/6$$

Similarly, the probability of death during a year is equal to the number of persons who die during the year divided by the <u>total</u> number at risk of dying (the number who die <u>plus</u> those who survive the year):

$$\text{Prob. (Death)} = \frac{\text{Number who die during year}}{\text{total number at risk of dying during year}} = \frac{\text{no. deceased}}{\text{no. deceased \& survivors}}$$

Probability, thus, can always be represented by a fraction where the numerator is included in (is part of) the denominator. Since the probability of any event is a fraction, it <u>can never be greater</u> than one, or less than zero: $0 \leq p \leq 1$. The limits of probability are 0 and 1.

There are two basic rules for the manipulation of probability: *addition rule* and *multiplication*

rule. Addition applies where the probability relates to: "this *or* that." Multiplication applies where the probability relates to: "this *and* that." Let us consider addition. If two events are mutually exclusive, such as turning up a one or a two on a die, what is the probability that in one toss either a one *or* a two will turn up? It is the *sum of the* probability of each event, $1/6 + 1/6 = 1/3$. Where the events are <u>not</u> mutually exclusive, such as the probability of drawing a heart or an ace from a deck of cards, then it becomes necessary to deduct the overlapping probability (i.e., the probability of an ace of hearts) <u>before</u> addition:

P (Heart <u>or</u> Ace)

(<u>not</u> mutually exclusive events)

P (H)   P (A)

P (H and A)

= P (H) + P (A) - P (H and A)

$= \dfrac{13}{52} + \dfrac{4}{52} - \dfrac{1}{52} = \dfrac{16}{52} = \dfrac{4}{13}$

FIGURE 2-1

PERCENT DISTRIBUTION OF HEADS AND TAILS
FOR ONE MILLION TRIALS OF 10 TOSSES

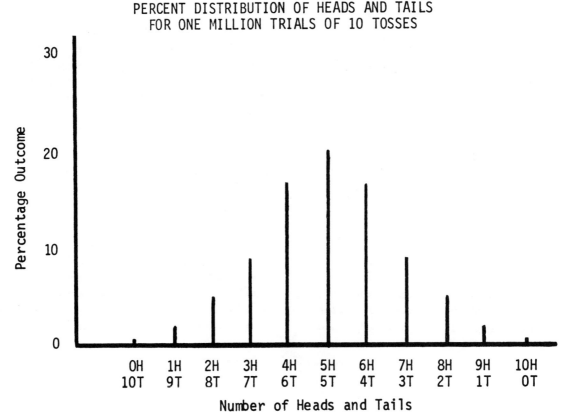

In the *multiplication rule* we have the joint occurrence (*joint or compound probability*) of two or more events, such as the probability of obtaining a head on the first toss of a coin *and* a head on the second. This is equal to the probability of a head on the first toss *multiplied* by the probability of a head on the second toss: $1/2 \times 1/2 = 1/4$. Note that this rule applies, as in coin tosses, where the probability of the first event in no way influences the probability of the second event (i.e., the probabilities are *independent*). As another example, suppose the average probability of death from a disease (i.e., case fatality rate) is 0.2, that is, 2 out of every 10 die. What is the probability of two successive fatal cases? Ans.: $0.2 \times 0.2 = 0.04$.

BINOMIAL PROBABILITY DISTRIBUTIONS — "TREE" DIAGRAM

Let us now use these probability rules to construct a few theoretical probability distributions. The first one we will generate is a *binomial population*. A "binomial population" is a population of two mutually exclusive categories, e.g., a population of 60 per cent males (proportion .60)[1] and 40 per cent females in a class, or a jar filled with 80 per cent green beads and 20 per cent yellow beads. The proportion of either of the two items can be called "p"[2] and the other "1-p" or "q". Note that "p" plus "q" must equal 1. In general we will assume either an infinitely large population, or that samples are replaced before the next draw so that the population proportions remain constant.

We toss one coin an infinite number of times and record each outcome. What will be the frequency or probability distribution of all possible outcomes of the toss of one coin? A single coin toss has only two outcomes — a head or a tail, and each is equally likely. Therefore, the binomial population generated consists of 50 per cent heads and 50 per cent tails ($p = q = 0.5$). Stated another way, the probability of drawing a head from the population is 1/2 and the probability of drawing a tail is 1/2. The population can be represented graphically as shown in Figure 2-2A.

Now let us consider probability distributions called *binomial distributions* generated by drawing

1. A proportion is the same as a percentage with the decimal point moved two places to the left.
2. We will use the label p to refer to the population (true) proportion, and $\hat{p}$ for the sample observed proportion.

samples from this binomial population. Let us first consider a sampling distribution where the sample size is two ($n = 2$). This is equivalent to tossing two coins in succession or drawing two coins from an infinite population of heads and tails. If we had a finite population, the same results would be obtained by sampling with replacement. Since the two events are thus independent, we can use the *multiplication rule*: the probability of obtaining two heads in successive drawings from the binomial population is equal to the probability of a head on the first coin multiplied by the probability of a head on the second: $1/2 \times 1/2 = 1/4$. Similarly, the probability of two successive tails is $1/4$.

The probability of obtaining a head followed by a tail is also $1/2 \times 1/2 = 1/4$, and the probability of obtaining a tail followed by a head is $1/4$. If we do not care in which *order* (*permutation*) the head and tail appear but will accept any *combination* of head and tail, we can then apply the *addition rule*: $1/4 + 1/4 = 1/2$. These probabilities are summarized symbolically in Table 2-1 by use of a "tree" diagram, and graphically in Figure 2-2. Similarly, the binomial distribution is shown for samples of size three ($n = 3$).

Note that all of these distributions, since they are sampling distributions from a binomial population, are called binomial (sampling) distributions. Table 2-2 and Figure 2-3 show binomial distributions where the two items in the binomial population are <u>not</u> in equal proportions, i.e., $p \neq 0.5 \neq q$.

BINOMIAL PROBABILITY DISTRIBUTIONS — BINOMIAL FORMULA

The "tree" method of building a binomial distribution is awkward when the size of the sample is large. We can make use, however of some familiar algebra. Remember "binomials" from high school: $(a+b)^2 = a^2 + 2ab + b^2$. If we call "b" the proportion p in the theoretical binomial population, and "a" the proportion of the remaining group or $q = 1-p$, then we have a formula for $(q + p)^n = q^n + npq^{n-1} + \ldots + p^n = 1$. This gives us the theoretical distribution of outcomes of random trials or samples from a binomial population (see Tables 2-1 and 2-2). Similarly, we can develop from "combinatorial" algebra, an equivalent expression which is very

FIGURE 2-2

PROBABILITY DISTRIBUTION OF OUTCOMES OF n TOSSES OF A COIN

(p = .5, q = .5)

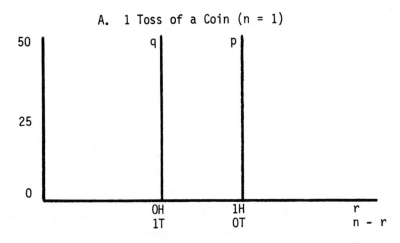

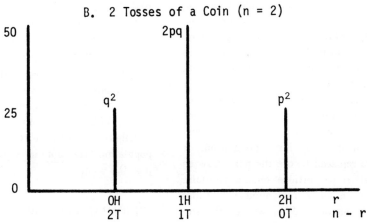

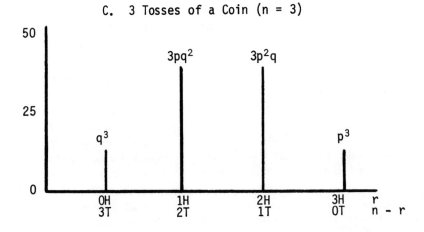

Number of Heads and Tails

TABLE 2-1

"Tree" Diagrams of Outcomes of n Tosses of a Coin
(p = .5, q = .5)

	Permutations (order)	Combinations	Probability

A. 1 Toss of a Coin (n = 1)

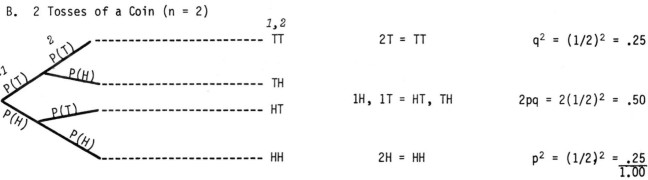

T	T	$q = 1/2 = .5$
H	H	$p = 1/2 = .5$
		$\overline{1.0}$

B. 2 Tosses of a Coin (n = 2)

TT	$2T = TT$	$q^2 = (1/2)^2 = .25$
TH		
HT	$1H, 1T = HT, TH$	$2pq = 2(1/2)^2 = .50$
HH	$2H = HH$	$p^2 = (1/2)^2 = .25$
		$\overline{1.00}$

C. 3 Tosses of a Coin (n = 3)

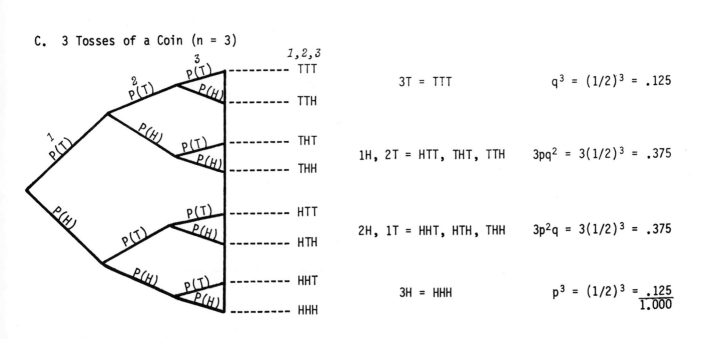

TTT	$3T = TTT$	$q^3 = (1/2)^3 = .125$
TTH		
THT	$1H, 2T = HTT, THT, TTH$	$3pq^2 = 3(1/2)^3 = .375$
THH		
HTT	$2H, 1T = HHT, HTH, THH$	$3p^2q = 3(1/2)^3 = .375$
HTH		
HHT	$3H = HHH$	$p^3 = (1/2)^3 = .125$
HHH		$\overline{1.000}$

FIGURE 2-3

PROBABILITY DISTRIBUTION OF OUTCOMES OF n DRAWS OF A BEAD

(p = .20 green beads, q = .80 red beads)

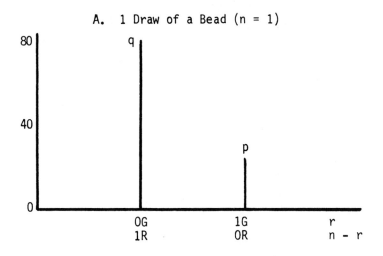

A. 1 Draw of a Bead (n = 1)

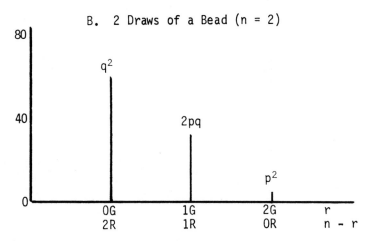

B. 2 Draws of a Bead (n = 2)

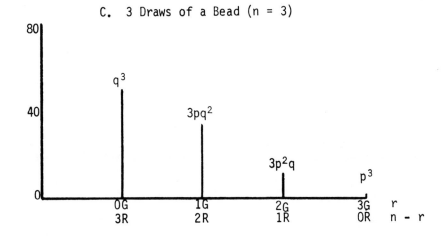

C. 3 Draws of a Bead (n = 3)

TABLE 2-2

"Tree" Diagrams of Outcomes of n Draws of a Bead
(p = .2 green beads, q = .8 red beads)

	Permutations (order)	Combinations	Probability

A. 1 Draw of a Bead (n = 1)

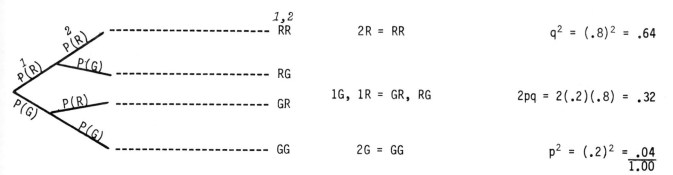

	1 R	R	q = .8
	G	G	p = .2
			1.0

B. 2 Draws of a Bead (n = 2)

	1,2 RR	2R = RR	$q^2 = (.8)^2 = .64$
	RG	1G, 1R = GR, RG	$2pq = 2(.2)(.8) = .32$
	GR		
	GG	2G = GG	$p^2 = (.2)^2 = .04$
			1.00

C. 3 Draws of a Bead (n = 3)

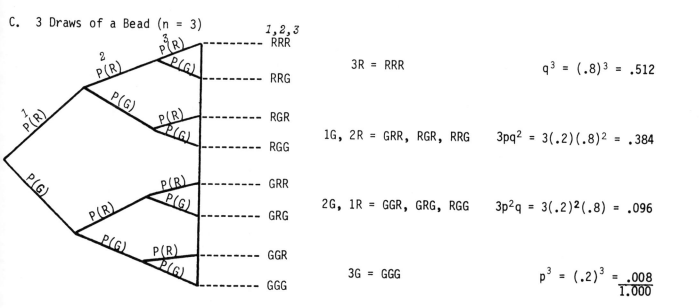

	1,2,3 RRR	3R = RRR	$q^3 = (.8)^3 = .512$
	RRG		
	RGR	1G, 2R = GRR, RGR, RRG	$3pq^2 = 3(.2)(.8)^2 = .384$
	RGG		
	GRR	2G, 1R = GGR, GRG, RGG	$3p^2q = 3(.2)^2(.8) = .096$
	GRG		
	GGR	3G = GGG	$p^3 = (.2)^3 = .008$
	GGG		1.000

easy to use: $\displaystyle\sum_{r=o}^{n} \frac{n!}{r!\,(n\text{-}r)!}\ p^r q^{n\text{-}r}$

  where n = the size of each sample (experiment or trial)

  r = the number of successes in one experiment or trial of size n

  n-r = the number of failures in one experiment or trial of size n

  p = the proportion of successes in the binomial population = probability of success

  q or (1-p) = the proportion of failures in the binomial population = probability of failure

  $\displaystyle\sum_{r=o}^{n}$ means: Sum all terms as r varies from o to n.

The exclamation point (!) is a factorial sign. The factorial of an integer is the product of that number and all successive lower integers (e.g. 3! = 3·2·1 note that 0! = 1).

The coefficient

$\dfrac{n!}{r!\,(n\text{-}r)!}$ of each term $\dfrac{n!}{r!\,(n\text{-}r)!}\ p^r q^{n\text{-}r}$

as it equals (or varies) from 0,1,2, . . . n indicates the number of permutations or ways that a specified outcome can occur. For example, there are three permutation (orders) in which one head and two tails can occur in three tosses of a coin (HTT, THT, TTH). Let us illustrate the use of this formula to determine the distribution of all possible outcomes of 3 tosses of a coin (n = 3). Here n, size of sample =3

  r, number of "successes" or heads, varies from 0 to 3

  n—r, number of "failures" or tails, varies from 3 to 0

  p, proportion of "successes" or heads in the binomial population = 0.5

  q = 1—p = proportion of "failures" or tails in the binomial population = 0.5

Note that "r" and "n-r" must always add to "n", and, as stated above, "p" and "q" must always add to 1.

This is a symmetrical distribution, e.g., P(1 H and 2 T) = P(2 H and 1 T) because p = q = 0.5 (i.e., the binomial population has equal proportions of the two items).

Suppose p and q are not equal. For example, 20% of the beads in a jar are green and 80% are red (p = proportion green = 0.2, and q = 1 — p, the proportion red = 0.8). Then from $\dfrac{n!}{r!\,n\text{-}r!}\ p^r q^{n\text{-}r}$, the terms in the binomial expansion are:

Prob. of 0G and 3R =

$\dfrac{3!}{0!3!}\ (.2)^0\,(.8)^3 = (.8)(.8)(.8) = .512$

Prob. of 1G and 2R =

$\dfrac{3!}{1!2!}\ (.2)^1\,(.8)^2 = 3(.2)(.8)(.8) = .384$

Prob. of 2G and 1R =

$\dfrac{3!}{2!1!}\ (.2)^2\,(.8)^1 = 3(.2)(.2)(.8) = .096$

Prob. of 3G and 0R =

$\dfrac{3!}{3!0!}\ (.2)^3\,(.8)^0 = (.2)(.2)(.2) = \dfrac{.008}{1.000}$

In this case, the distribution is not symmetrical, e.g., Prob. (1G and 2R) ≠ Prob. (1R and 2G) because the proportions of red and green beads differ.

Note that the binomial distribution, like the binomial population, is a series of discrete outcomes (one can have 2 green beads or 3 green beads, but not 2½).

A binomial population is a simple population to describe. If we know just one independent parameter, or constant, e.g., that the proportion (p) of green balls is .40, we can then determine that the proportion of red balls (q) is 1—.40, or .60 (see Figure 2-4). From this we can determine the complete binomial (probability) distribution of sample outcomes for any size of sample from this population. Assumptions of the sampling distribution are that (1) the probability or proportion (p) is constant from trial to trial, (2) the outcome

Prob. of If r=0 : 0 H and 3 T	=	$\dfrac{3!}{0!3!}$ (must agree)	$(.5)^0\,(.5)^3$	=	$\dfrac{\cancel{3}\cdot\cancel{2}\cdot\cancel{1}}{1\cdot\cancel{3}\cdot\cancel{2}\cdot\cancel{1}}\ (\cancel{5})^0\,(.5)^3 = (.5)^3$ Note: $(.5)^0 = 1$	=	.125
Prob. of If r=1 : 1 H and 2 T	=	$\dfrac{3!}{1!2!}$ (must add to 3)	$(.5)^1\,(.5)^2$	=	$\dfrac{3\cdot\cancel{2}\cdot\cancel{1}}{1\cdot\cancel{2}\cdot\cancel{1}}\ (.5)^1\,(.5)^2 = 3(.5)^3$ Note: exponents 1 & 2 add to 3	=	.375
Prob. of If r=2 : 2 H and 1 T	=	$\dfrac{3!}{2!1!}$	$(.5)^2\,(.5)^1$	=	$\dfrac{3\cdot\cancel{2}\cdot\cancel{1}}{\cancel{2}\cdot\cancel{1}\cdot 1}\ (.5)^2\,(.5)^1 = 3(.5)^3$	=	.375
Prob. of If r=3 : 3 H and 0 T	=	$\dfrac{3!}{3!0!}$	$(.5)^3\,(.5)^0$	=	$\dfrac{\cancel{3}\cdot\cancel{2}\cdot\cancel{1}}{\cancel{3}\cdot\cancel{2}\cdot\cancel{1}\cdot 1}\ (.5)^3\,(\cancel{.5})^0 = (.5)^3$ 1	=	$\dfrac{.125}{1.000}$

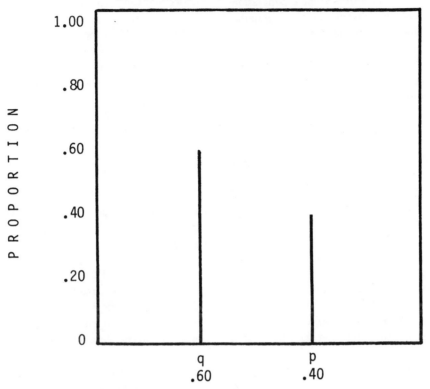

FIGURE 2-4

COMPLETE GRAPHIC DESCRIPTION
OF AN INFINITE BINOMIAL POPULATION

of each trial is independent, and (3) both successes and failures are counted.

By this method, one can obtain the probability of any single outcome readily. When the size of sample n is large, tables of factorials and tables of powers of numbers can assist in the calculations.

How can we use all this in medicine? The exercises provide a glimpse of some practical applications of binomial distributions to medicine and the next chapter continues this theme.

PROBLEM 2-1

2/3 of cardiac patients survive the first myocardial infarct. Of these survivors, 1/3 survive for 10 years. What proportion of all patients with myocardial infarct survive for 10 years?

ANSWER 2-1

This is a joint or compound probability = (Probability of surviving 1st infarct = 2/3) × (Conditional probability of surviving 10 years *if* one survives the first MI = 1/3) = $\frac{2}{3} \times \frac{1}{3} = \frac{2}{9}$

PROBLEM 2-2

Indicate *True* or *False* for each statement below: If *false*, state the reason.

(a) The hypothesis of no true difference is called the Null Hypothesis.

(b) Another way of stating this hypothesis is that the difference observed was caused by chance alone.

(c) In accepting the Null Hypothesis, it is concluded that a true difference does not exist.

(d) In testing the Null Hypothesis, a sample outcome is evaluated against a probability distribution of chance outcomes under the Null Hypothesis.

(e) A probability distribution of chance outcomes under the Null Hypothesis can be determined by experiment only.

ANSWER 2-2

(a) *True*. The hypothesis of no true difference is called the Null Hypothesis. Another way of stating this hypothesis is that two (or more) parameters are really equal. The

Null Hypothesis can be applied to a variety of situations, e.g., we can assert that the **means are equal for two populations; that a sample mean differs from a population mean only by chance; that two popula-tion proportions are equal, etc.**

(b) *True.*

(c) *False.* If the Null Hypothesis is accepted, it does not necessarily mean that there is no true difference but rather that there is insufficient evidence of it under the present experimental conditions.

(d) *True.*

(e) *False.* A probability distribution of chance outcomes under the Null Hypothesis can be determined on both an experimental and theoretical basis.

PROBLEM 2-3

Each of 60 student selects six beads from an infinitely large jar which has 80 per cent yellow beads and 20 per cent red beads.

Indicate *True* or *False* for each of the following statements: If *false*, state the reason:

(a) In this sampling situation the size of each sample (n) is 6.

(b) The number of trials or experiments is 360.

(c) The true proportion, p, is either .8 or .2.

(d) A sampling distribution is a distribution of true proportions around a sample proportion.

(e) In a sampling distribution, each sample is of the same size.

ANSWER 2-3

(a) *True.*

(b) *False.* The number of trials or experiments is 60.

(c) *True.*

(d) *False.* A sampling distribution is a distribution of sample proportions around a *true* proportion.

(e) *True.*

PROBLEM 2-4

The overall case fatality rate previously recorded for a particular disease has been .30. Three successive cases recently admitted to a hospital are fatal. Is it likely that there has been a true increase in fatality rate?

ANSWER 2-4

To answer this question it is necessary to determine the likelihood of three successive deaths under the Null Hypothesis that *there is no change,* i.e., $p = .30$.

In this problem the size of the sample, n, is 3; the outcome or number of deaths, r, is the same as $n = 3$; and p, the probability of death is .30. We then can apply the binomial formula

$$\frac{n!}{r!\ n\text{-}r!}\ p^r q^{n\text{-}r}$$

using the last term of the binomial series as r progresses from $0,1,2, \ldots n$ (i.e., where $r = n = 3$). Thus, $\frac{3!}{3!0!}\ (.3)^3\ (.7)^0 = (.3)^3 = .027$

Since the probability is so small (only 27 in 1,000 times would this occur given the case fatality rate of .30), it is likely that there has been a true increase in this rate.

PROBLEM 2-5

With standard treatment methods, five year survival in a large series of patients has been 50 per cent. Five patients with a particular type and stage of cancer were subjected to a new form of treatment.

(a) If survival under the new treatment were really the same as under the old, what is the probability that all 5 patients would be living at the end of five years?

(b) What is the probability that at least 4 will be living five years or more if the new treatment were really the same as the old treatment?

ANSWER 2-5

(a) The number of patients under study is $n = 5$. The proportion surviving under the old treatment is $p = .50$. The number of survivors is $r = 5$. We use the binomial formula $\frac{n!}{r!\ n\text{-}r!}\ p^r q^{n\text{-}r}$. Since $r = n$ we use the last term in the binomial series.
$\frac{5!}{5!0!}\ (1/2)^5\ (1/2)^0 = (1/2)^5 = \frac{1}{32} = .03$

(b) Since "at least" means 4 or more, we must add the probabilities of 4 and 5 survivors:
$= P(4) + P((5)\ \text{survivors}$
$= \frac{5!}{4!1!}\ (1/2)^4\ (1/2)^1 + \frac{5!}{5!0!}\ (1/2)^5$
$= 5\ (1/2)^5 + (\frac{1}{2})^5$
$= .16 + .03$
$= .19$

PROBLEM 2-6

Determine the distribution of all possible outcomes in 4 tosses of a coin

(a) by completing the "tree" diagram;

(b) by completing the binomial expansion.

A. Tree Diagram

Permutations (Order)*	Combinations	Probability
--TTTT	4T = TTTT	P(0H,4T) = 1/16
--TTTH --TTHT	1H, 3T = HTTT, THTT,	
--- ?	TTHT, TTTH	P(1H,3T) = ?
--THTT --THTH --THHT	2H, 2T = HHTT, HTHT, HTTH,	
--THHH	THHT, THTH, TTHH	P(2H,2T) = 6/16
-- ?		
--HTTH --HTHT --HTHH	? = HHHT, HHTH,	
--HHTT --HHTH	HTHH, THHH	P(3H,1T) = 4/16
--HHHT		
--HHHH	4H = HHHH	P(4H,0T) = 1/16

*16 equally likely outcomes

B. From the Binomial Expansion

$$\frac{n!}{r!(n-r)!} p^r q^{n-r} \text{ where } n = 4 \text{ and } p = 1/2, \ q = 1/2$$

$$P(0H,\ 4T) = \frac{4!}{4!0!} (1/2)^4 (1/2)^0 = (1/2)^4 = 1/16 = .0625$$

$$P(1H,\ 3T) = \frac{4!}{3!1!} (1/2)^3 (1/2)^1 = 4(1/2)^4 = 4/16 = .2500$$

$$P(2H,\ 2T) = \quad ? \quad (1/2)^2 (1/2)^2 = 6(1/2)^4 = 6/16 = .3750$$

$$P(3H,\ 1T) = \frac{4!}{1!3!} (1/2)^1 (1/2)^3 = 4(1/2)^4 = 4/16 = .2500$$

$$P(4H,\ 0T) = \frac{4!}{0!4!} (1/2)^0 (1/2)^4 = \quad ? \quad = 1/16 = \underline{.0625}$$

$$?$$

Problem 2-6 — Continued

Answer:

A. Tree Diagram

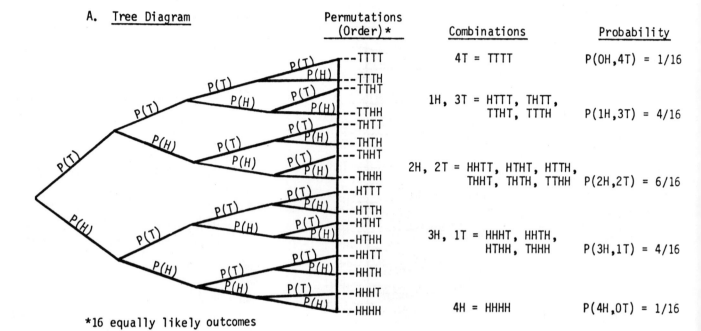

*16 equally likely outcomes

B. From the Binomial Expansion

$$\frac{n!}{r!(n-r)!} p^r q^{n-r} \text{ where } n = 4 \text{ and } p = 1/2, q = 1/2$$

$P(0H, 4T) = \frac{4!}{4!0!} (1/2)^4 (1/2)^0 = (1/2)^4 = 1/16 = .0625$

$P(1H, 3T) = \frac{4!}{3!1!} (1/2)^3 (1/2)^1 = 4(1/2)^4 = 4/16 = .2500$

$P(2H, 2T) = \frac{4!}{2!2!} (1/2)^2 (1/2)^2 = 6(1/2)^4 = 6/16 = .3750$

$P(3H, 1T) = \frac{4!}{1!3!} (1/2)^1 (1/2)^3 = 4(1/2)^4 = 4/16 = .2500$

$P(4H, 0T) = \frac{4!}{0!4!} (1/2)^0 (1/2)^4 = (1/2)^4 = 1/16 = \underline{.0625}$

$$1.0000$$

PROBLEM 2-7

From previous experience on a large series of allergy patients, it had been noted that 2/3 gave a positive reaction to a certain skin test. An allergy clinic tested an average of five patients per day.

What is the possibility that, among any five patients, (a) all will give a positive reaction? (b) three will give a positive reaction (c) two will give a negative reaction? (d) at least one will give a positive reaction?

ANSWER 2-7

The probabilities of outcomes among any 5 such allergy patients can be obtained by the use of the binomial formula $\dfrac{n!}{r!\,n\text{-}r\,!}\ p^r q^{n-r}$

where n = size of sample = 5

p = probability of a positive reaction 2/3

q = probability of a negative reaction 1/3

Therefore, the probabilities on any day are:

(a) P (all, i.e. 5, will give a positive reaction)

$$= \frac{5!}{5!0!}\,(2/3)^5\,(1/3)^0 = \frac{32}{243} = .132$$

(b) P (3 will give a positive reaction)

$$= \frac{5!}{3!2!}\,(2/3)^3\,(1/3)^2 = \frac{80}{243} = .329$$

(c) P (2 will give a negative reaction) This is the same question as (b):

$$= \frac{5!}{3!2!}\,(2/3)^3\,(1/3)^2 = \frac{80}{243} = .329$$

(d) P (that at least 1 will give a positive reaction) This is equivalent to determining the probability of zero positive reactions and subtracting this probability from 1.

$$= 1 - \left(\frac{5!}{0!5!}\,(2/3)^0\,(1/3)^5\right) = 1 - \frac{1}{243} = 1 - .004 = .996$$

PROBLEM 2-8

A virus suspension is prepared, and it is found that when a certain quantity is inoculated into eggs, 25% of the eggs become infected. If a random group of three eggs is inoculated, what are the probabilities that (a) none, (b) one, (c) two, and (d) three eggs become infected?

ANSWER 2-8

It is necessary to determine the probability distribution of outcomes for 3 inoculated eggs, when the probability (p) of an egg becoming infected is .25.

Use the binomial formula $\dfrac{n!}{r!\,(n\text{-}r)\,!}\ p^r q^{n-r}$

where n = size of sample = 3

p = probability that an egg will be infected = .25

q = probability that an egg will not be infected = .75

Then the respective probabilities are:

$$P(0\ \text{infected}) = \frac{3!}{0!3!}\,(.25)^0\,(.75)^3 = .4219$$

$$P(1\ \text{infected}) = \frac{3!}{1!2!}\,(.25)^1\,(.75)^2 = .4219$$

$$P(2\ \text{infected}) = \frac{3!}{2!1!}\,(.25)^2\,(.75)^1 = .1406$$

$$P(3\ \text{infected}) = \frac{3!}{3!0!}\,(.25)^3\,(.25)^0 = \frac{.0156}{1.0000}$$

SUMMARY OF CHAPTER 2

We have developed our first probability distribution, the binomial distribution:

— by experiment

— by theory

We demonstrated some uses of the distribution to evaluate clinical outcomes as well as to predict laboratory results.

CUMULATIVE GLOSSARY I: TERMS

Chapter 2

Sampling Distribution	Frequency distribution of all possible sampling outcomes indicating relative proportion of each.
Probability Distribution	A distribution which indicates the probability of all possible outcomes; the total area under the curve adds to <u>one</u>. May be a sampling distribution.
Probability of an event	Proportion of all possible events that are of the specified type.
Proportion	A fraction, expressed in decimals.
Binomial Population	Population of two mutually exclusive categories, e.g., those with and without specified attribute a.
Binomial Distribution	Frequency distribution (probability distribution) of all possible outcomes when sampling from a binomial population.
Permutation	A selection of terms (objects) arranged in a *specified* order.
Combination	A selection of terms (objects) arranged in *any* order.
Parameter	A fixed figure (quantity) which characterizes a given population.
Joint (Compound) Probability	Probability that two or more events $a, b, c \ldots n$ will occur simultaneously.
Conditional Probability	Probability of event b given that event a occurred.
Independent Events	Events either of whose occurrence in no way influences the probability of occurrence of the other.
Trial	Experiment or sample of specified size n.

CUMULATIVE GLOSSARY II: SYMBOLS

Chapter 2

p True proportion, in a binomial population, of specified attribute a.

q $1-p$ = remaining proportion, in the binomial population, without attribute a.

n Sample size.

r Number of successes, or elements with attribute a, in the sample.

n-r Number of failures, or elements without attribute a, in the sample.

P Symbol for probability (in Chapter 3, a special meaning will be assigned to P). Varies between 0 and 1.

$\hat{p}$ Observed proportion with attribute a in the sample.

$\hat{q}$ Observed proportion without attribute a, in the sample.

Σ (capital Greek letter sigma): take the sum of all terms indicated.

$!$ Factorial sign meaning: the product of that integer and all successive smaller integers. $3! = 3 \times 2 \times 1 = 6$

$\sim$ Approximately

∞ Infinity

$=$ Equals

$\neq$ Does not equal.

$a < b$ a is less than b

$a > b$ a is greater than b

$a \times b$ or $(a)(b)$ Product of a and b

$\therefore$ Therefore

3

Application of Binomial Distribution to Medicine: Comparison of One Sample Proportion with an Expected Proportion (for Small Samples)

Evaluation of a New Treatment • *Evaluation of a Risk Factor*

In the previous chapter, we began our discussion of qualitative data by describing a *binomial population* — a population consisting of only *two* categories — recessive or dominant alleles, living or dead animals, immunized or nonimmunized children.[1]

By drawing repeated samples of a specified size (n) from the binomial population, we generated a sampling distribution — a distribution of sample proportions ($\hat{p}$) around a true proportion (p). This frequency distribution of all possible sample outcomes from a binomial population is called a *binomial distribution*. Since all samples are drawn from the same population, they differ from each other only by chance and their relative frequencies sum to 1.

How can *binomial distributions* be put to use? We shall illustrate one application: to determine whether a proportion for a sample of small size differs significantly from an expected (population) proportion. The illustrations will be (1) the evaluation of a new treatment, and (2) the evaluation of a risk factor.

EVALUATION OF A NEW TREATMENT

Suppose for a particular disease the case fatality rate for many years with the standard treatment is 0.8 (that is, 80% die and 20% survive). A new treatment is tried on three cases and all (100%) survive. Is the new treatment superior to the old? We set up a "straw man", the null hypothesis, or hypothesis of zero difference between new and standard treatments, and see if it can be "knocked down."

How likely is it that <u>if</u> the true fatality rate is still 80% (proportion $0.\overline{8}$) as under the standard treatment, all three cases would have survived? We are dealing here with the binomial formula $\frac{n!}{r!\,(n\text{-}r)!}\,p^r q^{n\text{-}r}$ where

  n (size of sample) $= 3$

  p (probability of survival or success for any one case) $= 0.2$ [1]

  q (probability of death or failure for any one case) $= 0.8$ [1]

  r (number of survivals or successes) $= 3$

n-r (number of deaths or failures) $= 0$

The appropriate term in the binomial series is the last term:

$$\frac{3!}{3!0!}\,(.2)^3\,(.8)^0 = (.2)^3 = .008$$

---

[1]A *multinomial* population can be divided into *more than two* groups — such as a <u>trinomial</u> population of mild, moderate, or severely brain-damaged children. The formula for a trinomial expansion is:

$\frac{n!}{r!s!\,(n\text{-}r\text{-}s)!}\,p^r q^s z^{n\text{-}r\text{-}s}$; p, q and z refer to the proportions of the three terms in the trinomial population and r,s, and (n-r-s) refer to the number of each category in one trial of size n. We will discuss primarily binomial populations.

---

[1]Note that we can designate either probability as p or q. However, p usually refers to the probability of success and q to the probability of failure.

That is, under the standard treatment, in only 8 out of 1,000 trials of 3 cases would all 3 cases survive. The relatively low probability of such an outcome may seem surprising; it would be a very unusual event. Since it is so unlikely, the clinician may conclude that the standard treatment rate does not apply here, that the new treatment is different (better) than the standard, and he may proceed with its use for subsequent cases. The risk of error associated with this decision will be discussed in Chapter 8.

Suppose that out of the 3 experimental cases only 2 had survived. The appropriate "control comparison" then is the probability of <u>at least</u> 2 survivals, i.e., the probability that 2 survive ($r = 2$) or the probability that 3 survive ($r = 3$). By use of the addition rule, this probability is the sum of the last two terms in the binomial series:

$$\text{Prob.}_{(r=2)} \frac{3!}{2!1!}(.2)^2(.8)^1 + \text{Prob.}_{(r=3)} \frac{3!}{3!0!}(.2)^3(.8)^0 = 3(.2)^2(.8)^1 + (.2)^3 = .096 + .008 = .104$$

Thus, given the average survival of 20% ($p = 0.2$) an outcome of 2 or more survivals out of 3 cases is fairly common (occurs 10 times in 100 trials) and could likely be explained by chance, but an outcome of 3 survivals out of 3 cases is rare and suggests that the new treatment is likely to be different.

If the clinician had tested the new procedure on just 2 cases and both had survived, then the "control comparison" would be for $n = 2$ and $r = 2$:

$$\frac{2!}{2!0!}(.2)^2(.8)^0 = (.2)^2 = .04$$

Even this outcome is relatively rare (it occurs in only 4 in 100 trials). A probability of .05 ($P = .05$) arbitrarily may be considered significant. However, the clinician could have determined in advance that he would consider significant only values of $P = .01$ or less. In that case he would decide that .04 is not good enough evidence to change treatment methods. It is possible that with a larger sample, a difference significant at the .01 level may be found. On the other hand, a larger trial may show no difference, or a difference in the <u>opposite</u> direction. One cannot predict the outcome of increasing the size of the sample.

Suppose the standard case fatality rate is only 0.5 instead of 0.8. What would one conclude, then, about the superiority of the new treatment if there are 3 survivals among 3 experimental cases? The probability of such an event under the null hypothesis (that the new treatment is no different than the standard treatment) is $\frac{3!}{3!0!}(.5)^3(.5)^0 = (.5)^3$ or 0.125. Therefore, it would not be unusual to find 3 out of 3 cases surviving if the fatality percentage is only 50%. In contrast, if case fatality is essentially 100%, as in leukemia, then only <u>one</u> survival would demonstrate a superior treatment, since the probability of survival under the standard treatment is zero ($P = .00$).

We have just demonstrated how knowledge of probability can help the clinician evaluate an observed difference between a new treatment and a standard treatment. The question can be rephrased: given a binomial population with 80% deceased and 20% survivors, how unusual is it to find <u>in a sample of 3 from that population,</u> 2 survivors (67%) or 3 survivors (100%)? The binomial formula permits calculations of <u>exact</u> probabilities of such sample outcomes. These probabilities permit evaluation of chance as the explanation of the observed difference between the percent of survivors in the sample ($\hat{p}$) and the expected (population) survival percent, or $p = .20$.

EVALUATION OF A RISK FACTOR

Let us use the same method to evaluate a suggested sex difference in risk of cancer. In a county in one year, among 13 deaths from cancer for children under 1 year of age, there are more female than male deaths (8 vs. 5). Since approximately as many boys as girls are born, one would "expect" an equal sex distribution — theoretically $6\frac{1}{2}$ female and $6\frac{1}{2}$ male cancer deaths, or a probability of 0.5. Can the health officer conclude that there is a sex difference in the risk of dying from cancer among infants?

Let us obtain from the binomial formula, a theoretical (probability) frequency distribution of all possible outcomes of samples of size 13 taken from an infinite population of 50% boys and 50% girls (p and q each 0.5, $n = 13$, and r varies from 0 to 13) (Table 3-1 and Figure 3-1). We then assume the null hypothesis and rephrase the question: If a sample of n $=$ 13 is drawn from a population where the proportion of girls is the same as that of boys (p $=$ 0.5), how *unusual* is a sample outcome of 8 girls and 5 boys?

The term *unusual* involves two important con-cepts: (1) By unusual we really mean at least as unusual as the observed outcome, i.e., as far away from the center or expected value or further (more extreme). While we can determine the probability of any one outcome, e.g., exactly 8 girls

TABLE 3-1

Theoretical Distribution of Outcomes of Trials of Size n $=$ 13 Where p $=$ .5

(r) or (x) No. males	(n-r) or (n-x) No. females	$\dfrac{n!}{r!\,(n\text{-}r)!}\; p^r\, q^{n\text{-}r}$	Probability
0	13	$\dfrac{13!}{0!\,13!}\,(.5)^0\,(.5)^{13}$	$=$ .0001
1	12	$\dfrac{13!}{1!\,12!}\,(.5)^1\,(.5)^{12}$	$=$ .0016
2	11	$\dfrac{13!}{2!\,11!}\,(.5)^2\,(.5)^{11}$	$=$ .0095
3	10	$\dfrac{13!^{*}}{3!\,10!}\,(.5)^3\,(.5)^{10}$	$=$ .0349
4	9		.0873
5	8		.1571
6	7		.2095
7	6		.2095
8	5		.1571
9	4		.0873
10	3		.0349
11	2		.0095
12	1	$\dfrac{13!}{12!\,1!}\,(.5)^{12}\,(.5)^1$	$=$ .0016
13	0	$\dfrac{13!}{13!\,0!}\,(.5)^{13}\,(.5)^0$	$=$ .0001 1.0000

*Example of the calculation of a coefficient

$$\frac{13!}{3!\;10!} = \frac{13.\cancel{12}^{2}.11.\cancel{10!}}{\cancel{3}.\cancel{2}.1. \times \cancel{10!}} = 286$$

Remember

$$0! = 1$$
$$1! = 1$$

FIGURE 3-1

Probability Distribution of Outcomes For Samples of Size 13

$(p = .5, q = .5)$

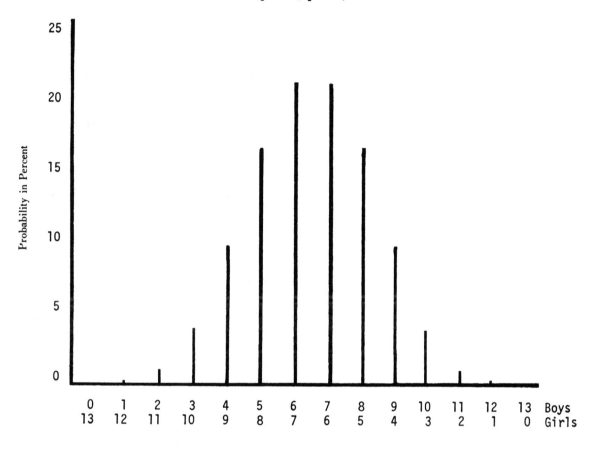

Number of Boys and Girls

in 13 boys and girls, this probability alone is not of interest to us since the outcome only suggests that a true difference might exist. Further, this probability does not provide a very satisfactory test of the null hypothesis because it can be seen from Figure 3-2 that as the sample size (n) increases and approaches infinity, the probability of any <u>one</u> outcome becomes smaller and smaller and approaches zero. Intuitively, therefore, it is necessary to add the probability of <u>all</u> outcomes as unusual as that observed or more unusual, i.e., the entire area of the "tail" <u>beyond</u> the observed outcome in order to test the suggested difference. (2) A second concept is that we must add the probabilities in both <u>tails</u> or directions (*two-tailed test*) when our question is phrased: *Is this difference significant?* The reason is that our question is <u>non-directional</u>. An example of a directional

question would be: Is the proportion of girls with cancer significantly *larger* than expected (0.5)? In the latter case, we would sum the probabilities of only one tail, the tail in which our observed outcome falls. This would be a *one-tailed test,* therefore.

To summarize then, to answer the non-directional question "What is the probability of an event as <u>unusual</u> as this?" we must add up all the probabilities which are as far away from the expected value or <u>further</u> in <u>both</u> directions. We designate this total probability value capital "P". P stands for the summed probability of a result as extreme as that observed or more extreme.[1]

[1]In some texts, this probability is designated p, and the probability of success for any one case or the proportion with an attribute in the population is given a designation other than p, such as Θ (theta) or π (pi).

FIGURE 3-2

Binomial Distribution Approaching Normal: Probability Distribution for Samples of Size n = 2, 4, 8, 16 where p = .5

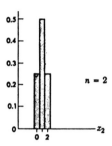

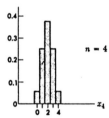

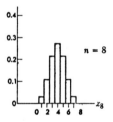

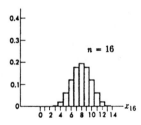

Adapted from Mosteller, Rourke, Thomas; Probability & Statistics Addison-Wesley Company, Inc. 1961

Let us apply this "construct" to our example: We obtain P by adding the probabilities of an outcome of 8, 9 . . . 13 females = .2905 (Table 3-2 and Figure 3-3) plus the probabilities of 5, 4 . . . 0 females = .2905 (note its equivalence to 5, 4 . . . 0 males, and 8, 9 . . . 13 males respectively).

For this problem then P = .58. Thus, in samples of size 13 from a binomial population of p = 0.5, more than one out of two times (exactly 58 out of 100 times), sample proportions as extreme as 8 females and 5 males, or more extreme, would occur just by chance. Therefore, one cannot rule out chance as the likely explanation of the observed outcome. There is insufficient evidence to reject the null hypothesis of equal cancer risk for males and females (p = q = 0.5).

Suppose, instead of 13 deaths in one county, we had 1795 cancer deaths under one year of age in a large state distributed as follows: 987 (55%) male and 808 (45%) female deaths. Note that in this larger sample, male deaths exceed female. Again, our question is: If approximately half of all infants are males, does 987 infant male deaths (or 55%) in a sample of 1795 represent an unusual event? Since actually 51%, rather than 50%, of all births are male, the sample percentage 55% will be compared with the population value of 51%.

But, we find that application of the binomial formula to a large sample is cumbersome. However, there is an offsetting fact: as the size of sample increases, the binomial distribution of sample outcomes approaches the normal distribution. In the next chapter, we will discuss the properties of the normal curve and illustrate how a table of its probability values can be used in place of the binomial probability distribution to evaluate large samples.

PROBLEM 3-1

Indicate *True* or *False* for each of the following statements: If *false*, state the reason.

a) A binomial population is a population of 2 or more mutually exclusive groups.

b) A sample proportion can be compared with an expected proportion using the binomial distribution.

c) The binomial distribution tells us the probability of all possible outcomes of samples drawn from the binomial population.

d) To determine how unusual the sample outcome is, by chance alone, we add the probabilities of all outcomes as extreme or less extreme. This sum is called P.

e) A two-tailed test assumes that if the Null Hypothesis is not true the sample proportion can

FIGURE 3-3

Probability Distribution of Outcomes For Samples of Size 13

(p = .5, q = .5)

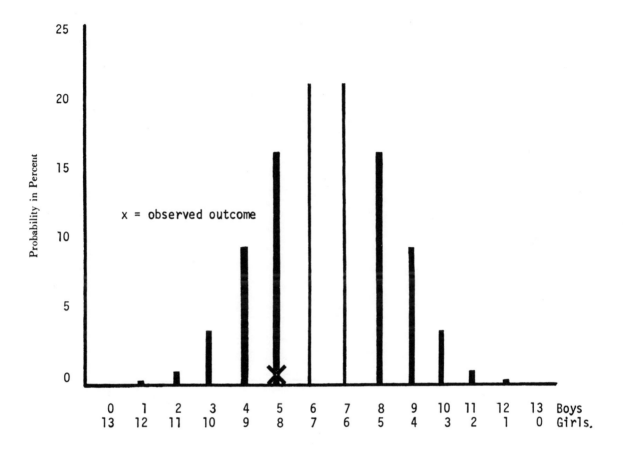

Number of Boys and Girls

Wide bars ▮ represent probabilities which when added = P

---

be *either* larger or smaller than the expected proportion.

f) In a one-tailed test, we assume that the sample proportion differs from the expected proportion in only one direction if the Null Hypothesis is not true.

ANSWER 3-1

a) *False.* A <u>binomial</u> population is a population of <u>only 2 groups.</u> If there are more than 2, we have a <u>multinomial</u> population.

b) *True.*

c) *True.*

d) *False.* To determine P, or how unusual the sample outcome is by chance alone, we add the probabilities of all outcomes *as extreme or more extreme.*

e) *True.*

f) *True.*

TABLE 3-2

Probability of x Male Deaths in 13 Deaths

If the Probability of a Death being Male is 0.5

No. of males in 13 (x)	No. of females in 13 (n-x)	Probability of a sample with x males and (n-x) females
0	13	.0001
1	12	.0016
2	11	.0095
3	10	.0349
4	9	.0873
5	8	.1571
6	7	.2095
7	6	.2095
8	5	.1571
9	4	.0873
10	3	.0349
11	2	.0095
12	1	.0016
13	0	.0001

.2905

.2905

$1 - P$ $= .5810 = P$

1.0000

PROBLEM 3-2

Classify the following questions as to whether they are "directional" or non-directional", i.e., whether the alternative hypothesis to the Null Hypothesis is two-tailed or one-tailed.

a) Is this proportion significantly different from the expected proportion?

b) Does treatment A result in the same proportion of cases as the standard treatment or in a significantly higher proportion?

c) Is $\hat{p}$ really equal to p or not?

d) Is .68 really equal to .80 (the previous proportion) or is it significantly lower?

ANSWER 3-2

a) two-tailed
b) one-tailed
c) two-tailed
d) one-tailed

PROBLEM 3-3

The usual case fatality rate for a disease is about 50%. In 4 successive cases, all but one dies. Can we conclude that there has been a significant increase in disease virulence and/or other factors?

ANSWER 3-3

We might rephrase the question: If we take repeated samples of size 4 from a binomial population where the true proportion (p) is .50 how unusual is an outcome as large as .75 ($\hat{p}$)? Thus we evaluate the sample outcome against one tail of the binomial distribution centered at p = .50 (or $\frac{1}{2}$) since the question is directional.

In Problem 2-6 we obtained the following probabilities from the binomial formula

$$\frac{n!}{r!\,(n-r)!}\ p^r q^{n-r} \text{ when } n=4 \text{ and } p=\frac{1}{2},\ q=\frac{1}{2}:$$

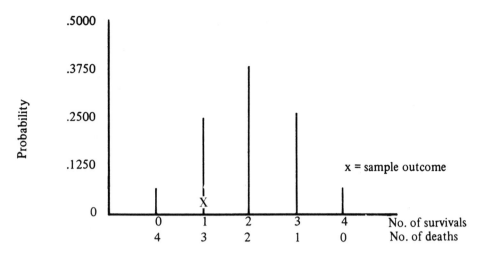

Our sample outcome is 1 survival and 3 deaths. The probability of such an outcome or one more extreme, is the sum of the probabilities of 1 or 0 survivals = .2500 + .0625 = .3125.

Thus P = .3125. This is a very likely event by chance alone (more than 31 in 100 trials of size 4). Therefore there is insufficient evidence of a true difference; i.e., sampling variation alone could account for the observed difference. The usual case fatality rate is still valid.

PROBLEM 3-4

Consider the same situation as Problem 3-3, but we observe that in 5 successive cases, all but one die. What conclusion can be reached?

ANSWER 3-4

Here n is 5 instead of 4, p and q are still $\frac{1}{2}$ each. We are interested in the probability of:

Prob. (1 survival and 4 deaths) =

$\frac{5!}{1!\,4!}$ $(\frac{1}{2})^1(\frac{1}{2})^4 = 5(\frac{1}{2})^5 = .156$

Prob. (0 survivals and 5 deaths) =

$\frac{5!}{0!\,5!}$ $(\frac{1}{2})^0(\frac{1}{2})^5 = (\frac{1}{2})^5 = .031$

Total $= 6(\frac{1}{2})^5 = .187$

P = .187, difference is still not significant. Chance alone can explain the outcome.

PROBLEM 3-5

In a report on the use of penicillin in skin grafting (Hirshfield, J. W., et al., Penicillin and Skin Grafting, *J.A.M.A.*, **125**: 1017-1019, 1944) a single graft was performed on each of 15 patients with third degree burns who was receiving penicillin intramuscularly. The take was satisfactory in all but one of these 15, so that the percentage of satisfactory takes was 93%.

Except for the intramuscular penicillin injections, the patients in this series received the same treatment as that used previously; the technique of preparation of the burn site for grafting was similar to that used before the advent of penicillin. In a previous large series, the take was unsatisfactory in "about one-third of the cases" and "satisfactory in two-thirds" ("unsatisfactory" is defined as a loss of 25% or more of the graft). Consider that these proportions represent the "true" parameters in the absence of penicillin.

We wish to compare the percentage (93%) of satisfactory takes in the sample of 15 penicillin-treated cases with two-thirds, or 66.7%, to see whether the difference might represent merely a chance fluctuation. The probabilities of finding 0, 1, 2, . . ., 15 satisfactory takes obtained from the binomial formula where n = 15, p = $\frac{2}{3}$ and q = $\frac{1}{3}$ are shown on the next page.

1. From the frequency distribution of the percentage of satisfactory takes expected by chance,
   a) Determine the probability of 93% or more satisfactory takes.
   b) Determine the probability of getting a deviation from the expected percentage of satisfactory takes as large as that observed, or larger.
   c) In view of these probabilities, does the percentage of satisfactory takes in skin grafting, when using penicillin, differ significantly from that experienced before its use?
   d) What can you say about the percentage of unsatisfactory takes as compared to that experienced previously?

2. Two other patients received two grafts each and had satisfactory takes on both sites. Does this influence your decision with respect to the value of penicillin?

Chance Distribution of Satisfactory Takes

Unsatisfactory Takes	Satisfactory Takes	% Satisfactory	Probability of Outcome
15	0	(0%)	.000
14	1	(7%)	.000
13	2	(13%)	.000
12	3	(20%)	.000
11	4	(27%)	.002
10	5	(33%)	.007
9	6	(40%)	.022
8	7	(47%)	.057
7	8	(53%)	.115
6	9	(60%)	.179
5	10	(67%)	.214
4	11	(73%)	.195
3	12	(80%)	.130
2	13	(87%)	.060
1	14	(93%) *	.017
0	15	(100%)	.002

(.000 through .022 bracketed as .031)

(.017 and .002 bracketed as .019)

1.000

*Sample outcome

Probability According to the Percentage of Satisfactory Takes

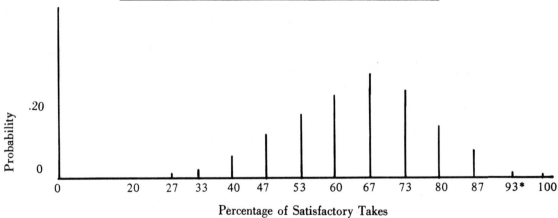

ANSWER 3-5

This problem is somewhat more difficult than the binomial problem of 13 cancer deaths because here our expected proportion (p) is .67 and not .50. Therefore, the binomial distribution is not symmetrical.

1. (a) The probability of getting 93% or more satisfactory takes is the probability of 14 satisfactory takes plus the probability of 15 satisfactory takes $= .017 + .002 = .019$.

(b) The question "a deviation as large as that expected . . . or larger" is a non-directional question, so we must consider the area in both tails. To the probability area obtained in answer to question (a) therefore, we must add the probability area in the other tail. Since 93% is 26% units from 67%

(our expected percentage) we deduct 26% from 67% to locate the deviation in the other direction. This value is 67% — 26% = 41% (or 40%) satisfactory takes which corresponds to 6 satisfactory takes out of 15. Thus we add the probabilities of 6, 5, . . .0 *or .022 + .007 + .002 = .031.* When added to the probability in the other tail, we get *.019 + .031 = .05.*

(c) The difference is just significant at the .05 level.

(d) The results are identical whether we consider "satisfactory takes" or "unsatisfactory takes." The expected % for unsatisfactory takes is 33% and the observed is 7%. The deviation between the observed and the expected is again 26% and again it is just significant at the 5% level.

2. The fact that both grafts were successful for each of the two patients does not influence my decision since two grafts on the same individual are not "independent" of each other. However, if the two patients had been included with the fifteen the proportion of successes would then have been increased to 16/17. My decision might then be influenced as significance was barely achieved previously at the 5% level. One graft from each of the 2 patients should have been chosen randomly and included in the series previous to the start of the experiment, and the experiment analyzed with regard to a single graft for each of 17 people.

SUMMARY OF CHAPTER 3

In this chapter, we answered the following types of questions:
—Is p̂ (the observed proportion) really different from p (the expected proportion)?
—Is p̂ really the same as p or is it larger?
In answering these questions, we used the concepts of
—"unusual" defined in a statistical sense as "extreme or more extreme"
—the probability, P, as the sum of an area
—two-tailed tests
—one-tailed tests
—binomial distribution for evaluating small samples

CUMULATIVE GLOSSARY I: TERMS

Chapter 3

Multinomial Population

Population of more than two mutually exclusive categories.

Two-Tailed Test

The alternative to the null hypothesis is a *non-directional* difference (A $\neq$ B). Therefore the probability of chance events as extreme or more extreme includes the area in <u>both</u> tails.

One-Tailed Test

The alternative to the null hypothesis is that A is smaller (or larger) than B. Therefore the probability of chance events as extreme or more extreme includes the area in only *one* tail.

CUMULATIVE GLOSSARY II: SYMBOLS

Chapter 3

P

Probability that an outcome as *unusual* as that observed will occur by chance alone *if* the null hypothesis is true. Therefore, it is the sum of the probabilities of all chance outcomes as extreme or *more* extreme.

4

The Normal Curve as an Approximation to the Binomial Distribution (for Large Samples)

Properties of the Normal Curve • Standardized Normal Curve • Application to a Large Binomial Sample • Standard Error of the Proportion

Up to now, we have discussed one type of probability distribution, the binomial, and shown how it could be used to determine whether an observed sample proportion is significantly different from an expected, or known, proportion. The binomial distribution enables one to calculate P, the exact probability that an outcome as extreme as that observed, or more extreme, is likely to arise by chance alone, if the null hypothesis is true.

The binomial formula is useful for evaluating small samples, but cumbersome for large samples. As the sample size (n) increases, however, the binomial distribution approaches the normal distribution, and the tabled probability values of the normal curve can be used in its place.

Look at the results of the binomial sampling experiments of the Biostatistics class at the Medical College of Pennsylvania in Figure 4-1. With small samples there are just a few possible (*discrete*) outcomes. As the size increases, however, so does the number of possible sample outcomes and the distribution becomes, in a sense, "less discrete". As the sample size approaches infinity, we have in effect a *continuous* distribution of outcomes. Furthermore, note that the shape of the curve changes. If $p \neq q$ as where $p = .2$ and $q = .8$, the distribution of outcomes is asym-

metrical (outcomes will tend to cluster around the p value). However, as the sample size (n) increases, the curve becomes more symmetric and begins to take a normal or "Gaussian" shape.

Even when the population is quite non-symmetrical (e.g. $p = .05$ and $q = .95$) as n approaches infinity the discrete binomial approaches the continuous normal. A guide is that the normal distribution is an adequate approximation to the binomial when both $n \times p$ and $n \times q$ (the size of sample multiplied by the population, or expected, proportions) = 5 or more: e.g., p or q of $0.1 \times n$ of 50, or p of $0.5 \times n$ of 10.

What are the properties of the normal distribution and how can it be used in place of the binomial?

PROPERTIES OF THE NORMAL CURVE

The normal distribution is the well-known "bell-shaped", Gaussian curve, or normal law of frequency of errors (Figure 4-2). It is an important curve in descriptive and inferential statistics, and its properties should be thoroughly understood: (1) it is a continuous, symmetrical curve with both tails extending to infinity; (2) all three common measures of central tendency —

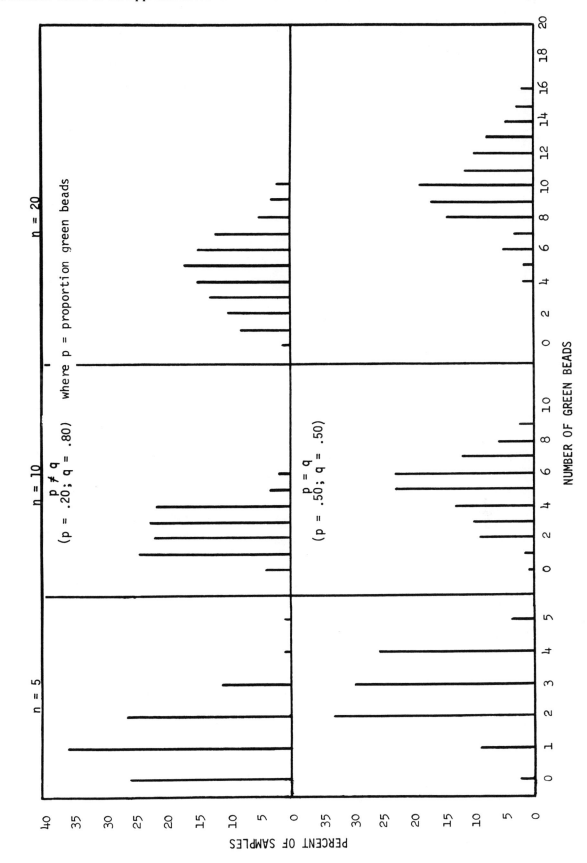

FIGURE 4–1

DRAWING BEADS FROM A JAR: EXPERIMENTAL RESULTS — CLASS OF 1971 OF MEDICAL COLLEGE OF PENNSYLVANIA

FIGURE 4-2

EXAMPLES OF NORMAL CURVES[1]

A. Normal curves with different means
but same standard deviation

B. Normal curves with same mean but
different standard deviations

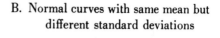

$$\mu_1 \neq \mu_2$$

$$\sigma_1 = \sigma_2$$

$$\mu_1 = \mu_2$$

$$\sigma_1 \neq \sigma_2$$

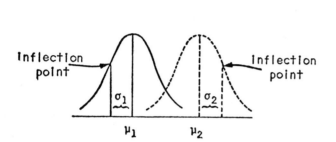

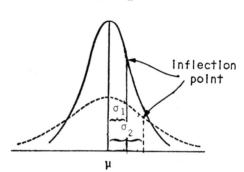

arithmetic mean, median, and mode — are identical[2]; (3) it is described by two parameters: arithmetic mean (μ) and standard deviation (σ); the arithmetic mean (μ) determines the location of the center of the curve; the standard deviation (σ) represents the "spread" or variation around the mean (σ is the distance along the x axis from the center μ to the inflection point or change in the direction of the curve); the larger the σ the greater the spread; (4) there exist an infinite number of normal curves depending upon the parameters μ and σ (Figure 4-2); and (5) all normal curves, however, have the property that between the mean and one standard deviation ($\mu \pm 1\sigma$) on either side is included 68%, between $\mu \pm 2\sigma$, 95%, and between $\mu \pm 3\sigma$, 99.7% of the total area under the curve (Figure 4-3).

STANDARDIZED NORMAL CURVE

Although each pair of mean (μ) and standard deviation (σ) defines a different normal curve,

the areas (probabilities) under the curve need be tabled for only one curve, the Standard normal curve (Table 4-1). This is because for any normal curve it is possible to relate the distance between any observed value x and the mean of the curve μ (x-μ distance) to the standard deviation of that curve. We obtain, by this transformation, a Standard normal deviate called $z = \dfrac{x\text{-}\mu}{\sigma}$. This may be rephrased: any observation from a normal distribution can be located on the normal curve in terms of the number of standard deviations it is from the center of the curve.

A simple example will illustrate. Suppose the mean (μ) of a normal distribution (population) of heights is 10 inches, an observed value (x) is 20 inches, and the standard deviation (σ) of the normal curve is 5 inches. Then

$$z = \frac{x\text{-}\mu}{\sigma} = \frac{20\text{-}10}{5} = \frac{2}{1} = 2.$$

This means that x can be located at 2 σ's (stan-

---

[1] Formula $y = \dfrac{1}{\sigma\sqrt{2\pi}}\ e^{-\frac{1}{2}\left[\frac{x\text{-}\mu}{\sigma}\right]^2}$ where y = ordinate value
x = abscissa value
π = 3.1416
e = 2.7183

[2] The arithmetic mean is the sum of all the observations divided by the number of observations, the median is the middle value in an ordered array from the lowest to the highest, and the mode is the most frequent value.

FIGURE 4-3

The Normal Frequency Distribution
and Proportionate Areas
Included Within Various Multiples of σ

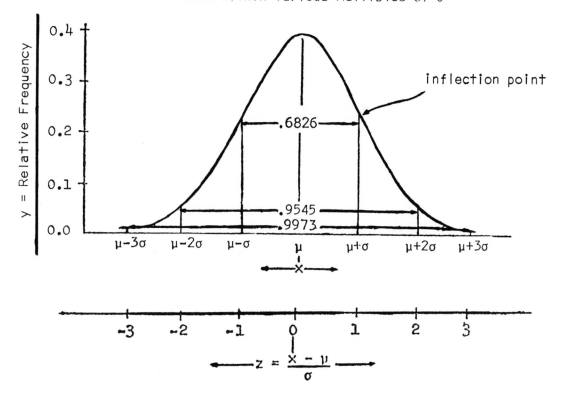

dard deviations) distance from the center of the curve.[1]

By referring to Table 4-1, we note that where z is approximately 2 (1.96, to be exact), 95% of the area under the curve falls between the center and the observation x in <u>either</u> direction. This area is called (1-P). Also, <u>5% of the area falls beyond</u> the observation x in either direction. This area is called (P). Thus any observation from a normal distribution can be located on the Standard normal curve, and (P), the probability of an outcome as extreme as x, or more extreme, determined (Figure 4-4).

APPLICATION TO A LARGE BINOMIAL SAMPLE

How can the normal distribution be used to evaluate large binomial samples? Let us investigate the problem posed in the previous article: among 1795 cancer deaths of persons under one year of age, 987 ($\hat{p} = .55$) were male, and 808 ($\hat{q} = .45$) were female. Is $\hat{p} = .55$ significantly different from $p = .51$, the population or expected proportion of male births?

Imagine an "infinitely large jar" filled in the proportion .51 red beads, representing boys, and .49 yellow beads, representing girls. If we took a million samples of size 1795, the sample outcomes would follow a binomial distribution and we could determine the exact probability of an outcome of 987 boys, 988 boys . . . 1795 boys, and sample outcomes as extreme in the other direction. Or we could compute these probabilities from the binomial formula (Table 4-2). Either method is not very practical. However, with a large n the discrete binomial distribution is approximated by

---

[1] The new variate "z", like the variate "x", also follows a normal distribution. The mean of the transformed distribution is zero (0) and the standard deviation (σ) is 1.

TABLE 4-1

SHORT TABLE OF AREAS OF THE STANDARD NORMAL CURVE

z	1 − P	P	z	1 − P	P	z	1 − P	P	z	1 − P	P
0.0	0.0000	1.0000	1.0	0.6827	.3173	2.0	0.9545	.0455	3.0	0.9973	.0027
0.1	.0797	.9203	1.1	.7287	.2713	2.1	.9643	.0357	3.1	.9981	.0019
0.2	.1585	.8415	1.2	.7699	.2301	2.2	.9722	.0278	3.2	.9986	.0014
0.3	.2358	.7642	1.3	.8064	.1936	2.3	.9786	.0214	3.3	.9990	.0010
0.4	.3108	.6892	1.4	.8385	.1615	2.4	.9836	.0164	3.4	.9993	.0007
0.5	0.3829	.6771	1.5	0.8664	.1336	2.5	0.9876	.0124	3.5	0.9995	.0005
0.6	.4515	.5485	1.6	.8904	.1096	2.58	.9901	.0099	3.6	.9997	.0003
0.7	.5161	.4839	1.64	.9000	.1000	2.6	.9907	.0093	3.7	.9998	.0002
0.8	.5763	.4237	1.7	.9109	.0891	2.7	.9931	.0069	3.8	.9999	.0001
0.9	.6319	.3681	1.8	.9281	.0719	2.8	.9949	.0051	3.9	.9999	.0001
			1.9	.9426	.0594	2.9	.9963	.0037			
			1.96	.9500	.0500						

$x - \mu =$ Deviation of a Variate from its Distribution Mean ($+$ or $-$)

$\sigma =$ Standard Deviation of the Distribution

$z = (x - \mu)/\sigma =$ The Deviation Expressed in Standard Units, the Normal Deviate

$1 - P =$ Corresponding Area under the Normal Curve between $-z$ and $+z$

$\doteq$ Probability according to the Normal Curve of Obtaining a Deviation Smaller than the Absolute Value of $x - \mu$

$P =$ Tail area of the Normal Curve or Area beyond $\pm z$

$=$ Probability of Obtaining a Deviation Equal to or Larger than the Absolute Value of $x - \mu$

Adapted from Fertig, John W. (mimeographed Lecture Notes, Columbia University School of Public Health and Administrative Medicine of the Faculty of Medicine)

a continuous normal distribution* whose probability values are tabled.

Let us locate our binomial sample outcome on the standard normal curve by the following translation to normal distribution values from binomial values:

	Normal distribution	Binomial distribution
Center of normal curve (mean)	μ	$p = .51$
Standard deviation of normal curve	σ	$\sqrt{\dfrac{pq}{n}} = \sqrt{\dfrac{(.51)\ (.49)}{1795}} = .012$
Observed sample outcome	x	$\hat{p} = .55$
Standard normal deviate (z)†	$\dfrac{x - \mu}{\sigma}$	$\dfrac{\hat{p} - p}{\sqrt{\dfrac{pq}{n}}} = \dfrac{.55 - .51}{\sqrt{\dfrac{(.51)\ (.49)}{1795}}} = 3.4$

* In the translation from the discrete binomial to the continuous normal a correction for continuity is made where n is small.

† In tests of significance, z is called the *critical ratio*, or test statistic, and P and 1-P refer to the specified areas under the condition that the Null Hypothesis is true.

FIGURE 4-4

ILLUSTRATION OF USE OF z SCALE
TO DETERMINE P FROM A STANDARD NORMAL CURVE

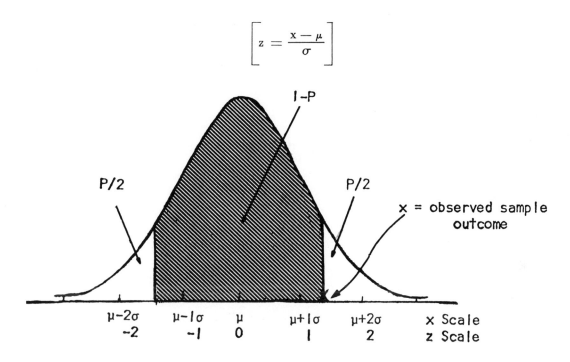

$$\left[z = \frac{x - \mu}{\sigma} \right]$$

Any x is located by determining $z = \frac{x - \mu}{\sigma}$ and then using the z scale.

Since $z = \frac{x - \mu}{\sigma}$ then $x = \mu + z\sigma$. By substituting values (0, 1, 2, etc.) for z, we can convert back to x, vice versa.

For our data, the standard normal deviate, z = 3.4. Thus, the observed proportion (.55) is more than 3 standard deviations from the expected proportion (.51) (Figure 4-5). The probability of this event or of one more extreme = P (the area beyond x). P is so small (less than .001) that it is very unlikely that the sample of .55 male deaths comes from a population where .51 is the true proportion. The null hypothesis that there is no true difference between the sample proportion (.55) and the expected population proportion (.51) is therefore rejected.

Since chance alone would very rarely explain the observed outcome if the null hypothesis were true, it appears likely that a true difference does exist, and that boys have a higher risk of cancer death than girls. We have rejected .51 as the true proportion of cancer deaths, but we are not certain that the true proportion is the observed proportion .55. It might be .55, but could it also be .54, .53, .56, .57, etc.? In Chapter 14 we will discuss methods of estimating confidence intervals on true (population) parameters.

STANDARD ERROR OF THE PROPORTION

The formula $\sqrt{\frac{pq}{n}}$ used above in place of σ is called the *Standard Error of the Proportion* ($SE_{\hat{p}}$). Like the binomial distribution, the normal distribution is centered around the population (or expected) proportion p (.51) and **not** the sample proportion $\hat{p}$ (.55). The normal curve in this illustration represents a probability distribu-

TABLE 4-2

THEORETICAL DISTRIBUTION OF OUTCOMES OF TRIALS
OF SIZE n = 1795 WHERE p = .51

$$\frac{n!}{r!(n\text{-}r)!} \quad p^r q^{n-r}$$

(r) or (x) No. Males	(n — r) No. Females	Probability of Outcome
0	1795	$\frac{1795!}{0!\ 1795!}\ (.51)^0\ (.49)^{1795}$
1	1794	$\frac{1795!}{1!\ 1794!}\ (.51)^1\ (.49)^{1794}$
2	1793	$\frac{1795!}{2!\ 1793!}\ (.51)^2\ (.49)^{1793}$
•	•	
•	•	
•	•	
•	•	
1795	0	$\frac{1795!}{1795!\ 0!}\ (.51)^{1795}\ (.49)^0$

TOTAL = 1.000

tion of sample outcomes drawn from a hypothetical population of .51 proportion boys and .49 proportion girls. Not all normal curves, however, are sampling distributions. They also represent continuous populations of measurements, such as height, blood pressure, etc. Continuous populations will be discussed in Chapter 9.

Note also that the Standard Error of the Proportion is a special form of a Standard Deviation of a normal curve where the normal curve does represent a sampling distribution. It is affected by (1) the proportion (p) in the population: the largest Standard Error is found when p = .5, and (2) n, the size of the sample: the larger the sample, the smaller the Standard Error — that is, the more closely the sample proportions ($\hat{p}$) will cluster around the true proportion (p).

To summarize, we have used both the binomial

FIGURE 4-5

LOCATION OF SAMPLE PROPORTION ON NORMAL CURVE OF SAMPLE PROPORTIONS
(n = 1795, p = .51, p̂ == .55)

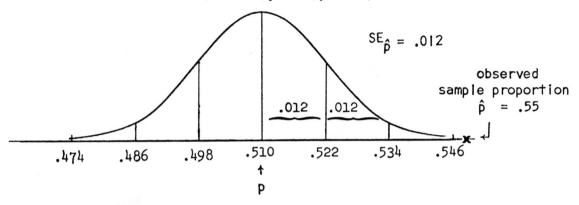

and the normal distributions to test whether a single, observed sample proportion (p̂) differs significantly from an expected, hypothetical or population proportion (p).[1] The binomial test is more exact and is useful for small samples. The normal deviate test (z) is adequate, and easier to use in the case of large samples. In the next chapter we will illustrate the use of the normal curve to test whether <u>two sample</u> proportions <u>differ significantly from each other.</u>

PROBLEM 4-1
There is only <u>one</u> normal curve. *True or False?*

ANSWER 4-1
False. There is an infinite number of normal curves depending upon μ (the mean) and σ (the Standard deviation). There is, however only <u>one</u> <u>standardized</u> normal curve.

PROBLEM 4-2
A point in any normal distribution can be located if the mean and Standard deviation are known. *True or False?*

ANSWER 4-2
True. A point, x, is located by transforming it to z (Standard Normal Deviate), that is, by (1) determining its distance from the center (μ), and (2) relating this distance (x — μ) to the Standard deviation of the curve (σ). This ratio, $\frac{x - \mu}{\sigma}$, is called z.

---

[1] When the Null Hypothesis is formally stated, the hypothetical proportion under H_0 is designated as p_0 (see Chapter 16).

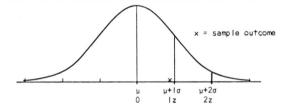

Conversely, given any point on the standardized normal curve (e.g., .9z from μ) we can determine its equivalent location on the original scale.

PROBLEM 4-3
(a) The mean ± 1 Standard deviation in a Normal curve of a sampling distribution of proportions around a population proportion will include what percent of the area?

(b) The mean ± 2 Standard deviations in a distribution of chance outcomes of samples of large size around a population proportion will include what percent of all the sample proportions?

(c) What is the Standard Deviation of the distributions in (a) and (b) called?

(d) What is the center of the curve?

ANSWER 4-3
Questions (a) and (b) are identical except for the number of Standard deviations.

A distribution of outcomes (p̂) of sample size n drawn from a binomial population with true proportion (p) will tend to follow the normal distribution as the size of sample increases. Therefore, the mean ± 1S.D. will include 68% of all sample outcomes (or 68% of the area under the curve) and the mean ± 2 S.D. will include approximately 95% of the outcomes or area.

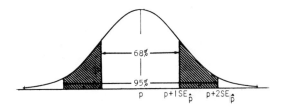

(c) The Standard Deviation of the chance distribution of sample proportions around the true proportion has the special name *Standard Error of the Proportion*.

(d) p, the expected or true proportion.

PROBLEM 4-4

Circle those characteristics that apply to the normal curve:

a) Symmetrical
b) Discrete
c) Median $=$ mean
d) Area adds to 1
e) Extends to infinity in either direction
f) Area between mean and both inflection point always $= .68$
g) Non-symmetrical
h) Continuous
i) Median $\neq$ mean
j) Area does not add to 1
k) Has only positive x (abscissa) values
l) Area between mean and both inflection points sometimes $= .68$

ANSWER 4-4

a,c,d,e,f,h. ————

PROBLEM 4-5

Using Table 4-1 together with Figures 4-3 & 4-4, answer the following questions:

(1) What area of the normal curve is included in
p $+ 1$ SE$_{\hat{p}}$?
p ± 1 SE$_{\hat{p}}$?
p ± 2 SE$_{\hat{p}}$?
p ± 3 SE$_{\hat{p}}$?
From $(-\infty)$ to $(+\infty)$? (∞ is the symbol for infinity)
From $(-\infty)$ to $(p - 2$ SE$_{\hat{p}})$?
From $(p + 2$ SE$_{\hat{p}})$ to $(+\infty)$?
(2) What is the effect of sample size (n) on SE$_{\hat{p}}$?

(3) How will (n) affect the shape of the normal curve of sample proportions?

ANSWER 4-5

(1) In translation of binomial sample data to the normal distribution, the expected proportion, p, is equivalent to μ, the center of the normal curve. The Standard error of the proportion, SE$_{\hat{p}}$, is equivalent to the Standard deviation of the Normal curve or σ. From the table of the Normal curve, therefore, we know the proportion of the total area of the normal curve included in the following:

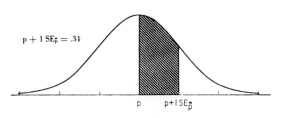

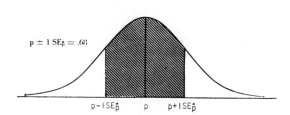

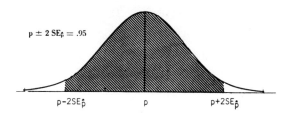

$$p \pm 3\,SE_{\hat{p}} = .997$$

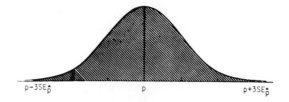

From $(-\infty)$ to $(+\infty) = 1$ or the whole curve

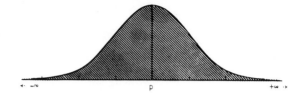

From $(-\infty)$ to $(p - 2\,SE_{\hat{p}}) = .023$. This is equal to half of P, or the area in one tail, where $z = 2$ or $P \sim .05$ ($\sim$ is a symbol for "approximately").

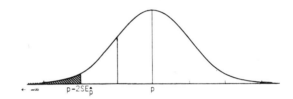

From $(p + 2\,SE_{\hat{p}})$ to $(+\infty) = .023$. Again, this is half of P, or the area in the other tail, where $z = 2$ or $P \sim .05$.

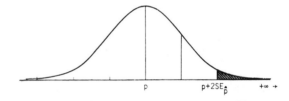

(2) As the sample size (n) increases the $SE_{\hat{p}}$ decreases since $SE_{\hat{p}} = \sqrt{\dfrac{pq}{n}}$

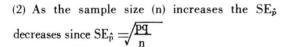

(3) As (n) *increases*, $SE_{\hat{p}}$ *decreases*, and therefore the curve will have less spread. The area of the curve close to the center (p) will increase because a greater proportion of the samples will have a value at or near the true p value. Conversely, as (n) *decreases*, $SE_{\hat{p}}$ will *increase*, and the curve will have more spread.

PROBLEM 4-6

Calculate the Standard Error of the Proportion $(SE_{\hat{p}})$ for
    (1) samples of size n = 25, p = .20
    (2) samples of size n = 100, p = .20
    (3) samples of size n = 25, p = .50
    (4) samples of size n = 100, p = .50

For each of these, sketch the (theoretical) normal curve of sample proportions (superimpose curves 1 and 2, and curves 3 and 4).

ANSWER 4-6

The Standard Error of the Proportion is calculated from the formula $SE_{\hat{p}} = \sqrt{\dfrac{pq}{n}}$ Values for n and p are given and q is 1-p. Therefore we obtain (see figures on next page):

(1) $\sqrt{\dfrac{(.20)\,(.80)}{25}} = \sqrt{\dfrac{.16}{25}} = \dfrac{.4}{5} = .08$

(2) $\sqrt{\dfrac{(.20)\,(.80)}{100}} = \sqrt{\dfrac{.16}{100}} = \dfrac{.4}{10} = .04$

(3) $\sqrt{\dfrac{(.50)\,(.50)}{25}} = \sqrt{\dfrac{.25}{25}} = \dfrac{.5}{5} = .10$

(4) $\sqrt{\dfrac{(.50)\,(.50)}{100}} = \sqrt{\dfrac{.25}{100}} = \dfrac{.5}{10} = .05$

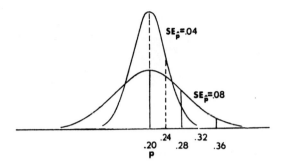

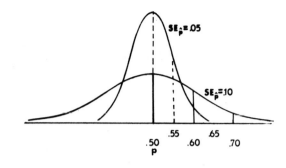

Note that

(a) The $SE_{\hat{p}}$ is larger for p = .50 than p = .20

(b) The $SE_{\hat{p}}$ varies *inversely* with the *square root* of the sample size. Thus if we increase the sample size to a number 4 times as large (i.e., from 25 to 100) we decrease the $SE_{\hat{p}}$ by ½.

PROBLEM 4-7

The case fatality rate for pneumonia in New York State for the three-year period, 1935-1937, is given as 20% (this figure is based on about 97,000 cases and for most purposes could be considered as a universe value).

(a) In a group of 36 cases during that year, what *percentage* could be expected to die?

What *number* could be expected to die?

(b) Since this is not the percentage that will actually die in each group of 36 cases, what is the standard deviation of the distribution of sample percentages which may be expected from successive groups of 36?

(c) Sketch a curve showing the expected distribution of sample percentages or proportions for groups of 36 cases.

ANSWER 4-7

(a) The *percentage* that could be expected to die for any sample is the average percent or 20%. In terms of proportion (p) = .20. The *number* that could be expected to die is the sample size (n) $\times$ p, or 36 $\times$ .20 = 7.2.

(b) The standard deviation of the distribution of sample percentages or proportions is the Standard Error of the Proportion ($SE_{\hat{p}}$) whose formula is

$$\sqrt{\frac{pq}{n}} = \sqrt{\frac{(.20)\,(.80)}{36}} = \sqrt{\frac{(.16)}{36}} = \frac{.4}{6} = .067$$

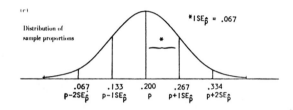

PROBLEM 4-8

The participation rate in a cancer detection program in a county has been 20% over the years. A new health educational program was tested on a sample of 100 residents of whom 40 subsequently participated in the cancer detection program. Is this sample participation rate significantly different from 20%?

ANSWER 4-8

Here we use the Normal curve to compare a sample proportion with an expected proportion because of the large n (100). The expected proportion, p, is .20. The sample proportion, p_o, is $\frac{40}{100} = .40$. To determine whether the sample participation rate (.40) is significantly different from the expected participation rate (.20) we must locate the sample on the chance distribution of sample outcomes. To do this, we use the test statistic $z = \dfrac{\hat{p} - p}{SE_{\hat{p}}}$ where $SE_{\hat{p}} = \sqrt{\dfrac{pq}{n}}$

Therefore, z =

$$\frac{.40 - .20}{\sqrt{\frac{(.20)\,(.80)}{100}}} = \frac{.20}{\sqrt{\frac{.16}{100}}} = \frac{.20}{\frac{.4}{10}} = \frac{.20}{.04} = 5$$

z = 5, P = << .0001

The difference between the sample and expected proportions is 5 times the $SE_{\hat{p}}$ on the chance distribution of sample outcomes. Therefore, it is very unlikely that such a sample would be drawn by chance from a population whose true proportion is .20 (less than 1 in 10,000 trials). Therefore, the sample participation rate is significantly different from 20%.

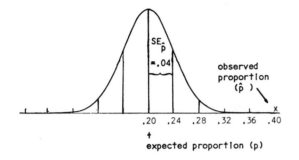

SUMMARY OF CHAPTER 4

The Normal Curve of Sample Proportions

—has characteristic areas.

—can approximate the binomial.

—is centered at p.

—if n is large, can be used to test whether $\hat{p}$ differs from p only by chance.

—has test statistic (Standard Normal deviate) z.

$$-z = \frac{x\text{-}\mu}{\sigma} = \frac{\hat{p}\text{-}p}{\sqrt{\dfrac{pq}{n}}}$$

The Standard Error of the Proportion ($SE_{\hat{p}}$)

—represents the Standard Deviation (σ) of the Normal Curve.

—is affected by p (or q) and n.

CUMULATIVE GLOSSARY I: TERMS

Chapter 4

Normal distribution

A bell-shaped (Gaussian) distribution of two parameters, mu, μ (mean) and sigma, σ (standard deviation). Some properties: (1) continuous, symmetrical, both tails extend to infinity; (2) arithmetic mean, mode and median are identical; (3) characteristic areas depend on distance of x from μ (in σ units); (4) the distance from μ to the inflection point represents σ.

Standard normal distribution

The normal distribution of the variate z with a mean (μ) of zero (0), and a standard deviation (σ) of 1.

Variate z

A new unit, the scale of the *standard* normal curve; it is created by transforming the distance any observation, x, is from the mean (or center) μ, of the normal curve, into *multiples of the standard deviation*, σ, of that curve, Thus, if x-μ is 10, and σ is 2, x is 5 multiples of σ from μ. In this case,

$$z = \frac{x\text{-}\mu}{\sigma} = \frac{10}{2} = 5$$

Standard Error

See SE in Glossary II: Symbols

CUMULATIVE GLOSSARY II: SYMBOLS

Chapter 4

x Any observed value.

μ (small Greek letter mu) The arithmetic mean of a distribution (usage generally restricted to the mean of a <u>population</u>).

σ (small Greek letter sigma) The standard deviation of a distribution (usage may be restricted to the standard deviation of a population).

z Standard normal deviate. A variate which expresses the distance of any observation (x) from the center (μ) of a normal curve, in relation to the standard deviation (σ) of that curve.

$$z = \frac{x - \mu}{\sigma}$$

1-P   Probability of a chance outcome *less extreme* than x under the null hypothesis. It is the total area under the curve (1) minus the area represented by P.

SE   Standard error. It is the special term for the standard deviation of a sampling distribution (reflects sampling or chance variation).

$SE_{\hat{p}}$ Standard Error of the proportion. It is the special term for the standard deviation of the distribution of sample proportions around a true proportion $=$

$$\sqrt{\frac{pq}{n}}$$

5

Comparison of Two Sample Proportions by the Normal Difference Test

Distribution of Chance Differences Between Two Sample Proportions • Standard Error of the Difference Between Two Sample Proportions • Location of a Sample Difference on the Distribution of Chance Differences

In the preceding chapter, we described the binomial probability distribution as a distribution of sample proportions ($\hat{p}$) around a true proportion (p). The distribution could be derived either by experiment or by theory. Since the sample proportions differ from the true proportion (p) only by chance, we can locate an observed sample proportion on this distribution and determine the exact probability of its occurrence (or of an outcome more extreme) by chance alone (P) under the null hypothesis.

Where the sample size (n) is large, the binomial distribution is cumbersome to calculate. However, for large (n) the binomial is approximated by the normal distribution, and therefore tabled areas (probabilities) under the Standard normal curve can be used instead (Table 4-1). These tests are summarized below:

Objective

1. to compare one sample proportion ($\hat{p}$) with an <u>expected</u> proportion (p)

Test

a) Small samples:
   use binomial distribution of sample proportions (based on p and n) to obtain exact probability (P)
   $$\frac{n!}{r!(n-r)!} \, p^r q^{n-r}$$

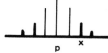

b) Large samples:
   use standard normal curve of sample proportions centered at p to obtain approximate probability (P)

$$z = \frac{\hat{p}-p}{\sqrt{\dfrac{pq}{n}}}$$

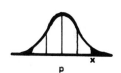

The tests of significance described thus far have been comparisons of <u>one</u> sample proportion ($\hat{p}$) with a population or expected proportion (p). Is it likely that this sample came from a population with the theoretical or expected p value? A more frequent problem involves the comparison of <u>two</u> sample proportions with each other or the difference between $\hat{p}_1$ and $\hat{p}_2$ ($\hat{p}_1$-$\hat{p}_2$) where there is no known or expected population value. Two treatments, or a treatment and a placebo, are tried on two randomized groups of patients, and a difference large enough to be of clinical interest is observed. For example, Table 5-1 presents the results of an experiment in which viosterol and cod-liver oil were given to two groups of children in a study on the prevention of rickets in infants. The proportion who developed rickets was .250 for viosterol and .182 for cod-liver oil, a difference of .068. Is this difference significant? What extension of statistical theory is necessary to answer this question? The solution to this problem is indicated in detail below and summarized in Table 5-6.

DISTRIBUTION OF CHANCE DIFFERENCES BETWEEN TWO SAMPLE PROPORTIONS

Let us return to our basic concepts about frequency distributions of sample outcomes and gen-

TABLE 5-1

Preventive Treatment for Rickets in Infants

Treatment	Rickets		Total	Proportion present
	Present	Absent		
Viosterol	21	63	84	.250
Cod Liver Oil	10	45	55	.182
Total	31	108	139	.223

difference = .068 (for .250 and .182)

Source: Johns Hopkins University School of Hygiene and Public Health lecture material.

erate experimentally an appropriate probability distribution. Instead of drawing a million single samples from an infinitely large binomial population or jar, we, draw repeatedly two samples from the same population and tabulate the difference in sample proportions $(\hat{p}_1 - \hat{p}_2)$.

We wish this experimental situation to be comparable to the data on rickets in Table 5-1. We do not know a priori the true proportion (p) of rickets in the binomial population. Our best estimate of (p) under the Null Hypothesis would be the overall proportion of rickets for the combined samples: $\frac{21 + 10}{84 + 55} = \frac{31}{139} = .223$. Let us call this estimate p'. Note that p' is not a simple average of $\hat{p}_1$ and $\hat{p}_2$ but a weighted average since the size of each sample influences (weights) the contributions of $\hat{p}_1$ and $\hat{p}_2$ to the overall p' value. Thus we shall assume that individuals with rickets are in the proportion .223 and that individuals without rickets are in the proportion (1-p) = .777. Also, let the size of the first sample (n_1) be 84 and that of the second sample (n_2) be 55.

Each time the two samples are drawn we record the respective proportions with rickets, $\hat{p}_1$ and $\hat{p}_2$, and calculate the difference $(\hat{p}_1 - \hat{p}_2)$. To be consistent, we always subtract $\hat{p}_2$ from $\hat{p}_1$, recording "+" for the difference if $\hat{p}_1$ is larger than $\hat{p}_2$

and "—" if $\hat{p}_1$ is smaller than $\hat{p}_2$ (Table 5-2). We thus generate a sampling distribution of differences between two sample proportions. These sample differences must be due solely to chance, since the samples are drawn from the same binomial population (Table 5-3).

What is the center of this distribution of sample differences? We would expect it to be the true difference: The average of all the sample proportions $(\hat{p}_1)$ for the first samples is the true proportion (p) of the binomial population. Similarly, the average of all the $\hat{p}_2$'s is the true proportion (p). Since both samples are drawn from the same population, (p) — (p) = 0. Stated in another way, by chance alone, there are likely to be as many "+" differences of a certain magnitude, where $\hat{p}_1$ is larger than $\hat{p}_2$, as there are "—" differences where $\hat{p}_2$ is larger than $\hat{p}_1$. Therefore, in the long run, these differences cancel and the average difference is zero. Also, from Table 5-3, we see that the frequency of outcomes is greatest around the expected difference of zero, and that the shape is that of a normal distribution.[1]

---

[1] As with the distribution of sample proportions: (1) "corrections for continuity" are needed when the normal distribution is used in place of the binomial, especially when n_1 and n_2 are small; (2) the binomial rather than the normal distribution is applicable when differences between proportions are based on very small samples (e.g. $n_1 \times p'$, $n_2 \times p'$, $n_1 \times q'$, or $n_2 \times q'$ is less than 5).

STANDARD ERROR OF THE DIFFERENCE BETWEEN TWO SAMPLE PROPORTIONS

The standard deviation of the normal curve of chance differences between two sample proportions is called the Standard Error of the Difference ($SE_{\hat{p}1-\hat{p}2}$). (As pointed out previously, the standard deviation of a distribution of sample outcomes is always designated a Standard Error.) Here the Standard Error formula is[1]

$$SE_{\hat{p}1-\hat{p}2} = \sqrt{\frac{p'q'}{n_1} + \frac{p'q'}{n_2}}$$

TABLE 5-2

Samples of 84 and 55, respectively, where probability of a success = .22

| Sample No. | n₁ = 84 | | n₂ = 55 | | Diff. |
	Number of successes (x_1)	$\hat{P}_1 = \dfrac{x_1}{n_1}$	Number of successes (x_2)	$\hat{P}_2 = \dfrac{x_2}{n_2}$	$\hat{P}_1 - \hat{P}_2$
1	22	.262	14	.255	.007
2	16	.190	11	.200	-.010
3	17	.202	10	.182	.020
4	18	.214	13	.236	-.022
5	17	.202	15	.273	-.071
6	9	.107	10	.182	-.075
7	20	.238	7	.127	.111
8	28	.333	7	.127	.206
:	:	:	:	:	:
:	:	:	:	:	:

Source: Johns Hopkins University School of Hygiene and Public Health lecture material.

TABLE 5-3

Distribution of 50 differences in proportions successful in samples of sizes 84 and 55 respectively, where probability of a success is .22.

Difference $\hat{P}_1 - \hat{P}_2$			Observed frequency	Theoretical frequency
−	(-.20) - (-.16)	minus differences	1	.9
	(-.15) - (-.11)		2	3.2
	(-.10) - (-.06)		11	8.1
	(-.05) - (-.01)		13	12.8
+	(0) - (+.04)	plus differences	13	12.8
	(+.05) - (+.09)		6	8.1
	(+.10) - (+.14)		2	3.2
	(+.15) - (+.19)		1	.8
	(+.20) - (+.24)		1	.1
	Total		50	50.0

Source: Johns Hopkins University School of Hygiene and Public Health lecture material.

---

[1]This is the SE formula for independent sample proportions. The samples are "independent" of each other because we have "drawn" them from an infinitely large population.

As stated before, the overall proportion of the two sample outcomes, or weighted average, p′, is used as the best estimate of the true population proportion under the hypothesis that both samples come from the same population. In this instance,

$$SE_{\hat{p}1-\hat{p}2} = \sqrt{\frac{(.223)(.777)}{84} + \frac{(.223)(.777)}{55}} = .072$$

Note that $SE_{\hat{p}1-\hat{p}2}$ is _larger_ than the Standard Error of either proportion: it is based on the _sum_ of two error variances (and not their difference), the variance of _each_ sample contributing to the overall variance (Figure 5-1).

LOCATION OF A SAMPLE DIFFERENCE ON THE DISTRIBUTION OF CHANCE DIFFERENCES

Now let us locate our observed difference of .068 on the normal distribution of chance differences. We use the general form for the Standard normal deviate (assuming that n is sufficiently large)

$$z = \frac{x-\mu}{\sigma}$$

observed outcome ← x
center of normal curve ← μ
standard deviation of normal curve ← σ

In this instance, x represents our observed difference $(\hat{p}_1-\hat{p}_2)$, μ is the center of the normal curve of differences or 0, and σ is the Standard Error of the Difference $(SE_{\hat{p}1-\hat{p}2})$. Thus, the critical ratio $z = \frac{(\hat{p}_1-\hat{p}_2) - 0}{SE_{\hat{p}1-\hat{p}2}}$. The calculation for our rickets problem is:

$$z = \frac{(.250 - .182) - 0}{.072} = \frac{.068}{.072} = 0.94.$$

Since z is only 0.94, the observed sample difference is less than 1 standard deviation (Standard Error) away from the center of the normal curve of chance differences (zero). From the standard normal table (Table 4-1) we find that when z is 0.94 the total area under the curve beyond our observation, x, on either side is between .3681 (z of 0.9) and .3173 (z of 1.0). In a complete table of the normal curve, we find that for a z of 0.94, P is .3472 or approximately .35. Thus a difference of the magnitude observed or greater is a very likely occurrence (35 in 100 trials) when two samples of sizes 84 and 55 are drawn from the same population (null difference) where p is .223. Since the difference is not significant, the Null Hypothesis cannot be rejected. One must conclude that there is insufficient evidence that a true difference does exist between the two treatment methods. (Chance alone could be a likely explanation of the difference observed.)

Let us use the normal curve of chance differences to evaluate another result. In an experiment comparing two types of sulfanilamide treatment on randomized groups of mice, the difference in percent dying is 16.7 (Table 5-4). Is there a true difference between the two treatment methods?

The weighted average (overall percent) dying for the two samples combined (p′) is 85.5%. We draw a million samples of size $n_1 = 60$ and $n_2 = 160$ from an infinitely large jar containing

TABLE 5-4

Experiment in which mice were given one "lethal dose" of staphylococcal injection and treated with sulfanilamide

Treatment group	Result			
	Lived	Died	Total	% Died
Group 1	16	44	60	73.3 } Difference
Group 2	16	144	160	90.0 } = 16.7%
Total	32	188	220	85.5

Group 1: 30 mg. sulfanilamide immediately after injection.
Group 2: 10 mg. immediately, 20 mg. 5 hours later.

Source: Johns Hopkins University School of Hygiene and Public Health lecture material.

FIGURE 5-1

NORMAL APPROXIMATION OF DISTRIBUTIONS OF SAMPLE VALUES AROUND A TRUE VALUE

<u>Samples From Two *Different* Populations:</u>

A. Distributions of sample proportions around a *true proportion*

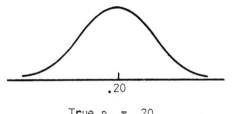

.20

True p_2 = .20

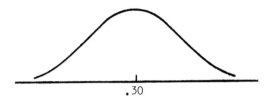

.30

True p_1 = .30

B. Distribution of sample differences between two proportions around a *true difference* of .10.

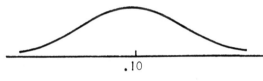

.10

True $p_1 - p_2$ = .10

<u>Samples from The *Same* Population:</u>

A. Distributions of sample proportions around a *true proportion*.

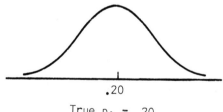

.20

True p_1 = .20

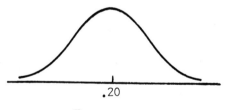

.20

True p_2 = .20

B. Distribution of sample differences between two proportions around a *true difference* of 0.

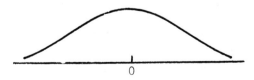

0

True $p_1 - p_2$ = 0

TABLE 5-5

Repeated samples of size 60 and 160 respectively, where p = .855

| Sample No. | $n_1 = 60$ | | $n_2 = 160$ | | Diff. |
	Number of deaths (x_1)	$\hat{P}_1 = \dfrac{x_1}{n_1}$	Number of deaths (x_2)	$\hat{P}_2 = \dfrac{x_2}{n_2}$	$\hat{P}_1 - \hat{P}_2$
1	52	.867	140	.875	-.008
2	51	.850	138	.862	-.012
3	48	.800	133	.831	-.031
4	49	.817	134	.838	-.021
5	46	.767	132	.825	-.058
6	47	.783	131	.819	-.036
7	54	.900	132	.825	.075
8	50	.833	142	.888	-.055
9	56	.933	137	.856	.077
10	52	.867	132	.825	.042
.	.	.	.	.	.
.	.	.	.	.	.
.	.	.	.	.	.

Source: Johns Hopkins University School of Hygiene and Public Health lecture material.

85.5% yellow beads representing deceased individuals, and 14.5% green beads representing survivors (Table 5-5). The distribution of differences in proportion of yellow and green beads between samples 1 and 2 approximates the normal distribution. The calculation for the critical ratio, z (Standard normal deviate) is shown in % form:

$$z = \frac{(\hat{p}_1 - \hat{p}_2) - 0}{SE_{\hat{p}1 - \hat{p}2}} = \frac{(73.3 - 90.0) - 0}{\sqrt{\dfrac{(85.5)\,(14.5)}{60} + \dfrac{(85.5)\,(14.5)}{160}}} = \frac{-16.7\%}{5.3\%} = -3.1$$

In this case, $|z|^* = 3.1$. That is, the observed difference of -16.7 in percent dying is more than 3 Standard Deviations (Standard Errors) away from the center of the curve (0 difference). P associated with this z value is only .0019. Thus a difference of this magnitude or greater would occur in only 19 out of 10,000 trials, if the two samples were drawn from the same population (i.e., if the Null Hypothesis of no difference between the two treatments is true). Since .0019 is such a small probability (rare event), we can reject the Null Hypothesis and accept the alternative hypothesis that there is a true difference between the two treatments. In Chapter 14, the method of estimating confidence intervals on the true difference will be presented.

The tests on the two examples in this chapter are summarized in Table 5-6. In the next chapter, we will describe an alternative procedure for comparing sample proportions, the Chi Square test.

TABLE 5-6

SUMMARY OF TESTS OF
TWO SAMPLE PROPORTIONS

A. Viosterol vs. Cod Liver Oil

A test using the normal curve is always the critical ratio, $z = \dfrac{x - \mu.}{\sigma}$

Specifically, in this instance:

observed difference → center of normal curve of differences

$$z = \frac{(\hat{p}_1 - \hat{p}_2) - 0}{SE_{\hat{p}_1 - \hat{p}_2}} = \frac{(.068) - 0}{.072} = 0.94$$

↑ Standard Error of the Difference

*| | = absolute value.

where $SE_{\hat{p}1-\hat{p}2} = \sqrt{\dfrac{p'q'}{n_1} + \dfrac{p'q'}{n_2}} = \sqrt{\dfrac{(.223)(.777)}{84} + \dfrac{(.223)(.777)}{55}} = .072$

and p' is the overall proportion, and $q' = 1 - p'$.

Since $z = .94$, $P \sim .35$, difference is not significant.

Thus for A on the distribution of sample differences (where $n_1 = 84$, $n_2 = 55$, and $p = .223$), z tells us that the observed sample difference is located less than 1 Standard Error from 0.

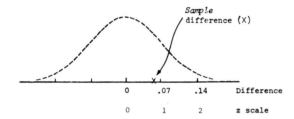

B. Sulfanilamide Treatment (Groups I and II)

$z = \dfrac{(\hat{p}_1 - \hat{p}_2) - 0}{SE_{\hat{p}1-\hat{p}2}} = \dfrac{(-16.7\%) - 0}{5.3\%} = -3.1$

where $SE_{\hat{p}1-\hat{p}2} = \sqrt{\dfrac{(85.5)(14.5)}{60} + \dfrac{(85.5)(14.5)}{160}} = 5.3\%$

Since $z = -3.1$, $P = .0019$, difference is significant.

Thus for B on the distribution of sample differences (where $n_1 = 60$, $n_2 = 160$, and $p = 85.5\%$), z tells us that the observed sample difference is located 3.1 Standard Errors from 0.

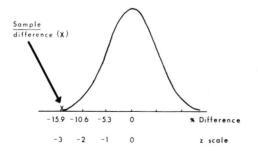

PROBLEM 5-1

Indicate *True* or *False* for the following statements: If *false*, state the reason.

a) The mean $\pm$ 2 Standard deviations in a normal curve of differences between two sample proportions from the same population will include 68% of the area.

b) The theoretical mean of the above sampling distribution is .5.

c) The area, P, in a normal curve of sample differences represents the probability of a sample difference as extreme as that observed or more extreme under the Null Hypothesis.

d) The area $1 - P$ in a normal curve of sample differences represents the probability of a difference less extreme than that observed.

e) The standard deviation of the normal curve of sample differences has the special name Standard Error of the Difference.

ANSWER 5-1

a) *False.* The mean $\pm$ 2 standard deviations in a normal curve of differences between two sample proportions will include 95% of the area; 68% of the area will be included between the mean $\pm$ 1 standard deviation.

b) *False.* The theoretical mean of the above sampling distribution is 0.

c) *True.*

d) *False.* The area $1 - P$ in a normal curve of sample differences represents the probability of a difference less extreme than that observed only if the *Null Hypothesis* is true (i.e. chance is the only factor operating.)

e) *True.*

PROBLEM 5-2

Indicate *True* or *False* for the following statements: If *false*, state the reason.

a) The z value or critical ratio in a normal difference test relates the observed difference to the Standard Error of the Difference.

b) A z of 2 means that the size of the observed difference is 2 times the size of the Standard Error of the Difference.

c) A z of 2 is associated with a P value of .01.

d) Usually with a P value of .05 or less, we accept the Null Hypothesis.

ANSWER 5-2

a) *True.*

b) *True.*

c) *False.* A z of 2 is associated with a P value of .05.

d) *False.* Usually with a P value of .05 or less, we *reject* the Null Hypothesis and call such a difference "significant".

PROBLEM 5-3

The Standard Error of the Difference in a sampling distribution of chance differences between two independent sample proportions is equal to the <u>difference</u> between the Standard Errors of the Proportions for the two samples. *True or False?*

ANSWER 5-3

False: The Standard Error of the Difference is the square root of the sum of, and is larger than, either of the two Standard Errors of the Proportions.

PROBLEM 5-4

a) What area of the normal curve of sample differences under the Null Hypothesis is included in the following?

$$0 \pm 1 \ SE_{\hat{p}1-\hat{p}2} \mid \text{From } (-\infty) \text{ to } (+\infty)$$
$$0 \pm 2 \ SE_{\hat{p}1-\hat{p}2} \mid \text{From } (-\infty) \text{ to } (0 - 2 \ SE_{\hat{p}1-\hat{p}2})$$
$$0 \pm 3 \ SE_{\hat{p}1-\hat{p}2} \mid \text{From } (0 + 2 \ SE_{\hat{p}1-\hat{p}2}) \text{ to } (+\infty)$$

b) What is the effect of sample sizes (n_1 and n_2) on $SE_{\hat{p}1-\hat{p}2}$ and on the shape of the normal curve of sample differences?

ANSWER 5-4

a) Most of these areas are identical to those in Problem 4-5. However for μ we substitute 0 (rather than p) and for σ we substitute $SE_{\hat{p}1-\hat{p}2}$ (rather than $SE_{\hat{p}}$):

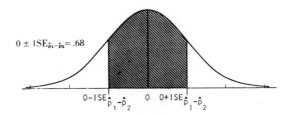

$$0 \pm 1SE_{\hat{p}_1-\hat{p}_2} = .68$$

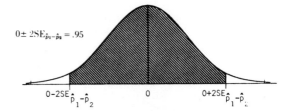

$$0 \pm 2SE_{\hat{p}_1-\hat{p}_2} = .95$$

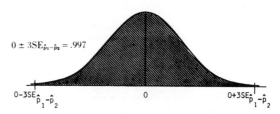

$$0 \pm 3SE_{\hat{p}_1-\hat{p}_2} = .997$$

From $(-\infty)$ to $(+\infty) = 1$
or the whole curve:

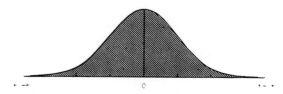

From $(-\infty)$ to $(0 - 2 \ SE_{\hat{p}1-\hat{p}2}) = .023$
= half of P or the area in one tail (where z = 2 or P $\sim$ .05):

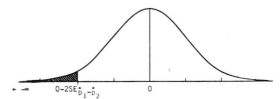

From $(0 + 2 \ SE_{\hat{p}1-\hat{p}2})$ to $(+\infty) = .023$
= half of P or the area in the other tail (where z = 2 or P $\sim$ .05):

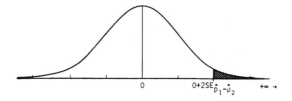

b) As n_1 and n_2 increase, the Standard Error decreases since $SE_{\hat{p}_1-\hat{p}_2} = \sqrt{\dfrac{p'q'}{n_1} + \dfrac{p'q'}{n_2}}$.

As a result, the height of the curve at 0 and the area of the curve close to 0 will increase because a greater proportion of the sample differences will have a value at or near the true difference of 0.

PROBLEM 5-5

1. In the interpretation of a difference $(\hat{p}_1-\hat{p}_2)$ in the percentage surviving in two treatment groups, what importance should be attached to*:

(a) the size of the difference $(\hat{p}_1-\hat{p}_2)$?

(b) the size of the critical ratio $\dfrac{(\hat{p}_1-\hat{p}_2) - 0}{SE_{\hat{p}_1-\hat{p}_2}}$
and the probability P associated with it?

2. Is it possible to have the situation

(a) where $(\hat{p}_1-\hat{p}_2)$ is small in a practical sense, but the critical ratio is large?

(b) where $(\hat{p}_1-\hat{p}_2)$ is large enough to be of interest, but the critical ratio is small?

3. State in your own words the meaning of P (the probability associated with the critical ratio) and of 1-P.

ANSWER 5-5

1.(a) The size of the observed difference $(\hat{p}_1-\hat{p}_2)$ and the possible true difference "behind" it, is the point of interest in the study.

(b) The size of the critical ratio $\dfrac{(\hat{p}_1-\hat{p}_2) - 0}{SE_{\hat{p}_1-\hat{p}_2}}$
indicates the number of standard errors away from zero the observed difference is. This enables one to determine the probability (P) of obtaining a chance difference as large or larger. If the probability is smaller than a predetermined level (e.g., .05 or .01), the difference is considered significant, that is, unlikely to be due to chance.

2.(a) This is the situation where $(\hat{p}_1-\hat{p}_2)$ is small or even trivial, but the sample is large which reduces the size of $SE_{\hat{p}_1-\hat{p}_2}$. Therefore, $(\hat{p}_1-\hat{p}_2)$ divided by this small $SE_{\hat{p}_1-\hat{p}_2}$ will give a large ratio and a significant result.

(b) This is the situation where in contrast to (a) the samples are small. As a result, the size of $SE_{\hat{p}_1-\hat{p}_2}$ is large. Therefore, although the observed difference is large, it is small

relative to its standard error. A larger sample is necessary to provide evidence that there is a true difference *if* one exists.

3. P is the probability that, if the Null Hypothesis is true, a difference between $\hat{p}_1$ and $\hat{p}_2$ as large as that observed or larger would occur just due to chance.

4. 1-P is the probability that, if the Null Hypothesis is true, a difference between $\hat{p}_1$ and $\hat{p}_2$ smaller than that observed would occur as a result of chance alone.

Note that, in both instances there is the basic assumption in calculating P, that the samples are drawn from the same population (i.e., the Null Hypothesis is true).

PROBLEM 5-6

The following table presents hypothetical data on the investigation of the effect of two bacteriostatic agents, sulfanilamide and sulfathiazole, in the prevention of hemolytic staphyloccus aureus infection of the peritoneum of dogs:

Mortality from Peritonitis Among Dogs Treated With Sulfanilamide or Sulfathiazole

Treatment	Deaths	Survivors	Total
Sulfanilamide	50	50	100
Sulfathiazole	60	40	100

1. Is there a significant difference in the proportion of deaths among dogs treated with sulfanilamide and those treated with sulfathiazole?

2. Does sulfanilamide significantly *decrease* the proportion dying from peritonitis compared with the proportion dying among dogs that received sulfathiazole?

ANSWER 5-6

1. This is a two-tailed test since the question is non-directional. (See Chapter 3.)

The Critical Ratio, $z = \dfrac{(\hat{p}_1-\hat{p}_2) - 0}{SE_{\hat{p}_1-\hat{p}_2}} =$

$$\dfrac{(\hat{p}_1-\hat{p}_2) - 0}{\sqrt{p'q'\left(\dfrac{1}{n_1} + \dfrac{1}{n_2}\right)}}$$

where $\hat{p}_1$ and $\hat{p}_2$ refer to the proportion dying in the two treatment groups, p' is the overall proportion and $q' = 1\text{-}p'$.

---

*We refer here in all instances to absolute values (i.e., without regard to sign).

$$\hat{p}_1 = \frac{50}{100} = .50 \qquad \hat{p}_2 = \frac{60}{100} = .60 \qquad \hat{p}_1 - \hat{p}_2 = -.10$$

$$p', \text{ the overall proportion} = \frac{50 + 60}{100 + 100} = \frac{110}{200} = .55 \qquad q' = 1 - .55 = .45$$

$$p'q' = (.55)\ (.45) = .2475$$

$$z = \frac{-.10}{\sqrt{.2475\left(\frac{1}{100} + \frac{1}{100}\right)}} = \frac{-.10}{\sqrt{.0049}} = \frac{-.10}{.07} = -1.43$$

$$z = -1.43, P \sim .16$$

The difference is not significant. Note that it does not matter whether z is "+" or "−" in a two tailed test.

2. The second question is directional since it asks whether there is a significant *decrease* in the proportion dying in one treatment group. This is a one-tailed test, therefore. One carries out the test in the same manner since z locates the sample outcome on the distribution of chance differences centered around 0. In this case, however, we want the P value to represent the area in the one-tail only. Since in the Standardized Normal Table 4-1, P represents the area in both tails asociated with a z value, we must ask the question: What P value when *divided in half* will be .05? *Obviously, that P is .10* and the z associated with it is 1.64. Note that this is smaller than the z (1.96) required for a two-tailed test. Our observed z value of 1.43 is lower than the z of 1.64 required even for a one-tailed test. Therefore, sulfanilamide treatment does not produce a significantly lower proportion of deaths than sulfathiazole.

Note that a directional question ordinarily would not be asked unless it is, a priori, "impossible" for sulfanilamide to be worse than sulfathiazole.

PROBLEM 5-7

The famous epidemiologic investigation in England by Dr. Alice Stewart and colleagues studied factors in the occurence of leukemia and other malignant disease in children.

---

[1]Stewart, Alice, et al., Malignant Disease in Childhood and Diagnostic Radiation in Utero, *Lancet*, September 1, 1956, Vol. 2, p. 447.

The following was taken from an interim report (Lancet, September 1, 1956)[1] describing the study and presenting results for 547 children and their matched controls: The addresses of all children certified as dying from leukemia or malignant disease during the three years 1953-55 were collected and the attendant doctors asked for permission to approach the parents. Where the request was approved, the mother was invited to cooperate by allowing a doctor from the local-authority health department to call and interview her. An interview by the same doctor was also arranged with the mother of a control, a child of the same age and sex, chosen at random from a list of births in the town or rural district in which the affected child's parents were living when the death occurred. In addition to eliciting information about the child's health the questionnaire asked about the mother's health and medical procedures, treatment, etc., before and during the relevant pregnancy. All investigations and treatments were recorded and wherever possible x-ray data checked with hospital notes.

The table below shows the reported radiation experience of the mothers and children in the study.

a) Analyze the data in the antenatal abdominal x-ray group (group 1) to see whether the difference between cases and controls is one that is likely to arise by chance alone. Select any other group in the table and analyze the difference between cases and controls in the same way. What is your interpretation of these comparisons?

b) Comment on the problem of recall re: x-ray history.

c) Why was it desirable for the same physician to interview both case and matched control child?

History of X-ray Examinations
Children with Malignant Disease and Controls
Matched for age, sex, and locality

Classification of child	Total	(1) Abdominal X-ray of mother (diagnostic) before birth of survey child		(2) Other X-ray of mother (diagnostic) before birth of survey child		(3) Abdominal X-ray of mother (diagnostic) before conception of survey child		(4) Other X-ray of mother (diagnostic) before conception of survey child		(5) Post natal X-ray of child (diagnostic)	
		Yes	No or unk.	Yes	No or unk.	Yes	No or unk.	Yes	No or unk.	Yes	No or unk.
Malignant disease	547	85	462	58	489	45	502	211	336	91	456
Control	547	45	502	55	492	54	493	207	340	99	448
Total	1094	130	964	113	981	99	995	418	676	190	904

Table from Stewart, Alice, et al., loc. cit.

ANSWER 5-7

a) The proportion with antepartum x-rays was 7.3 percentage points higher for the case than the control children. The z value is 3.7 which is significant at the .0002 level. This difference is very unlikely to occur by chance alone. No other x-ray group is significant:

Group (1) Abdominal X-ray of mother (diagnostic) before birth of survey child:

The critical ratio $z = \dfrac{(\hat{p}_1 - \hat{p}_2) - 0}{SE_{\hat{p}_1 - \hat{p}_2}}$

$$\hat{p}_1 = \frac{85}{547} = .155 \qquad \hat{p}_2 = \frac{45}{547} = .082 \qquad \hat{p}_1 - \hat{p}_2 = .073$$

$$p' = \frac{85 + 45}{547 + 547} = \frac{130}{1094} = .119$$

$$q' = 1 - .119 = .881 \qquad p' \times q' = .1048$$

$$z = \frac{(\hat{p}_1 - \hat{p}_2) - 0}{\sqrt{p'q'\left(\dfrac{1}{n_1} + \dfrac{1}{n_2}\right)}} = \frac{.73}{\sqrt{.1048\left(\dfrac{1}{547} + \dfrac{1}{547}\right)}} = \frac{.073}{\sqrt{.000383}} = \frac{.073}{.0196}$$

$$z = 3.72 \qquad P \sim .0002$$

Groups (2), (3), (4), and (5) Similar computations for these groups give:

(2) $z = \dfrac{.005}{.018} = .28 \qquad P \sim .80$

(3) $z = \dfrac{-.017}{.0173} = -.98 \qquad P \sim .34$

(4) $z = \dfrac{.008}{.029} = .28 \qquad P \sim .80$

(5) $z = \dfrac{-.015}{.023} = -.65 \qquad P \sim .50$

} Difference is not Significant

Although the difference between cases and controls in the proportion who had received antepartum x-rays is highly significant, the observed difference is not very large. While the evidence of association between malignancy of the child and antepartum x-ray suggests that this practice is inadvisable, most of the cancer cases did not have antepartum x-rays and a sizeable proportion of the controls had such x-rays, Additional explanations of childhood malignancy should be sought although such x-rays may be a contributing factor.

The finding that the differences between case and control children for other types of x-ray is not significant adds weight to the belief that the significant difference for antepartum x-rays has not been due to selective factors. Selection would probably affect the findings of all types of x-ray similarly.

b) There is a definite problem of recall. The mother of a child with leukemia may be more or less likely to remember an x-ray than the mother of a child without leukemia. However, the fact that there was only one group (antenatal abdominal) which showed a significant difference between case and control groups would tend to make one less concerned about differential recall. It is not clear from this excerpt whether all mothers' medical records were searched even if they did not report x-rays. If feasible to obtain, such information would be more reliable than self-reports.

c) Of necessity a large number of doctors conducted the interviews, but they all followed the same convention and used standard schedules. Since the same doctor interviewed each case control pair (provided the parents of the dead child had not moved out of the area) this would tend to minimize interviewer differences re: the case-control comparison.

SUMMARY OF CHAPTER 5

The Normal Curve of chance differences between two sample proportions under the *Null Hypothesis*
- - is centered at 0.
- - can be used to test whether $p_1 = p_2$, or $(p_1 - p_2) = 0$, i.e., the true proportions are equal.
- - has test statistic (Standard Normal deviate) z.

$$- \cdot z = \frac{x - \mu}{\sigma} = \frac{(\hat{p}_1 - \hat{p}_2) - 0}{SE_{\hat{p}1 - \hat{p}2}} = \frac{(\hat{p}_1 - \hat{p}_2) - 0}{\sqrt{\dfrac{p'q'}{n_1} + \dfrac{p'q'}{n_2}}}$$

The Standard Error of the Difference $(SE_{\hat{p}1 - \hat{p}2})$
- - represents the Standard Deviation (σ) of the above Normal Curve.
- - is larger than the $SE_{\hat{p}}$ of either sample.

CUMULATIVE GLOSSARY I: TERMS

*Critical
ratio*

A test statistic, formed from the sampling outcome, which indicates the significance of the sampling result.

*Standard
normal
deviate
(z) test*

Any significance test using the standard normal curve.

The critical
ratio is:

observed outcome
center of normal curve
standard deviation of normal curve

$$z = \frac{x - \mu}{\sigma}$$

The specific interpretation of x, μ and σ depends upon the specific normal distribution and test.

Normal difference test	A z test based on the normal curve of chance differences between 2 random samples from the same binomial population. The test assumes the Null Hypothesis is true (a 0 difference exists).

$$z = \frac{(\hat{p}_1 - \hat{p}_2) - 0}{SE_{\hat{p}_1 - \hat{p}_2}}$$

Standard Error of the difference	See $SE_{\hat{p}_1 - \hat{p}_2}$ in Glossary II.
Weighting	Multiplying a value by some factor such as n, the size of the sample, in order to give it proper importance in obtaining a combined value.

CUMULATIVE GLOSSARY II: SYMBOLS

Chapter 5

p_1	true proportion with attribute a in binomial population 1
p_2	true proportion with attribute a in binomial population 2
q_1	$1-\hat{p}_1$, true proportion without attribute a in binomial population 1
q_2	$1-\hat{p}_2$, true proportion without attribute a in binomial population 2
$\hat{p}_1$	proportion with attribute a in sample 1
$\hat{p}_2$	proportion with attribute a in sample 2
$\hat{q}_1$	$1-\hat{p}_1$, or proportion without attribute a in sample 1
$\hat{q}_2$	$1-\hat{p}_2$, or proportion without attribute a in sample 2
p'	common estimate of true proportion, p, with attribute a in the binomial population. Obtained either from a weighted average of sample proportions, $\hat{p}_1$ and $\hat{p}_2$, with n_1 and n_2 as weights or from the total proportion of successes for the combined samples.
q'	$1-p'$, or common estimate of the true proportion, $1-p$, without attribute a, in the binomial population.
$SE_{\hat{p}_1 - \hat{p}_2}$	Standard Error of the Difference between two sample proportions. The special term for the standard deviation of the distribution of differences between 2 random samples from the same binomial population.

$$= \sqrt{\frac{p'q'}{n_1} + \frac{p'q'}{n_2}} \quad \text{or} \quad \sqrt{p'q'\left(\frac{1}{n_1} + \frac{1}{n_2}\right)}$$

CUMULATIVE REVIEW I

(Chapters 1-5)

BINOMIAL AND NORMAL DEVIATE TESTS FOR QUALITATIVE DATA

To date, we have described the use of the binomial and normal probability distributions for tests of qualitative (enumerative) data. The highlights of these tests are given below:

Objective   Test

1. to compare one sample proportion ($\hat{p}$) with an <u>expected proportion</u> (p)

    a) use binomial distribution of sample proportions centered around p to obtain exact probability (P)* (for *small* samples)

$$\frac{n!}{r!(n\text{-}r)!} \, p^r q^{n-r}$$

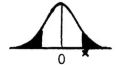

    b) use standard normal curve of sample proportions centered at p to obtain approximate probability (P)* (for *large* samples)

$$z = \frac{\hat{p} - p}{\sqrt{\dfrac{pq}{n}}}$$

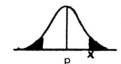

2. to compare <u>two</u> sample proportions ($\hat{p}_1$ and $\hat{p}_2$) with <u>each other</u>

    a) use standard normal curve of sample differences centered at 0 to obtain approximate probability (P)* (for *large* samples)

$$z = \frac{(\hat{p}_1 - \hat{p}_2) - 0}{\sqrt{\dfrac{p'q'}{n_1} + \dfrac{p'q'}{n_2}}}$$

where p' is overall p observed (common estimate of p)

*P is the probability of a chance outcome as far away from the expected (center) value as that observed or further, under the assumption that the Null Hypothesis is true. It is therefore, the area indicated in black.

6

Chi Square Test
(2 × 2 Contingency Tables)

Chi Square Distribution • Concept of 2 × 2 Contingency Tables • Expected Numbers • Calculation of χ^2 • Evaluation of χ^2 • Yates' Correction for Continuity

---

We have used the binomial and normal probability distributions for determining whether, under the Null Hypothesis, an outcome <u>as unusual</u> as that observed (i.e., as extreme or more extreme) is likely to occur by chance alone. An alternative test for enumerative or binomial data is the Chi Square test. Most Chi Square tests can be called tests of association because they answer the question: Is there an association between a factor or attribute and an outcome? The Chi Square test also is important and useful because of its versatility: it can be used with multinomial data, i.e., data classified into *more* than 2 categories. In order to apply the Chi Square test, the physician should be familiar with some of the properties of the Chi Square probability distribution.

CHI SQUARE DISTRIBUTION

The Chi Square distribution is one of a series of statistical distributions whose shape varies with the number of independent values contributing to the distribution. These independent contributions are called *degrees of freedom*, and are abbreviated as "df." Examples of Chi Square distributions are shown in Table 6-1; also in Figure 6-1 for df =

1, 2, 3, and 6. The term "degrees of freedom" will be explained more fully when the appropriate number of df is determined for each example below.

CONCEPT OF 2 × 2 CONTINGENCY TABLES

Let us use the Chi Square distribution to test whether there is an association between the treatment regimens, viosterol or cod-liver oil, and the presence of rickets. We will use the data presented in Chapter 5 (see Tables 5-1 and 6-2.) The data can be visualized as a typical contingency table with 2 rows and 2 columns forming 4 cells:

GROUPS

		A	B
DISEASE	Yes		
PRESENT	No		

The approximate formula for any Chi Square is:

$$\chi^2_{df} = \Sigma \left[\frac{(\text{observed number} - \text{expected number})^2}{\text{expected number}} \right]$$

for all cells.*

---

*χ, Chi. Σ, capital Sigma meaning "take the sum of"

TABLE 6-1

SHORT TABLE OF CHI-SQUARE CORRESPONDING TO SELECTED VALUES OF P

P

df	.50	.10	.05	.02	.01
1	0.45	2.71	3.84	5.41	6.63
2	1.39	4.61	5.99	7.82	9.21
3	2.37	6.25	7.82	9.84	11.34
4	3.36	7.78	9.49	11.67	13.28
5	4.35	9.24	11.07	13.39	15.09
6	5.35	10.64	12.59	15.03	16.81
7	6.35	12.01	14.07	16.62	18.48
8	7.34	13.36	15.51	18.17	20.09
9	8.34	14.68	16.92	19.68	21.67
10	9.34	15.99	18.31	21.16	23.21

P = Probability of attaining or exceeding χ^2, through chance alone, if the null hypothesis is true.

Abridged from more complete table (see Appendix, Table C).

This implies that for each cell: (1) an expected number is determined under the null hypothesis, (2) the expected number is subtracted from the observed number, (3) this deviation is then squared, and (4) the squared deviation is divided by the expected number. The sum of these terms = χ^2. Since a 2 row by 2 column contingency table has 4 cells, there are 4 terms.

EXPECTED NUMBERS

How is the expected number determined? The null hypothesis assumes that the two samples are drawn from the same binomial population and differ only by chance. As noted in Chapter 5, our best estimate of the proportion (p) of the binomial population from which the two samples are drawn is the overall, or weighted average (p') of the sample proportions $\hat{p}_1$ and $\hat{p}_2$. This can be obtained from the total row line: p' = 31/139 or .223. Thus we expect .223 of the total 84 viosterol children (or 18.7) and .223 of the total 55 cod-liver oil children (or 12.3) to have rickets.[1]

[1]Expected numbers could also be computed by calculating p' and q' in the other direction, i.e., the overall proportions given viosterol or cod-liver oil. E.g., since 84/139, or 60% of the children were given viosterol, under the null hypothesis 60% of the 31 ricket and 60% of the 108 non-ricket children could be expected to have been given viosterol (18.7 and 65.3, respectively).

These expected numbers are entered in parentheses in the corner of each cell in Table 6-2. Similarly, the overall proportion without rickets (q') is 108/139 or .777. Therefore, the expected numbers without rickets can be determined by multiplying the totals 84 and 55 by .777.

TABLE 6-2

CHI SQUARE TEST FOR EXAMPLE ON PREVENTIVE TREATMENT FOR RICKETS IN INFANTS

Treatment	Rickets		Total
	Present	Absent	
Viosterol	21$^{(18.7)}$	63$^{(65.3)}$	84
Cod Liver Oil	10$^{(12.3)}$	45$^{(42.7)}$	55
Total	31	108	139

$$\chi^2 = \Sigma \left[\frac{(\text{Observed number}-\text{Expected number})^2}{\text{Expected number}} \right]$$

(Continued at bottom of next page)

FIGURE 6-1

Distribution of Chi-Square with 1, 2, 3 and 6 Degrees of Freedom (df)

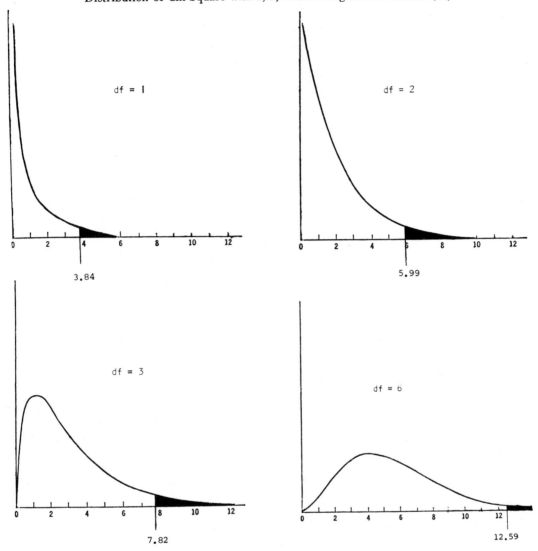

CHI SQUARE VALUE

Shaded Portion = Zone of Significance (.05 Level). The total area under each curve is unity.

TABLE 6-2 (Continued):

Expected numbers shown in parentheses are obtained as follows:

$$\frac{31}{139} \text{ (or .223)} \times 84 = 18.7, \frac{108}{139} \text{ (or .777)} \times 84 = 65.3$$

$$\frac{31}{139} \text{ (or .223)} \times 55 = 12.3, \frac{108}{139} \text{ (or .777)} \times 55 = 42.7$$

$$\chi^2_{1df} = \frac{(21-18.7)^2}{18.7} + \frac{(63-65.3)^2}{65.3} + \frac{(10\text{-}12.3)^2}{12.3} + \frac{(45-42.7)^2}{42.7}$$

$$= .91, P \sim .35 \text{ difference is not significant}$$

Note that once we obtain the expected number for <u>any one</u> of the four cells, the expected numbers for the remaining three cells are automatically determined (constrained). For example, after the expected number of 18.7 is entered, the remaining three expected numbers can be obtained by subtracting 18.7 from the respective row or column total[1]. Therefore, there is only <u>one</u> independent difference (degree of freedom or <u>df</u>) in a 2 x 2 table.

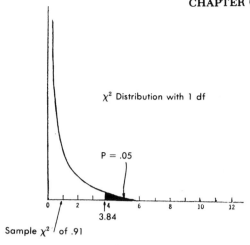

χ^2 Distribution with 1 df

P = .05

0   2   4   6   8   10   12
3.84

Sample χ^2 of .91

CHI SQUARE VALUE

CALCULATION OF χ^2

The computations for χ^2 for this experiment are shown below:

$$\chi^2{}_{1df} = \Sigma \frac{(\text{observed number} - \text{expected number})^2}{\text{expected number}}$$

$$= \frac{(21-18.7)^2}{18.7} + \frac{(63-65.3)^2}{65.3} + \frac{(10-12.3)^2}{12.3} + \frac{(45-42.7)^2}{42.7}$$

Since there is only one independent difference (df) the numerator of all four fractions is the same $(2.3)^2$ and can be factored out[2]:

$$= (2.3)^2 \left[\frac{1}{18.7} + \frac{1}{65.3} + \frac{1}{12.3} + \frac{1}{42.7} \right]$$

Table E of the Appendix (p. 246) can then be used to simplify the fractions inside the parentheses:

$$= (2.3)^2 (.053 + .015 + .081 + .023) = .91$$

EVALUATION OF χ^2

To evaluate a χ^2 of .91 for 1 df we look at the first row of Table 6-1. (This abbreviated table indicates the χ^2 associated with common P values for df 1 through 10.) A χ^2 of .91 falls between a P value of .50 and .10. In an unabridged Chi Square table, P is approximately .35. Since P of .35 is considerably greater than .05, χ^2 is not sig-

nificant: the observed χ^2 of .91 is considerably less than the χ^2 (3.84) associated with a P of .05. (The more unusual the outcome, the <u>larger</u> will be the χ^2 value.)

Note that 3.84 is the square of 1.96, the z or Normal deviate value associated with a P of .05.

Similarly, χ^2 of .91 in this example is $\sim$ square of .94, the z from the Normal difference test for the same data (Chapter 5). Both values are associated with a P $\sim$ .35. Thus, in all 2×2 contingency tables, or tables with 1 df, $\chi^2 = z^2$, and identical P values are obtained; the Chi Square and Normal difference tests are equivalent.[1]

Table 6-3 shows the χ^2 calculations for the sulfanilamide experiment discussed in Chapter 5. As with the z test, the resulting χ^2 of 10.2 is associated with a P considerably less than .01. Therefore, the difference is significant.

YATES' CORRECTION FOR CONTINUITY

For tables with only 1 degree of freedom, Yates' correction[2] is required to compensate for the fact that a continuous distribution like the Chi Square distribution is applied to discrete (qualitative) data. The correction is: reduce the

---

[1] It is best to compute all four expected figures by the procedure described in the preceeding paragraph and then check these calculations by verifying that the sums of the expected numbers equal the row and column totals.

[2] Since the square of a + or − difference is the same, the sign can be ignored.

---

[1] Except for rounding errors.

[2] This correction is similar to a continuity correction for small numbers required when the Normal test is applied to qualitative (binomial) data.

absolute magnitude of each (observed − expected) difference by 0.5 or ½ before squaring. This correction reduces χ^2 and therefore the P or significance of the result:

$$\chi_c^2 = \Sigma \; \frac{(|O\text{-}E| - \frac{1}{2})^2}{E}$$

TABLE 6-3

CHI SQUARE TEST FOR EXAMPLE ON SULFANILAMIDE TREATMENT FOR STAPHYLOCOCCUS

Experiment in which mice were given one "lethal dose" of staphylococcal injection and treated with sulfanilamide.

Result

Treatment Group	Lived	Died	Total
Group 1	16 (8.7)	44 (51.3)	60
Group 2	16 (23.3)	144 (136.7)	160
Total	32	188	220

Group 1: 30 mg. sulfanilamide immediately after injection.

Group 2: 10 mg. immediately, 20 mg. 5 hours later.

$$\chi^2 = \Sigma \; \frac{(O-E)^2}{E} = \frac{(16-8.7)^2}{8.7} + \frac{(44-51.3)^2}{51.3} + \frac{(16-23.3)^2}{23.3} + \frac{(144-136.7)^2}{136.7}$$

$$= (7.3)^2 \left[\frac{1}{8.7} + \frac{1}{51.3} + \frac{1}{23.3} + \frac{1}{136.7}\right] = (7.3)^2 \, (.011 + .019 + .043 + .007) = 10.2$$

$\chi^2_{\,1df} = 10.2, P < .01$, difference is significant

Yates' correction tends to overcorrect and it is trivial when numbers are large. Furthermore, if a χ^2 is not significant one need not bother with this correction because the corrected χ^2 will be less significant. However, if the χ^2 is borderline in significance, an adjusted χ^2 should be computed, especially if numbers are small.

In the next chapter we will conclude our discussion of Chi Square tests.

PROBLEM 6-1

Indicate *True* or *False* for the following statements: If *false*, state the reason.

a) A Chi Square test compares observed with expected numbers.

b) Expected numbers are obtained on the assumption that there is a true difference between the groups.

c) In a table of two rows and two columns since there is 1 independent difference there are 2 degrees of freedom.

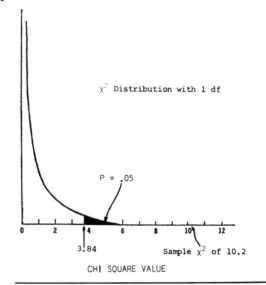

d) In a contingency table with 1 df it is desirable to use Yates' correction for continuity particularly when numbers are small and the results are of borderline significance.

e) In this procedure 1 is substracted from each (Observed − Expected) difference in the computation of χ^2.

f) Use of Yates' correction results in a smaller χ^2 value.

ANSWER 6-1

a) *True.*

b) *False.* The expected numbers are obtained on the assumption that there is no true difference between the groups.

c) *False.* If there is only 1 independent difference there is only 1 degree of freedom.

d) *True.*

e) *False.* Using Yates' procedure ½ or 0.5 is substracted from each (Observed—Expected) difference before squaring.

(f) *True.*

PROBLEM 6-2

In a test between two treatment groups the ratio of the observed difference to the Standard Error of the Difference is 1.96. A Chi Square test for the same data gives a result of 3.84 (1 df).

(a) What hypothesis is being tested?

(b) What is the P value associated with the observed difference?

ANSWER 6-2

(a) The Null Hypothesis — that there is *no true* difference.

(b) P = .05

PROBLEM 6-3

Strickland, B. A., and Hahn, J. L., in a report on the effectiveness of Dramamine® in the prevention of airsickness[1], obtained the following results:

ference in percentages not becoming airsick?

(3) Test the statistical significance of the association between treatment and airsickness by comparing the proportion receiving Dramamine among those who became airsick with the proportion receiving Dramamine among those who did not become airsick. How do the results compare with the above?

(4) Below are the details of the experiment whose data you have just tested. If you had read the experimental design before carrying out the tests, would you have considered the calculations worth doing?

"A procedure was devised whereby one-hour flights simulating flight through turbulent air in a C-47(DC-3) airplane were utilized. Volunteers were obtained from among individuals stationed at Randolph Air Force who were not on flying duty. No other selection factors were utilized within this group since it was desired to have as a test group a cross-section of young adult males who had not become conditioned or adapted to aircraft motion.

"Twelve flights of 18 individuals each have been carried out to date. On each flight conditions encountered in flying through gentle and moderately turbulent air were simulated. All variable factors were either controlled or 'randomized'. Methodology was as follows:

"a) Each group of 18 men on a flight was subdivided by random allocation into a group of nine who received a 100-mg tablet of Dramamine and another nine who received a placebo identical in appearance. Care was taken to prevent each individual from knowing whether he received drug or placebo.

"b) The drug or the placebo was administered

TABLE 1

| Preflight Medication | Airsick | | Not Sick | | |
	Number	Percentage	Number	Percentage	Total Number
Dramamine	31	28.7	77	71.3	108
Placebo	60	55.6	48	44.4	108

(1) Test the statistical significance of the difference in the percentage becoming airsick under the two treatments by two methods. Are the results similar?

(2) What do these tests tell you about the dif-

concurrently from 25 to 45 minutes before each flight.

"c) Seating arrangement in the airplane was carefully controlled so that an equal number of individuals who received the drug were distributed symmetrically in the forepart and the afterpart of the cabin. The same procedure was used in seating the individuals who received the placebo. In addi-

[1] Effectiveness of Dramamine® in Prevention of Airsickness, Science, 109: 359, 1949

tion, drug and placebo subjects were symmetrically distributed on the right and left sides of the cabin. "d) All flights were made at an altitude of 5,000 feet above mean sea level. The pilots had previously developed methods of simulating flight through gentle and moderately turbulent air . . . "e) As in previous studies carried out on motion sickness at the School of Aviation Medicine,

the incidence of airsickness in the subjects was judged on a purely objective basis, i.e., whether or not vomiting occurred.

"Twelve flights were made under the conditions described and a total of 216 subjects were tested. One-half of the subjects received Dramamine and the other half a placebo. The results are shown in Table 1."

ANSWER 6-3

(1) Test of significance by the Normal difference method.

$$z = \frac{(\hat{p}_1 - \hat{p}_2) - 0}{SE_{\hat{p}1 - \hat{p}2}} \text{ in }\%$$

where $p_1 = 31/108 = 28.7\%$
$p_2 = 60/108 = 55.6\%$

average $p' = \frac{31 + 60}{108 + 108} = \frac{91}{216} = 42.1\%$

$$SE_{\hat{p}1 - \hat{p}2} = \sqrt{\frac{p'q'}{n_1} + \frac{p'q'}{n_2}}$$

$1 - p' = q' = 100\% - 42.1\% = 57.9\%$

$$= \sqrt{\frac{(42.1)(57.9)}{108} + \frac{(42.1)(57.9)}{108}} = \sqrt{2\frac{(2438)}{108}} = \sqrt{45.14} = 6.7\%$$

$$\therefore z = \frac{(28.7 - 55.6) - 0}{6.7} = \frac{-26.9\%}{6.7\%} = -4.02, P < .01$$

The difference between the two groups in the percentage becoming airsick is significant at <.01 level.

Test of Significance by Chi Square

	Sick	Not Sick	Total
Dramamine	31 (45.5)	77 (62.5)	108
Placebo	60 (45.5)	48 (62.5)	108
Total	91	125	216

Expected numbers are obtained by using the average proportions sick and not sick multiplied by the total number of cases in each treatment group, under the assumption of no difference between groups (Null Hypothesis).

$\frac{91}{216}$ (or 42.1%) $\times$ 108 = 45.5 $\frac{125}{216}$ (or 57.9%) $\times$ 108 = 62.5

Note that since the total number (108) is the same for each group, the expected numbers also are the same.

$$\chi^2_{1df} = \Sigma\left[\frac{(O-E)^2}{E}\right] = \frac{(31-45.5)^2}{45.5} + \frac{(60-45.5)^2}{45.5} + \frac{(77-62.5)^2}{62.5} + \frac{(48-62.5)^2}{62.5}$$

All O—E differences are the same (14.5) in absolute value

therefore $\chi^2 = (14.5)^2\left[\frac{1}{45.5} + \frac{1}{45.5} + \frac{1}{62.5} + \frac{1}{62.5}\right] = 15.96$

For 1 df, a χ^2 of 15.96 is significant at <.01 level. Note that χ^2 of 15.96 is approximately the same as z^2 or $(4.02)^2$ (values are not identical because of rounding). The P values also are the same by both methods. methods.

(2) The results would be exactly the same if the difference in <u>not</u> becoming airsick were tested. For example:

$$\hat{p}_1 = \frac{77}{108} = 71.3\% \qquad \hat{p}_1 - \hat{p}_2 = 26.9\%$$

$$\hat{p}_2 = \frac{48}{108} = 44.4\% \qquad p' = 57.9, q' = 42.1\%$$

$$SE_{\hat{p}_1 - \hat{p}_2} = \sqrt{\frac{2\ (57.9)\ (42.1)}{108}} = \sqrt{45.14} = 6.7\%$$

$$z = \frac{(\hat{p}_1 - \hat{p}_2) - 0}{SE_{\hat{p}_1 - \hat{p}_2}} = \frac{26.9\%}{6.7\%} = 4.02 \quad P < .01$$

The χ^2 test would involve the same numbers also.

(3) If the tests were carried out by comparing the proportion receiving Dramamine among those who became sick and among those who did not become sick ($\hat{p}_1 = \frac{31}{91} = .34$, and $\hat{p}_2 = \frac{77}{125} = .62$ respectively) again the same z and χ^2 values would be obtained, e.g. $p' = \frac{108}{216} = .50$;

$$q' = \frac{108}{216} = .50$$

$$z = \frac{(.34 - .62) - 0}{\sqrt{\frac{(.50)\ (.50)}{91} + \frac{(.50)\ (.50)}{125}}} = -4.02$$

The expected numbers for the χ^2 test would be the same as before.

(4) *Yes.* On the whole, the experiment is well designed. However, the following questions arise: Were the pilots able to simulate flight through turbulence adequately? Is vomiting the only valid criterion of airsickness?

PROBLEM 6-4

Among 200 hypertensive hospitalized patients, 100 were selected at random and given a new drug. The remainder were given a placebo. Of the 100 receiving the drug 80 improved, compared with 60 of the 100 who received a placebo. What would you conclude?

ANSWER 6-4

The Chi Square test is carried out below:

	Drug	Placebo	Total
Improved	(70) 80	(70) 60	140
Did not Improve	(30) 20	(30) 40	60
Total	100	100	200

Expected numbers (in parentheses) are obtained as follows:

$$\frac{140}{200} \times 100 = 70 \qquad \frac{140}{200} \times 100 = 70$$

$$\frac{60}{200} \times 100 = 30 \qquad \frac{60}{200} \times 100 = 30$$

$$\chi^2 = \Sigma\ \frac{(Obs. - Exp.)^2}{Exp.} = \frac{(80-70)^2}{70} + \frac{(60-70)^2}{70} + \frac{(20-30)^2}{30} + \frac{(40-30)^2}{30}$$

$$= (10)^2 \left[\frac{1}{70} + \frac{1}{70} + \frac{1}{30} + \frac{1}{30} \right]$$

$$= (10)^2\ (.014 + .014 + .033 + .033)$$

$$\chi^2_{\ 1df} = 9.4 \qquad P < .01$$

Difference is Significant. (Such a difference would occur by chance less than 1 in 100 trials if the Null Hypothesis were true.)

PROBLEM 6-5

The following are hypothetical results on five year survivals after treatment of a given type of cancer with surgery alone and with combined therapy (surgery plus radiation). You may assume that patients were assigned to the two groups with proper randomization and that the two groups were comparable with respect to all pertinent characteristics except treatment.

Outcome

Treatment	Survived 5 years	Did not survive 5 years	Totals
Surgery Alone	64	36	100
Combined Therapy (Surgery plus radiation)	216	84	300
Totals	280	120	400

Note that 72% of the group that received combined therapy survived 5 years while the survival rate for the surgical group was only 64%. Is there a significant difference in the results of treatment?

ANSWER 6-5

Outcome

Treatment	Survived 5 years	Did not survive 5 years	Totals
Surgery Alone	(70) 64	(30) 36	100
Combined Therapy (Surgery plus radiation)	(210) 216	(90) 84	300
Totals	280	120	400

Expected Numbers (in parentheses) are obtained as follows:

$$\frac{100}{400} \times 280 = 70 \qquad \frac{100}{400} \times 120 = 30$$

$$\frac{300}{400} \times 280 = 210 \qquad \frac{300}{400} \times 120 = 90$$

$$\chi^2 = \Sigma \; \frac{(O-E)^2}{E} = \frac{(64-70^2)}{70} + \frac{(36-30)^2}{30} + \frac{(216-210)^2}{210} + \frac{(84-90)^2}{90}$$

$$\chi^2 = (6)^2 \left[\frac{1}{70} + \frac{1}{30} + \frac{1}{210} + \frac{1}{90} \right] = 36 \; (.014 + .033 + .005 + .011)$$

$$\chi^2 {}_{1df} = 2.27 \qquad P > .10$$

Difference is not Significant. (Chance alone can explain the difference.)

PROBLEM 6-6

Because of an outbreak of acute sore throats following a charity luncheon, an investigation was made of the food eaten by those who became sick and those who did not become ill. Which of the two foods below, egg salad or macaroni and cheese, appears more "suspect" as the possible vehicle?

	Ate				Did Not Eat			
	Ill	Not Ill	Total	Attack Rate	Ill	Not Ill	Total	Attack Rate
Egg Salad	38	27	65	58%	3	18	21	14%
Macaroni and Cheese	20	14	34	59%	21	31	52	40%

ANSWER 6-6

We arrange the data to form two Chi Square tests of association between food eaten and becoming ill.

Egg Salad

	Ill	Not Ill	Total
Ate	(31.2) 38	(33.8) 27	65
Did Not Eat	(9.8) 3	(11.2) 18	21
Total	41	45	86

( ) = Expected Numbers

$$\chi^2_{1df} = (6.8)^2\left[\frac{1}{31.2} + \frac{1}{33.8} + \frac{1}{9.8} + \frac{1}{11.2}\right] = 11.7$$

$P < .01$

Difference is Significant

Macaroni and Cheese

	Ill	Not Ill	Total
Ate	(16.3) 20	(17.7) 14	34
Did Not Eat	(24.7) 21	(27.3) 31	52
Total	41	45	86

( ) = Expected Numbers

$$\chi^2_{1df} = (3.7)^2\left[\frac{1}{16.3} + \frac{1}{17.7} + \frac{1}{24.7} + \frac{1}{27.3}\right] = 2.66$$

$P > .10$

Difference is not Significant

Note: Because the numbers are fairly small, we apply Yates' Correction for continuity to the data on egg salad and determine if the χ^2 is still significant after adjustment. The correction reduces the (Obs.—Exp.) difference by 0.5:

$$\chi^2_{c\ 1df} = (6.8 - 0.5)^2\left[\frac{1}{31.2} + \frac{1}{33.8} + \frac{1}{9.8} + \frac{1}{11.2}\right] = 10.44 \quad P < .01$$

The difference is still significant.

The data suggest an association between eating egg salad and development of disease that is unlikely to be due to chance. Association between macaroni and cheese and illness has not been demonstrated. Some or all of the people who ate macaroni and cheese and became ill may have eaten egg salad. Further analysis of the data (not available here) would indicate whether or not this is so.

SUMMARY OF CHAPTER 6

Chi Square Test
- - is an alternative test for a difference between two sample proportions.
- - is a test of association between a factor or attribute and an outcome.
- - requires the calculation of Expected numbers based on the Null Hypothesis.
- - is equal to $\Sigma\left[\frac{(\text{Obs. No.} - \text{Exp. No.})^2}{\text{Exp. No.}}\right]$ term for each cell of a table.

Chi Square test for a 2 row $\times$ 2 column table
- - has 1 degree of freedom
- - has a χ^2 value equal to the square of z, the Standard Normal deviate.

CUMULATIVE GLOSSARY I: TERMS

Chapter 6

Chi Square (χ^2)
Distribution

A distribution used in tests of significance on qualitative data. It can be used to compare sample distributions or a sample distribution with a theoretical distribution. The approximate formula for χ^2 is

$$\Sigma \left[\frac{(\text{Observed number} - \text{expected number})^2}{\text{expected number}} \right] \quad \text{or} \quad \Sigma \; \frac{(O - E)^2}{E}$$

Shape of the distribution depends on the number of degrees of freedom. df.

Yates' Correction

A correction for continuity, to compensate for the application of a continuous distribution to discrete (qualitative) data, used in Chi Square tests with 1 df. The correction is to subtract ½ from each (Observed − Expected) difference before squaring:

$$\chi_c^2 = \Sigma \; \frac{(|O - E| - \frac{1}{2})^2}{E}$$

Degrees of freedom (df)

Number of independent contributions to a theoretical sampling distribution (such as χ^2, t, and F distribution).

Contingency table

A classification of qualitative data into r rows and c columns (to which a Chi Square test of association can be applied.)

Expected number

Number expected in a particular category in a sample under the assumption of the Null Hypothesis (no true difference exists).

CUMULATIVE GLOSSARY II: SYMBOLS

Chapter 6

χ	small Greek letter Chi
χ^2	Chi Square $= \Sigma \left[\dfrac{(O - E)^2}{E} \right]$. See Glossary I: Terms
χ_c^2	Chi Square with Yates' correction. See Glossary I: Terms
df	degrees of freedom. See Glossary I: Terms
r	number of rows in a table
c	number of columns in a table
$\|\|$	absolute value, i.e., without regard to sign

7
Chi Square Test (Concluded)

r × c Contingency Tables (Larger than 2 × 2) • Test for Goodness of Fit • Summary Notes on Chi Square Test

In Chapter 6, we described the Chi Square test for a contingency table consisting of 2 rows and 2 columns of data. The test, which can be called a test of association, serves as an alternative to the normal test for a difference between two sample proportions. In this chapter, we present other applications of Chi Square.

r × c CONTINGENCY TABLES (LARGER THAN 2 × 2)

An important use of Chi Square is the comparison of more than 2 treatment groups or more than 2 outcomes categories.[1] An example of 3 rows and 3 columns of data (3 × 3) is given in Table 7-1 for an ecological study of Baltimore City.

are applied to each total group under the assumption of no true difference between ranks (Null Hypothesis). The expected numbers are shown in parentheses and the calculation of χ^2 carried out in Table 7-1.

With respect to the number of degrees of freedom (df) it can be shown that for a table of 3 rows and 3 columns (9 cells) there are only 4 independent expected values. Once these 4 are specified, the remaining 5 are "constrained" by the row and column totals, that is they can be obtained by substracting the first 4 values from the totals. A general method of determining the number of degrees of freedom for any r × c table is given by the formula:

$$\text{Degrees of freedom} \quad (\text{df}) = (\text{number of rows} - 1) \times (\text{number of columns} - 1)$$
$$\text{df} = (r - 1) \times (c - 1).$$
$$\text{Thus, for a } 3 \times 3 \text{ table: df} = (3 - 1) \times (3 - 1) = 4.$$

One hundred and fifty-eight census tracts were ranked according to the proportion of persons in the tract who were on public assistance. The tracts were then placed, in order of rank, into four approximately equal groups (quartiles). The two middle quartiles were then combined to make three final groups. Each tract was grouped also according to psychiatric admission rate, ending with a 3 × 3 cross classification.

The principles of analysis are the same as for the 2 × 2 contingency table. To obtain the expected number for each cell, overall proportions

Recall from Chapter 6 that a Chi Square test can be called a test of association. Our question here is: is there an association between Factor A (public assistance) and Factor B (psychiatric admission rate) for Baltimore City census tracts? In this example, the observed χ^2 of 4 df is 63.2. Reference to Table 6-1 for 4 df shows that for this χ^2 value P is considerably less than .01 ($\chi^2_{.01}$ is only 13.28). Therefore, one can conclude that there is an association between the two factors, i.e., the variation in psychiatric admission rate among census tracts grouped according to propor-

---

[1] The outcome categories can be collected in discrete form originally, such as "mild," "moderate," "severe" dysfunctioning, or, as illustrated in the example below, can be derived from measurement data which have been subsequently grouped into categories.

TABLE 7-1

Distribution of Baltimore City Census Tracts by Quartile Ranking of Three-Year
Psychiatric Admission Rate and of Proportion of Persons on Public Assistance.[1]

Number of tracts ranked in quartiles by: Three-year total psychiatric admission rate	Number of tracts ranked in quartiles by: Proportion of persons on public assistance			
	I Lowest quartile	II and III Middle quartiles	IV Highest quartile	Total No. of tracts
IV Highest quartile	2 (10.37)*	15 (19.73)	23 (9.90)	40
II and III Middle quartiles	14 (20.50)	50 (39.00)	15 (19.50)	79
I Lowest quartile	25 (10.13)	13 (19.27)	1 (9.60)	39
Total Tracts	41	78	39	158

*( ) Expected numbers: e.g., $10.37 = \left(\frac{41}{158}\right) \times 40$; $19.73 = \left(\frac{78}{158}\right) \times 40$

$$\chi^2 = \Sigma \left[\frac{(O - E)^2}{E} \right]$$

$$= \frac{(2 - 10.37)^2}{10.37} + \frac{(15 - 19.73)^2}{19.73} + \frac{(23 - 9.90)^2}{9.90}$$

$$+ \frac{(14 - 20.50)^2}{20.50} + \frac{(50 - 39.00)^2}{39.00} + \frac{(15 - 19.50)^2}{19.50}$$

$$+ \frac{(25 - 10.13)^2}{10.13} + \frac{(13 - 19.27)^2}{19.27} + \frac{(1 - 9.60)^2}{9.60}$$

$$\chi^2_{4df} = 63.2 \qquad P < .001$$

[1]Klee, G., Spiro, E., Bahn, A.K., and Gorwitz, K.: An Ecological Analysis of Diagnosed Mental Illness in Baltimore, in Psychiatric Epidemiology and Mental Health Planning. Psychiatric Research Report 22, American Psychiatric Association, April, 1967, Washington, D.C.

tion of persons on public assistance is very unlikely to be explained by chance if the Null Hypothesis is true. Note that the Chi Square test does not indicate the strength of the association. The correlation coefficient (to be discussed in Chapter 13) provides a quantitative measure of degree of association.

Another example of a Chi Square test of association for 4 rows and 2 columns of data is presented in Table 7-2.

Note that Yates' correction for continuity is not used for contingency tables larger than 2×2.

TABLE 7-2

Chi Square Test of Association for 4 × 2 Table

Survival data on 193 patients with bundle branch block

Below is an example of data on a controversial topic —

Is there an association between age and prognosis in bundle branch block acquired after the age of 39 years or can the variation in survival be explained by chance?

Age at diagnosis	Outcome 1 year after diagnosis		Total
	Dead	Alive	
40-49.9 years	3 (5.74)	24 (21.26)	27
50-59.9 years	15 (11.68)	40 (43.31)	55
60-69.9 years	9 (13.59)	55 (50.40)	64
70-79.9 years	14 (9.98)	33 (37.01)	47
TOTAL	41	152	193

4 × 2 table $\therefore$ df = (r—1) (c—1) = (4—1) (2—1) = 3 independent differences

Null Hypothesis: Prognosis is independent of age.

Expected numbers (in parentheses) obtained as follows:

$$\frac{41}{193} \times 27 = (5.74) \qquad \frac{152}{193} \times 27 = (21.26)$$

$$\frac{41}{193} \times 55 = (11.68) \qquad \frac{152}{193} \times 55 = (43.31) \text{ etc.}$$

$$\chi^2_{3df} = \frac{(3 - 5.74)^2}{5.74} + \frac{(24 - 21.26)^2}{21.26} + \cdots \frac{(14 - 9.98)^2}{9.98} + \frac{(33 - 37.01)^2}{37.01} = 6.883$$

P > .05 since critical $\chi^2_{.05}$ for 3df = 7.82

Therefore the prognosis does not differ significantly with the patient's age. Note that since each expected number is 5 or more, the χ^2 test is valid.

Source of data: Johns Hopkins University School of Hygiene and Public Health. See also Cochran, W., Biometrika 10:417, 1954, for an alternative test which can be more powerful when one axis (e.g., age) is orderable.

TEST FOR GOODNESS OF FIT

Up to now we have used Chi Square to compare sample distributions with each other. Another very useful application of Chi Square is a comparison of an observed distribution with some theoretical distribution, called a "goodness of fit" test. The theoretical or expected distribution could be the normal, binomial, or any other statistical distribution, for example, the distribution of the general population by blood group type. This test is equivalent to comparing a sample value with a population value, whereas the previous test (r × c Contingency Chi Square test) is analogous to comparing values from two or more samples with each other.

We will compare an observed distribution with the uniform or rectangular distribution. The latter is a theoretical distribution which assumes the same relative frequency for all groups (Figure 7-1). A survey is made on 2,000 persons given unlabelled cigarettes representing 4 different brands, and their first preference is determined. (The order in which individuals are given the cigarettes is randomized to offset any carry-over effect.) Column 1 of Table 7-3 shows the observed distribution of respondents by preferred brand. Since the expected distribution is the uniform distribution, one would expect equal preference among the 4 brands, or 500 preferences for each brand (Column 2). Could the difference between the observed and expected numbers be explained by chance alone?

Several additional columns are added to Table 7-3 to aid in the χ^2 calculation: in Column 3, the difference between the observed and expected numbers is entered (these entries must add up to zero). In Column 4, each deviation is squared, and in Column 5 the squared deviation is divided by the expected number. The sum of the last column gives us directly the χ^2 value of 2.0.

Figure 7-1

**COMPARISON OF AN OBSERVED DISTRIBUTION
WITH THE UNIFORM DISTRIBUTION**

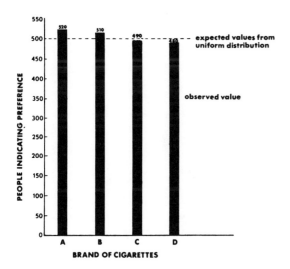

*Same as Rectangular Distribution

What is the appropriate number of degrees of freedom for a Goodness of Fit Test of this type? Since the "Observed — Expected" column must total to zero, there is one constraint or a loss of 1 df for the total, i.e., the first 3 entries are independent of each other but the 4th is automatically determined. Since there is only one column of data df is simply the (number of rows — 1) = (4 — 1) = 3.

For a P of .05, 3 df, the χ^2 must be at least 7.82 (see Table 6-1 of Chi Square Values). Our experimental result, $\chi^2 = 2.0$, is well below this "critical" χ^2 (7.82). It is associated with a P of approximately .50. Therefore, one can conclude that the observed distribution does not deviate significantly from the expected distribution — there is insufficient evidence of a real preference for any brand (Figure 7-2).

Another application of a Goodness of Fit Test is the following data from Science, September 30, 1949 (Lucia, S. P., Hunt, M. L., and Talbot, J. C.: On The Relationship of Blood Group A to Rh Immunization and the Occurrence of Hemolytic Disease of the Newborn, pp. 309-330.)

Among 11,649 pregnant women, there were observed 228 sensitized Rh-negative women. Of these 124 had an Rh+ child with hemolytic disease. The distribution of these women by blood group was:

Blood Group	No. of Women
O	43
A	66
B	11
AB	4
TOTAL	124

TABLE 7-3

Chi Square Test for Goodness of Fit:

Observed Distribution of Preference for Cigarette Brand Compared with Uniform Distribution

Brand	(1) Observed	(2) Expected[1]	(3) O—E	(4) (O—E)^2	(5) (O—E)^2/E
A	520	500	+20	400	0.8
B	510	500	+10	100	0.2
C	490	500	—10	100	0.2
D	480	500	—20	400	0.8
TOTAL	2,000	2,000	0		2.0 = χ^2

[1]Expected numbers obtained from the Uniform (Rectangular) distribution

$$\chi^2_{3df} = \Sigma \left[\frac{(O—E)^2}{E} \right] = 2.0 \qquad P \sim .50, \text{ difference not significant}$$

In a large random sample of the population of the area, the percentages of O, A, B and AB were respectively 44.8%, 39.7%, 11.3%, 4.2%. Is the distribution of the 124 women by blood group significantly different from the blood group distribution in the general population?

To answer the question, we compare the observed numbers for the 124 Rh-negative women by blood group with expected numbers based on the general population.

Blood Group	(1) Obs. No.	(2) Exp. No.	(3) (O—E)	(4) (O—E)^2	(5) (O—E)^2/E
O	43	55.6	—12.6	158.76	2.86
A	66	49.2	+16.8	282.24	5.74
B	11	14.0	— 3.0	9.00	.64
AB	4	5.2	— 1.2	1.44	.28
TOTAL	124	124.0	0		9.52

$\chi^2_{3df} = 9.52$ $P < .05$

The "expected" number of Rh-negative in each blood group category (Col. 2) is obtained by multiplying the <u>percentages</u> in each group in the general population by the total number of Rh-negative women. Thus, the expected number of type O, Rh-negative women is 44.8% $\times$ 124 = 55.6. In a similiar manner we compute the "expected" number for the remaining three groups and check that the sum of the expected numbers is 124. We then compute each Observed—Expected difference (Col. 3) and check that these differences add to zero. In Column 4, we compute (O—E)^2 and in Column 5 (O—E)^2/E, for each row. The sum of Col. 5 entries, 9.52, is our observed χ^2 value. The degrees of freedom is (number of rows — 1) or (4 — 1) = 3. The critical χ^2 (.05) is 7.82. Therefore, P is less than .05 and we can conclude that the Rh-negative women differ significantly from the general population in blood group distribution (Figure 7-2).

Note that an observed distribution could also be fitted to a theoretical distribution such as the binomial or normal distribution. In such cases where the parameters (p), or (μ) and (σ), are estimated from the data it is necessary to subtract an additional degree of freedom for <u>each</u> parameter estimated. Thus, just as we lose a df for the constraint of the "total", each parameter that must be estimated from the sample adds a further restric-

tion and reduces the number of independent differences.

SUMMARY NOTES ON CHI SQUARE TEST

The Chi Square test is a versatile and important test for the physician. Principles and limitations are summarized below:

1. It can be used only for qualitative (enumerative) data.[1]
2. It is applicable to samples of any size

FIGURE 7-2 CHI SQUARE TEST FOR GOODNESS OF FIT

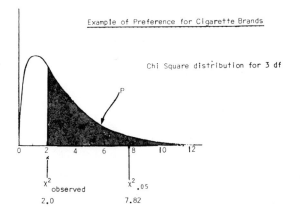

Example of Preference for Cigarette Brands

Chi Square distribution for 3 df

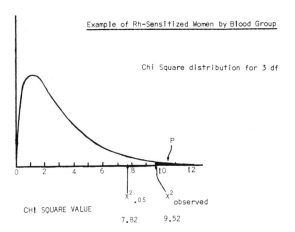

Example of Rh-Sensitized Women by Blood Group

Chi Square distribution for 3 df

CHI SQUARE VALUE

---

[1]It can also be used for quantitative (measurement) data after transformation (e.g., by ranking) into discrete categories.

(except as noted in 9 and 10 below) or any number of categories.

3. The final computation always involves actual <u>numbers</u> of items, <u>not percents</u> or <u>proportions.</u>

4. For each category, the <u>difference is obtained between the number observed and the number expected on the basis of the Null Hypothesis.</u> This difference is then squared, and divided by the expected number: $\dfrac{(O-E)^2}{E}$. The <u>sum</u> of all such terms, one for each category, is χ^2.

$$\chi^2 = \Sigma \left[\frac{(O-E)^2}{E} \right]$$

5. For any percentage deviation of observed from expected, the larger the sample size, the larger will be $\dfrac{(O-E)^2}{E}$. Therefore, χ^2 will tend to be larger with larger samples.

6. The <u>number of categories,</u> however, affects the number of independent differences or degrees of freedom (df) and therefore the shape of the theoretical distribution of χ^2.

7. The larger the number of df, the larger must be χ^2 for a given level of significance.

8. When two or more *sample* distributions are compared, the appropriate test is the r × c Contingency Chi Square Test. The data are arranged in *r* rows and *c* columns (contingency table) and df = (r − 1) × (c − 1). The expected numbers are obtained by multiplying the total number in each sample by the respective proportions in the <u>total</u> distribution. When a *sample* distribution is compared with a *population* distribution, the appropriate test is a Goodness of Fit Chi Square Test. In this case, the expected numbers are obtained from the proportions in the <u>population distribution</u> and df = (r − 1).

9. The sampling distribution of χ^2 will conform to the theoretical distribution of χ^2 only if the <u>expected</u> number for each cell is 5 or more.[1] Small cells can be combined to form large cells (if appropriate). Otherwise exact binomial probabilities should be computed using Fisher's Exact Test in place of the Chi Square test.

10. For χ^2 with only 1 degree of freedom:

   (a) Yates' correction is required to compensate for the fact that a continuous distribution (χ^2) is applied to discrete (qualitative) data. <u>Yates' correction for continuity reduces the absolute magnitude of each difference by 0.5 or $\frac{1}{2}$ before squaring.</u> This reduces the χ^2 value and therefore the P or significance of the result.

$$\chi^2_c = \Sigma \frac{(|O-E| - \frac{1}{2})^2}{E}$$

Yates' correction is trivial, however, when numbers are large.

   (b) The P value associated with χ^2 is the same as the P value for the Normal deviate test (since $\chi^2 = z^2$).

11. The ordinary Chi Square test can be used for comparing independent (non-correlated) samples only. For example, it cannot be used without modification where the data represent response to different drugs administered to the <u>same</u> patient.[2]

This concludes our presentation of significance tests on qualitative data. In the next chapter, we will review the decision making process and then begin the analysis of quantitative data.

PROBLEM 7-1

Indicate *True* or *False* for the following statements:

a) The number of independent differences that contribute to a χ^2 test determines the number of degrees of freedom.

b) In a table of two rows and two columns, there is only one degree of freedom. After we determine one expected value, the remaining three are constrained.

c) All four of the observed—expected differences in a 2 × 2 table are the same except for the sign of the difference.

d) A χ^2 test is applicable to more than two rows and two columns.

e) In an r × c table there are (r) × (c) degrees of freedom.

f) A Goodness of Fit test compares a sample distribution with a population or theoretical distribution.

g) A Goodness of Fit test has a table of r rows and 1 column.

h) In a Goodness of Fit test there are always r − 1 degrees of freedom.

---

[1] An expected value as low as 1 is acceptable under certain conditions. See Cochran, W., *loc. cit.*

[2] For paired observations, use McNemar's test (see Prob. 13-18) or later modification (Gart, J., Biometrika 56:75, 1969).

ANSWER 7-1

a) *True.*

b) *True.*

c) *True.* All four of the observed—expected differences have the same absolute value in a 2×2 table but two of the differences will be negative and the other two positive.

d) *True.*

e) *False.* In an r $\times$ c table there are $(r - 1) \times (c - 1)$ degrees of freedom. Thus, in a 3×2 table there are $(3 - 1) \times (2 - 1)$ or 2 degrees of freedom. If we are given any two values we can determine the others using the row and column totals.

f) *True.*

g) *True.*

h) *False.* In a Goodness of Fit test, there are at the *most* (r — 1) degrees of freedom since "1" is always subtracted from the total. An additional df must be subtracted for each additional parameter of the theoretical distribution which is estimated from the data (e.g., p).

PROBLEM 7-2

Indicate *True or False* for the following statements: If *false*, state the reason.

a) The shape of the Chi Square Distribution is independent of the number of degrees of freedom which contribute to it.

b) The larger the number of degrees of freedom, or categories, the larger is the critical χ^2 value associated with a P of .05.

c) Using the χ^2 table, we note that for 1 df, the χ^2 value associated with a P of .05 is 5.99 and for 2 df it is 11.07.

d) For 1 df, the χ^2 value is sometimes the square of the z value obtained from the normal difference test.

ANSWER 7-2

a) *False.* The shape of the Chi Square Distribution depends upon the number of degrees of freedom which contribute to it.

b) *True.*

c) *False.* For 1 df, the χ^2 value associated with a P of .05 is 3.84 while for 2 df it is 5.99.

d) *False.* For 1 df, the χ^2 value is always the square of the z value obtained from the normal difference test.

PROBLEM 7-3

In a study of the relation of tonsillectomy to the type of poliomyelitis (JAMA. July, 1954)[1] the following data were obtained:

Poliomyelitis Patients Aged 10-14, by Type of Infection and History of Tonsillectomy

Type	No. of Patients	Tonsils		% Absent
		Present	Absent	
Bulbar	115	16	99	86.1
Severe spinal	135	77	58	43.0
Mild spinal	161	76	85	52.8
Nonparalytic	50	24	26	52.0
Total	461	193	268	58.1

Is the difference in history of tonsillectomy for the bulbar and other forms of poliomyelitis one that chance would frequently produce?

---

[1]Anderson, G. W., and Rondeau, J. L.: The Absence of Tonsils as a Factor in the Development of Bulbar Poliomyelitis (JAMA, **154**:1123-1130, 1954).

ANSWER 7-3

Here we have a 4×2 contingency table. We obtain the expected number Present and expected number Absent for each type of poliomyelitis assuming that there is no true difference (the Null Hypothesis). Thus for each type we expect 58.1% absent and 41.9% present (the overall percentages); $58.1\% \times 115 = 48.2$, $41.9\% \times 115 = 66.8$, etc. The expected numbers are shown in parentheses below:

Type	Total No.	No. Present	No. Absent
Bulbar	115	16 (48.2)	99 (66.8)
Severe spinal	135	77 (56.6)	58 (78.4)
Mild Spinal	161	76 (67.5)	85 (93.5)
Nonparalytic	50	24 (20.9)	26 (29.1)
Total	461	193 (193)	268 (268)

We then compute the $\dfrac{(O-E)^2}{E}$ for the 8 cells. Note that the (Obs.—Exp.) difference for each type is the <u>same</u> for "Present" and "Absent" categories:

$$\chi^2 = \frac{(16-48.2)^2}{48.2} + \frac{(99-66.8)^2}{66.8}$$
$$+ \frac{(77-56.6)^2}{56.6} + \frac{(58-78.4)^2}{78.4}$$
$$+ \frac{(76-67.5)^2}{67.5} + \frac{(85-93.5)^2}{93.5}$$
$$+ \frac{(24-20.9)^2}{20.9} + \frac{(26-29.1)^2}{29.1}$$

$$= \frac{(-32.2)^2}{48.2} + \frac{(32.2)^2}{66.8}$$
$$+ \frac{(20.4)^2}{56.6} + \frac{(-20.4)^2}{78.4}$$
$$+ \frac{(8.5)^2}{67.5} + \frac{(-8.5)^2}{93.5}$$
$$+ \frac{(3.1)^2}{20.9} + \frac{(-3.1)^2}{29.1}$$

Carrying out the computation we find that $\chi^2 = 52.3$, $df = (4-1)(2-1) = 3$, since if we know 3 independent expected numbers, e.g., 3 "Present" or 3 "Absent" expected numbers, we know all the 5 remaining expected numbers. The χ^2 of 52.3 is highly significant: $P < .001$. There is an excess of tonsillectomies in the bulbar group.

Note that, in this example, because we are dealing with the categories "Present" and "Absent", it is very easy to forget to compute (Obs. — Exp.) differences for <u>both</u> categories. In that case we would have erroneously obtained only part of the correct χ^2 value (in this instance, about one-half of the correct value).

PROBLEM 7-4

The following quotation modified from an article by Maes, V., Boyce, F., et al. in the Annals of Surgery (Postoperative Evisceration with an Analysis of Forty-four Cases, **100**: 968-982, November, 1934) summarizes certain aspects of a comparative study:

"The mortality, like the incidence, seems to us another point on which considerable confusion exists. The reported figures vary very widely. White reports sixteen deaths in thirty cases (53%). Meleney and Howes report twenty-two deaths in fifty cases (44%). Grace reports fifteen deaths in forty cases (38%). Colp reports seven deaths in thirty cases (23%)."

While there may be reasons other than those of chance why the mortality percentages among the series of cases reviewed by Maes differ, it is of interest to inquire as to whether or not the variability among the percentages could be explained by chance alone. Set up the problem showing how you would answer this inquiry.

ANSWER 7-4

Table of Observed Frequencies

Reported by:	No. of Deaths	No. of Survivors	Total	Fatality %
White	16	14	30	53
Meleney and Howes	22	28	50	44
Grace	15	25	40	38
Colp	7	23	30	23
Total	60	90	150	40

This is a 4 row × 2 column Chi Square table.[1] Under the Null Hypothesis of no difference between investigators we would "expect" each investigator to have 40% deaths and 60% survivors among his cases. Therefore, we can compute the expected numbers of deaths and survivors for each surgeon,

$$\text{e.g.: } 40\% \times 30 = 12 \text{ expected deaths} \atop 60\% \times 30 = 18 \text{ expected survivors} \Bigg\} \text{ for White.}$$

These numbers are shown in parentheses below, and the calculation of χ^2 is illustrated.

	No. Deaths	No. Survivors	Total
White	16 (12)	14 (18)	30
Meleney and Howes	22 (20)	28 (30)	50
Grace	15 (16)	25 (24)	40
Colp	7 (12)	23 (18)	30
Total	60 (60)	90 (90)	150

$$\chi^2 = \left. \begin{array}{l} \dfrac{(16-12)^2}{12} + \dfrac{(14-18)^2}{18} \\[2mm] + \dfrac{(22-20)^2}{20} + \dfrac{(28-30)^2}{30} \\[2mm] + \dfrac{(15-16)^2}{16} + \dfrac{(25-24)^2}{24} \\[2mm] + \dfrac{(7-12)^2}{12} + \dfrac{(23-18)^2}{18} \end{array} \right\} = \left\{ \begin{array}{l} \dfrac{(4)^2}{12} + \dfrac{(-4)^2}{18} \\[2mm] + \dfrac{(2)^2}{20} + \dfrac{(-2)^2}{30} \\[2mm] + \dfrac{(-1)^2}{16} + \dfrac{(1)^2}{24} \\[2mm] + \dfrac{(-5)^2}{12} + \dfrac{(5)^2}{18} \end{array} \right\} = \left\{ \begin{array}{l} 1.33 + .89 \\[2mm] + .20 + .13 \\[2mm] + .06 + .04 \\[2mm] + 2.08 + 1.39 \end{array} \right\} = 6.12$$

Note that for each row there is only 1 independent difference and that once 3 of these row differences are obtained the fourth is "constrained". Therefore, there are only 3 degrees of freedom:

$$(4-1)(2-1) = 3 \times 1 = 3 \text{ df}$$

Carrying out the χ^2 calculation, $\chi^2_{3df} = 6.12$, $P > .05$, Difference not significant.

---

[1]See also Ryan, T. A., Significance Tests for Multiple Comparisons of Proportions, Variances and Other Statistics, Psychol. Bull. 47:318, 1960.

PROBLEM 7-5

Given the following data on blood group distributions[1]:

Blood Group Distribution of Normal Individuals by Nationality

	O	A	B	AB	Total
			Number		
Canada	447	408	116	29	1000
Germany	462	490	121	27	1100
New York City	456	357	140	47	1000
Total	1365	1255	377	103	3100
			Percent		
Canada	44.7	40.8	11.6	2.9	100.0
Germany	42.0	44.5	11.0	2.5	100.0
New York City	45.6	35.7	14.0	4.7	100.0
Total	44.0	40.5	12.2	3.3	100.0

Is there a significant difference by nationality in distributon by blood group type? (It will be sufficient to indicate how the Expected numbers are obtained and the number of degrees of freedom.)

ANSWER 7-5

This is a large table of three rows and four columns (3×4) but simply analyzed by the Chi Square test. On the assumption that the overall percentages for blood groups (44.0, 40.5, 12.2, and 3.3) apply to each nationality, expected numbers are computed as follows:[2]

O	A	B	AB	Total
$44.0 \times 1000 = 440$	$40.5 \times 1000 = 405$	$12.2 \times 1000 = 122$	$3.3 \times 1000 = 33$	1000
$44.0 \times 1100 = 484$	$40.5 \times 1100 = 445$	$12.2 \times 1100 = 133$	$3.3 \times 1100 = 37$	1100
$44.0 \times 1000 = 440$	$40.5 \times 1000 = 405$	$12.2 \times 1000 = 122$	$3.3 \times 1000 = 33$	1000
1364	1255	377	103	3100

$$df = (r - 1)(c - 1) = (3 - 1)(4 - 1) = (2)(3) = 6$$

[1]Source: Fertig, John: (Mimeographed Notes) Columbia University School of Public Health and Administrative Medicine of the Faculty of Medicine.

[2]Numbers do not add to total because of rounding.

PROBLEM 7-6

The hypothetical distribution of 100 child patients according to number of siblings is:

0	siblings — 15%
1-3	siblings — 30%
4 or more	siblings — 55%

(a) Suppose in the total school population of comparable age and socio-economic status the percentage distribution of children according to number of siblings (0, 1-3, and 4 or more) is 5%, 50%, and 45% respectively. Determine whether there is a significant difference between patients and the general population in the number of siblings.

(b) Suppose the patients were compared with a sample of 100 school children with percentages 5%, 50% and 45%. Is the difference significant?

ANSWER 7-6

This is a "tricky" problem requiring recognition of the difference between the situations in (a) and (b). In (a) we compare the sample of child patients with the total school population. Therefore, a Goodness of Fit test of 3 rows and only 1 column is appropriate. In (b) the comparison is between 2 samples — the sample of child patients and a sample of school children. Therefore, we have a contingency Chi Square test, in this case, of 3 rows and 2 columns. The calculations are carried out below.

(a)

No. Siblings	Obs. No.	Exp. No.	O — E	(O — E)²	(O — E)²/E
0	15	5	10	100	100/5 = 20.0
1-3	30	50	—20	400	400/50 = 8.0
4+	55	45	10	100	100/45 = 2.2
	100	100	0		30.2 = χ^2

df = (3 — 1) = 2 df
Observed χ^2_{2df} = 30.2   P $\sim$ .001
Difference is Significant.

(b)

No. Siblings	Patients	School Children	Total	Expected Proportion
0	15 (10)*	5 (10)	20	20/200 = .10
1-3	30 (40)	50 (40)	80	80/200 = .40
4+	55 (50)	45 (50)	100	100/200 = .50
	100	100	200	

*( ) = Expected number

$$\chi^2 = \Sigma \left[\frac{(O-E)^2}{E}\right] = \frac{(5)^2}{10} + \frac{(-5)^2}{10} \left.\begin{array}{c} \\ \\ \end{array}\right\} \qquad \left\{\begin{array}{c} 2\frac{(25)}{10} = 5 \\ \end{array}\right.$$

$$+ \frac{(-10)^2}{40} + \frac{(10)^2}{40} \left.\begin{array}{c} \\ \end{array}\right\} = \left\{\begin{array}{c} + 2\frac{(100)}{40} = 5 \\ \end{array}\right.$$

$$+ \frac{(5)^2}{50} + \frac{(-5)^2}{50} \left.\begin{array}{c} \\ \end{array}\right\} \qquad \left\{\begin{array}{c} + 2\frac{(25)}{50} = 1 \\ \end{array}\right.$$

Total   = 11

df = (3 — 1) (2 — 1) = 2
Observed χ^2_{2df} = 11,   P $\sim$ .01
Difference is Significant.

SUMMARY OF CHAPTER 7

Chi Square distribution
- - can be used to test 2 or <u>more</u> groups and/or categories.
- - has values which will increase as df increase.

Chi Square Contingency Test
- - compares two or more samples with each other.
- - has (r — 1) $\times$ (c — 1) df.

Chi Square Goodness of Fit Test
- - compares a sample (observed) distribution with a *population* (theoretical) distribution.
- - has (r — 1) df.

CUMULATIVE GLOSSARY I: TERMS

Chapter 7

Chi Square contingency test   A Chi Square test of qualitative data in which two or more sample distributions are compared with each other (contingency table). Has (r — 1) $\times$ (c — 1) df.

Goodness of Fit test   A Chi Square test of qualitative data in which a sample distribution is compared with a theoretical or population distribution. Has (r — 1) df. An additional df is substracted for each parameter of the theoretical distribution estimated from the sample itself.

CUMULATIVE REVIEW II

(Chapters 1-7)

SIGNIFICANCE TESTS ON QUALITATIVE DATA

(Samples from Binomial Populations = two categories, e.g., alive or dead; or from Trinomial Populations = three categories, e.g., mild, moderate, severe; etc.)

Objective	Test

1. to compare <u>one</u> sample proportion ($\hat{p}$) with an <u>expected</u> proportion (p)

   a) use binomial distribution based on p and n (small samples)

$$\frac{n!}{r!\,(n\text{-}r)!}\,p^r q^{n-r}$$

   b) use standard normal curve of sample proportions centered at p (large samples)

$$z = \frac{\hat{p} - p}{\sqrt{\dfrac{pq}{n}}}$$

   c) use Chi Square Goodness of Fit test (1df) (large samples)

2. to compare <u>two</u> sample proportions ($\hat{p}_1$ and $\hat{p}_2$) with <u>each other</u>

   a) use standard normal curve of sample differences centered at 0

$$z = \frac{(\hat{p}_1 - \hat{p}_2) - 0}{\sqrt{\dfrac{p'q'}{n_1} + \dfrac{p'q'}{n_2}}}$$

where p′ is overall p observed (weighted average)

   b) use Chi Square test (2 × 2) (1df). Use p′, overall p observed (weighted average), as <u>expected proportion</u>

3. to compare <u>more than two</u> sample proportions (more than <u>two</u> treatments or more than two categories) (multinomial)

   a) use Chi Square Contingency test (r × c) where df = (r − 1) (c − 1)

4. to compare an <u>observed</u> (sample) distribution with a <u>theoretical</u> (population) distribution

   .a) use Chi Square Goodness of Fit test where df = (r − 1)

NOTE:

1. z test is always $= \dfrac{x - \mu}{\sigma}$

   ┌ observed outcome

   ← center of normal curve

   └ standard deviation of normal curve   (= Standard Error of curve of sample outcomes)

2. Chi Square test is always $\Sigma \left[\dfrac{(O - E)^2}{E} \right]$ for <u>all</u> cells where O and E are observed and expected frequencies.

   df is number of <u>independent</u> differences (degrees of freedom)

3. The hypothesis being tested is always the <u>Null Hypothesis</u>. $H_o : \mu_1 = \mu_2$

   or $(\mu_1 - \mu_2) = 0$

8

Review of the Decision Making Process; the Error Risks

The Objective • The General Procedure for Decision Making • Type I Error • Type II Error • Summary of Error Risks

We have now completed the high points of tests of significance on qualitative (enumerative) data. Before proceeding to descriptive and analytic methods for quantitative (measurement) data, let us review the formal steps in the decision making process and the risks of error involved.

THE OBJECTIVE

Ordinarily we do not know the true (population) parameters such as the true proportion (p) or whether $(\mu_1 - \mu_2) = 0$. In the face of uncertainty, however, we make a decision based upon a "negative" type of statistical evidence. It is possible that any two samples were actually drawn from the same population and just by chance produced the observed difference. Therefore, before we are willing to assume that a real difference exists, we attempt to rule out chance as a likely cause of the observed difference. However, we do so with a predetermined risk of error.

Examples where the decision making procedure is followed:

1. A sample proportion is observed which differs from some previously observed proportion or expected value. Could the difference be explained by chance variation?

2. The means or proportions for two samples, one a treated group and the other a control group, differ. Is it likely that this difference is due to chance alone?

THE GENERAL PROCEDURE FOR DECISION MAKING

1. Determine whether a two-tailed test or a one-tailed test will be made. If the alternative hypothesis specifies the direction of the difference (e.g., $\mu_1 > \mu_2$), it is a one-tailed test. If the alternative hypothesis specifies only a non-directional difference or inequality (e.g., $\mu_1 \neq \mu_2$), or $(\mu_1 - \mu_2) = 0$, it is a two-tailed test. It is customary to apply a two-tailed test (because it is more conservative) unless there are special circumstances, such as where deviations can occur in only one direction.

2. Choose α (alpha), *the arbitrary level of significance* (usually .05 or .01).

3. Assume the *Null Hypothesis* (i.e., no true difference).

4. Calculate the appropriate *test statistic*, e.g., z or χ^2 for enumerative data.

5. Determine, by reference to tabled values for that statistic, the probability (P) of the observed value or of a more extreme value *if* the Null Hypothesis is true.

6. If P is less than the predetermined α level (.05 or .01, by convention) the probability that the event will occur, given that there is no true difference, is considered small. That is, chance alone is an unlikely explanation. Therefore, we reject the Null Hypothesis and accept the alternative hypothesis that a true difference exists.

7. If P is greater than .05 this indicates that more than 5 in 100 times such a difference or one more extreme could likely arise by chance if the Null Hypothesis were true. Thus, although a true difference <u>may</u> exist, <u>chance alone</u> could also explain the occurrence. Therefore, there is "insufficient evidence of a difference," and the Null Hypothesis is accepted. If a true difference does exist, a larger sample <u>may</u> provide evidence of its existence (i.e., we have <u>not proved</u> that there is no true difference).

TYPE I ERROR

It was pointed out that these rules assist the clinician in making a decision in the face of uncertainty and that there is a risk of error depending upon (1) the *actual situation* and (2) the *decision made.*

Let us imagine first the situation where unknown to us the Null Hypothesis is actually *true.* Two samples of size $n_1 = 60$ and $n_2 = 30$ are drawn from the same binomial population (with a p of 0.20). The two normal curves[1] in Figure 8-1A represent distributions of a million random samples of sizes n_1 and n_2 around the true proportion. Note that the Standard Deviation of the distribution (Standard Error) is <u>larger</u> for the distribution of samples of <u>smaller</u> size $(n_2 = 30)$.

We draw a third normal curve in Figure 8-1B to represent the distribution of <u>differences</u> between these sample proportions. Note: (1) The Standard Deviation (Standard Error) of this curve is larger than that for either of the two curves above. (2) The curve represents a distribution of sample differences occurring solely by chance. The center of this curve of differences is therefore zero, the true difference $(\mu_1 - \mu_2) = 0$.

Since the curve follows the normal distribution the probability of a sample difference falling within the region $(0 \pm 1.96 \text{ SE}) = .95$. If the predetermined alpha (α) level of significance is .05, then 95 out of 100 times the sample outcome will fall within the $(1-\alpha)$ or *acceptance region* of the curve and the Null Hypothesis is accepted. No error will be made since the Null Hypothesis is actually true. However, 5 out of 100 times, just by chance alone, the sample outcome will fall in the *rejection region* (beyond $0 \pm 1.96 \text{ SE}$) and the Null Hypothesis will be rejected incorrectly. This is called the Type I Error.

[1]Because $(n \times p)$ and $(n \times q) > 5$, we can use the normal approximation to the binomial distribution.

FIGURE 8-1

ACTUAL SITUATION: Null Hypothesis
$H_0 : \mu_1 = \mu_2$, is TRUE

A. Distribution of Sample Proportions Around a True Proportion where $\mu_1 = \mu_2 = \mu$.

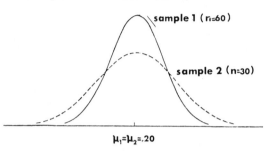

$\mu_1 = \mu_2 = .20$

B. Distribution of Differences Between Two Sample Proportions where True Difference $(\mu_1 - \mu_2) = 0$.

TWO TAILED TEST

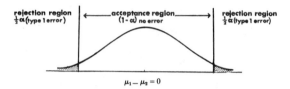

$\mu_1 - \mu_2 = 0$

Note: All sample outcomes are tested against the Null Hypothesis Curve. Here, the Null Hypothesis is actually TRUE. Therefore:

All of the actual sample area falling within the Acceptance Region $(1-\alpha)$ of the Null Hypothesis Curve represents no error.

Stippled area is the actual sample area falling within the Rejection Region of the Null Hypothesis Curve $=$ Type I Error (α). Since the Null Hypothesis is True, there is no Type II (β) Error.

TYPE II ERROR

Now suppose the actual situation is that the Null Hypothesis is *false.* For example, sample 1 is drawn from a binomial population with a true p of .50 and sample 2 from a binomial population with a true p of .20. In Figure 8-2A the distributions of a million such random sample proportions are shown. Note that although the true proportions are different, the two sampling distributions overlap. The extent of overlap depends on sample sizes n_1 and n_2, the population variances, and the size of the true difference.

FIGURE 8-2

ACTUAL SITUATION: Null Hypothesis

$H_0 : \mu_1 = \mu_2$, is FALSE

A. Distribution of Sample Proportions Around a True Proportion Where $\mu_1 \neq \mu_2$.

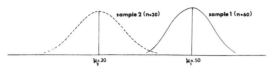

B. Distribution of Differences Between Two Sample Proportions Where True Difference $(\mu_1 - \mu_2) = .30$.

ONE TAILED TEST

Distribution Under Null Hypothesis   *True Distribution*

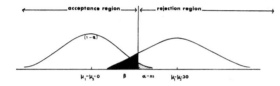

Note: Here, the Null Hypothesis is actually FALSE (i.e., a true difference does exist, in this case .30). However, all sample outcomes are tested against the Null Hypothesis Curve.

The predetermined $\alpha = .05$ area (*Stippled*) of the Null Hypothesis Curve determines its Acceptance and Rejection Regions.

The probability of an actual sample (a sample from the true distribution of differences on the right) falling within this predetermined <u>Acceptance Region</u> is β (Type II Error) (*Shaded*).

The actual sample area (of the true distribution) falling within the <u>Rejection Region</u> of the Null Hypothesis Curve represents no error $(1 - \beta)$.

Since the Null Hypothesis is False, there is no Type I Error.

FIGURE 8-3

FACTORS REDUCING SIZE OF β

(TYPE II) ERROR RISK

ONE TAILED TEST

Distribution Under Null Hypothesis   *True Distribution*

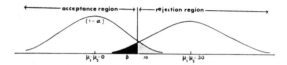

A. $\underline{\alpha}$ Level Chosen: e.g. α is .10 instead of .05 therefore $(1 - \alpha)$ or the Acceptance Region of the Null Hypothesis curve is smaller.

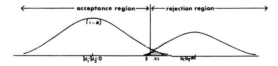

B. <u>Size of Samples</u>: e.g. $n_1 = 100$, $n_2 = 50$ instead of $n_1 = 60$, $n_2 = 30$; therefore, the Standard Error is smaller and curves further apart compared to original curves

or <u>Population Variance</u>: The Variance is smaller and, therefore, so is the Standard Error.

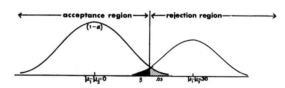

C. <u>Size of True Difference</u>: e.g. $\mu_1 - \mu_2 = .40$ instead of .30; therefore, curves are further apart compared to original curves.

See Note for Figure 8-2 above.

In Figure 8-2B two normal curves are drawn. The one on the right represents the true distribution of differences between our sample proportions, centered at the true difference of .30 (or .50 − .20). On the left is the theoretical curve of sample differences under the Null Hypothesis, $H_0 : (\mu_1 - \mu_2) = 0$, (there is no difference). A sample outcome is <u>always</u> evaluated against the *Rejection Region* and the *Acceptance Region* of <u>this</u> Null Hypothesis curve. The Type II (or β) Error occurs when a sample from the distribution on the right (the curve of true differences) falls within the Acceptance Region of the curve on the left (the hypothetical curve of chance differences under the Null Hypothesis). The β Error is illustrated in Figure 8-2B for a one-tailed test.

It can be seen in Figure 8-3 that the probability of a Type II (β) Error will depend upon several factors (1) <u>the α level chosen</u>: the larger α is (e.g., .10 instead of .05 as in Figure 8-3A), the smaller the β error is, (2) <u>the size of the samples and of the population variances</u> (Figure 8-3B): these factors affect the Standard Error of the curves and therefore the extent of their overlap; and (3) <u>the true difference</u> between the populations from which samples were drawn (Figure 8-3C): the larger the true difference the further apart are the two curves.

In setting up an experiment, the β (Type II) Error is often overlooked. Unless the sample sizes are large enough, one may too often fail to reject the Null Hypothesis because a true difference falls in the Acceptance Region of the Null Hypothesis curve. "Power" curves are available which assist in estimating the β Error risk for various assumed true differences (*alternative hypotheses*) and sample sizes.

SUMMARY OF ERROR RISKS

Type I Error

(α): the Null Hypothesis is *true* (the samples come from the same population) but is *rejected* because the result falls in the α (alpha) region of the Null Hypothesis curve. The error risk is α, the level of significance arbitrarily adopted (e.g., .05). If $\alpha = .05$, then <u>in the long run</u> 5 in 100 times the Null Hypothesis will be rejected when actually true. Such an error risk is not very great and can be lowered by selecting α at .01 or smaller.

Type II Error

(β): the Null Hypothesis is *false* (a real difference exists) but is *accepted* because the result falls within the $(1-\alpha)$ acceptance region of the Null Hypothesis curve. The probability of this error, called β (beta), depends on: (1) the true difference, (2) the sample size and population variance, and (3) the level chosen for α (the smaller α is, the larger β is, see Figure 8-3). Not only are many values of β possible, but β is <u>unknown</u> since we do not know the true difference. There may be a high probability of saying "no difference has been demonstrated" when there is a true difference.

		DECISION MADE	
		Null Hypothesis is *accepted*	Null Hypothesis is *rejected*
ACTUAL	Null Hypothesis is *true*	NO ERROR	TYPE I ERROR (α)
SITUATION	Null Hypothesis is *false*	TYPE II ERROR (β)	NO ERROR

We have presented a systematic approach to inference and the decision making process as applied to qualitative data. In the next chapters we will apply these concepts and procedures to quantitative data. In Chapter 9, we will indicate how quantitative populations can be described by the use of various summary measures.

PROBLEM 8-1

Before accepting that a true difference exists, it is first necessary to rule out chance as the likely explanation of the observed outcome. This decision making process involves a number of steps. Indicate *True* or *False* for the following statements as to procedure:

a) Choose the appropriate two-tailed test.

b) Choose the 0.05 level of significance.

c) Assume the Null Hypothesis.

d) Calculate the appropriate test statistic from the data.

e) Determine the P value associated with that statistic.

f) Accept or reject the Null Hypothesis depending on whether P is larger or smaller than .05.

ANSWER 8-1

a) *False.* Determine whether a two-tailed or one-tailed test is appropriate.

b) *False.* Select the <u>arbitrary</u> level of significance, i.e., .05 is not <u>sacrosanct</u> and it may <u>better</u> suit your purposes to select another level of significance.

c) *True.*

d) *True.*

e) *True.*

f) *False.* Accept or reject the Null Hypothesis based on the P value <u>and the level of significance determined previously.</u> This may or may not be .05.

PROBLEM 8-2

State in your own words the meaning of P = .30, P = .05, P = .01. What action would you take in each case?

ANSWER 8-2

All three probability values refer to the probability of occurrence of an event as extreme as that observed or more extreme by chance alone under the Null Hypothesis (no true difference).

Graph for Problem 8-2

DISTRIBUTION OF CHANCE DIFFERENCES UNDER THE NULL HYPOTHESIS

Shaded Area = P

P = .30   P = .05   P = .01

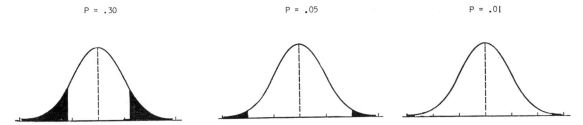

That is, *if* the Null Hypothesis is true, then —

P = .30 means that the event will occur by chance in 30 out of 100 trials. Since this event is very likely, chance cannot be ruled out as the explanation of the sample outcome. Therefore, the Null Hypothesis of no true difference cannot be rejected.

P = .05 means that by chance alone the event will occur only 5 in 100 times. Since this event is relatively rare, chance is an unlikely explanation of the sample outcome. Therefore, the Null Hypothesis of no true difference is rejected, provided that .05 is the level of significance (or α) arbitrarily chosen in advance.

P = .01 means that the chance event will occur very rarely, only 1% of the time, if no true difference exists. Usually the decision is made to reject the Null Hypothesis in such a case.

PROBLEM 8-3

(a) If P < .05, does this *prove* that a drug is more effective than the placebo? Explain.

(b) If P is > .05 does this *prove* that a drug is no more effective than the placebo? Explain.

ANSWER 8-3

(a) No! P < .05 means that the outcome observed or one more extreme would occur by chance less than 5 in 100 times if the Null Hypothesis is true. Thus it is an unlikely event. If α has been set at .05 we reject the Null Hypothesis and accept the alternative hypothesis of a true difference. Nevertheless, the fact is that

such an extreme outcome does occur by chance (5 in 100 trials) when there is no true difference. In such a case we have made a Type I Error, i.e., we rejected the Null Hypothesis when actually true.

(b) No! P > .05 means that more than 5 in 100 times a difference as large as that observed or larger would occur by chance alone when the Null Hypothesis is true. Since this is a frequent event, chance is a likely explanation of the outcome and cannot be ruled out. Because we cannot reject the Null Hypothesis, we accept it. However, acceptance of the Null Hypothesis merely states that there is insufficient evidence of a true difference. If a true difference does exist we have made a Type II Error. A larger sample will be necessary to show a significant difference *if* one exists.

PROBLEM 8-4

(a) What are the two types or error we might make in testing hypotheses?

(b) How is the size of the risk of one type of error related to the size of the other error risk?

ANSWER 8-4

(a) Type I Error: Rejection of the Null Hypothesis when true (determined by α).

Type II Error: Acceptance of the Null Hypothesis when false (represented by β).

(b) The larger α is, the smaller β is.

PROBLEM 8-5

Indicate *True* or *False* for the following statements:

a) The risk of accepting the Null Hypothesis of no true difference when a true difference actually exists is called the β (or Type II) Error.

(b) Three factors affecting the size of the error risk are the size of the true difference, the α level of significance chosen, and the size of the sample.

c) The β (or Type II) Error risk can be determined precisely but the Type I Error risk is generally not known.

ANSWER 8-5

a) *True.*

b) *True.*

c) *False.* The Type I Error risk can be deter-

mined precisely but the Type II Error risk depends upon the true difference. This is generally not known in a sampling situation.

SUMMARY OF CHAPTER 8

The test statistic can be incorporated into a formal decision making process.

This process defines two types of error:
- - rejecting the Null Hypothesis when true (Type I or α)
- - accepting the Null Hypothesis when false (Type II or β)

Only the Type I Error risk can be determined precisely.

CUMULATIVE GLOSSARY I: TERMS

Chapter 8

Type I (α) *Error*	The Null Hypothesis is *true* (the true difference is zero) but is *rejected* because the observed result falls in the α (alpha) or rejection region of the Null Hypothesis curve. The error risk is therefore α, the arbitrary level of significance, and is predetermined.
Type II (β) *Error*	The Null Hypothesis is *false* (a true difference does exist) but is *accepted* because the observed result falls within the $1-\alpha$ region (acceptance region) of the Null Hypothesis curve. Error risk cannot be readily determined. Also called the β Error (see Glossary II for β).
Acceptance Region	$1-\alpha$ region of the Null Hypothesis curve.
Rejection Region	α region or tail(s) of the Null Hypothesis curve.
Null Hypothesis (significance) Test	A test of the Null Hypothesis (zero difference). If the Null Hypothesis is *rejected* the specific alternative hypothesis is *accepted*. See H_o in Glossary II.
Alternative Hypothesis	The hypothesis that is accepted when the Null Hypothesis is rejected. See H_a in Glossary II.
Null Hypothesis Curve	Theoretical sampling distribution under assumption of no true difference.

CUMULATIVE GLOSSARY II: SYMBOLS

Chapter 8

H_o

Null Hypothesis (zero difference) :
$H_o : \mu_1 = \mu_2$ or $(\mu_1 - \mu_2) = 0$

H_a

Alternative Hypothesis:
$H_a : \mu_1 \neq \mu_2$ (non directional, a two-tailed test) , or
$H_a : \mu_1 > \mu_2$ or $\mu_1 < \mu_2$ (directional, one-tailed test)

α

alpha or predetermined *arbitrary* level of significance
(usually .05 or .01). Determines the Type I Error risk or risk of a
false claim of a true difference.

β

beta, equivalent to the Type II Error risk or risk of failing to detect a true difference. Inversely related to the factors: α level, true difference, and size of sample. Directly related to population variance.

9

Description
of a Quantitative Population

*Types of Quantitative (Continuous) Populations • Measures of
Central Tendency • Measures of Dispersion or Variability*

Previous chapters discussed populations of qualitative or categorical data (also called binomial or multinomial) and inferences about such populations based on samples. Tests of significance applicable to binomial and multinomial qualitative populations were illustrated. Descriptions and inferences about such populations are relatively simple. A binomial population, for example, can be completely described by *one* parameter p, since the proportion of the other category, q, must be 1-p.

We now begin the topic of quantitative populations, typically data involving measurements of a continuous variable, such as blood pressure or weight. Such populations are usually more complex, requiring *more* than one parameter for adequate description — at least an average value and some measure of variation in the population.

In this chapter, we shall describe the most common types of continuous populations and some of the summary measures (parameters) used to characterize them. In the next chapter, we will continue our discussion with analysis of the data ordered in a cumulative fashion.

TYPES OF QUANTITATIVE (CONTINUOUS) POPULATIONS

It is important to note that the population of a continuous variable may have *any* shape: skewed, uniform, etc. (Figure 9-1). One possible shape is that of a *normal distribution*.

Normal distribution

A normal distribution can be completely described by mean (μ) and standard deviation

(σ), and has other unique characteristics shown in Figure 9-1A. Quantitative populations which follow the normal distribution include: (1) many populations of measurements on plants and animals which represent the sum of large numbers of independent components (e.g., intelligence quotients of school children and blood pressures of healthy young men) and (2) measurement errors produced by the additive effects of a large number of elementary errors (e.g., errors in titration of pH.)

Many natural phenomena are <u>not</u> normally distributed, however. *Parametric* tests and measures[1] which assume that the underlying population is normally distributed should not be applied to such data. *Nonparametric* (distribution-free) tests should be used instead, or the data may be transformed to a normal population, e.g., to log doses.

Table 9-1 and Figure 9-2 present data on mouth temperatures of 205 presumably healthy young men. It can be seen that the shape of the distribution is approximately that of a normal curve. Although it represents a finite number of individuals for purposes of illustration let us consider it a population. Some principles of presentation of such data, including summarization of the data by grouping into class intervals, is discussed in Table 9-1. In Figure 9-2 the data grouped in class intervals of 0.4°F are presented graphically both in the form of a histogram and as a frequency (line) polygon.

[1]For example, the *t*-test, and certain applications of the correlation coefficient, r. (See Chapters 11 and 15).

Figure 9-1

HYPOTHETICAL EXAMPLES OF CONTINUOUS DISTRIBUTIONS

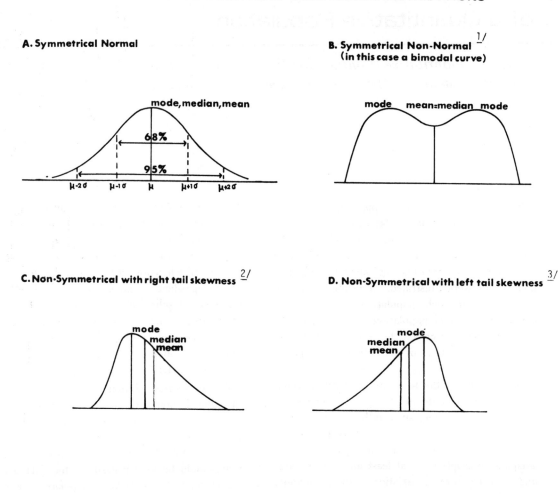

A. Symmetrical Normal

B. Symmetrical Non-Normal [1]
(in this case a bimodal curve)

C. Non-Symmetrical with right tail skewness [2]

D. Non-Symmetrical with left tail skewness [3]

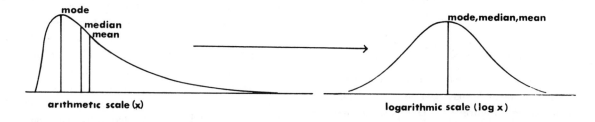

E. Non-Symmetrical Log Normal

F. Transformation of Log Normal

arithmetic scale (x)

logarithmic scale (log x)

[1] The bimodality of this population suggests that it is not homogeneous and should be divided into subgroups for analysis.

[2] Same as positive skewness.

[3] Same as negative skewness.

TABLE 9-1
Mouth Temperature at Physical Examination
Population of Healthy Young Men (C. W. Heath, 1945) *

Temp. °F[1]	No. of Men	0.2° Grouping Temp. °F	No. of Men	0.4° Grouping Temp. °F	No. of Men	0.6° Grouping Temp. °F	No. of Men
97.0	2	97.0- 97.1	2	97.0- 97.3	4	97.0- 97.5	10
97.2	2	97.2- 97.3	2	97.4- 97.7	16	97.6- 98.1	53
97.4	3	97.4- 97.5	6	97.8- 98.1	43	98.2- 98.7	109
97.5	3	97.6- 97.7	10	98.2- 98.5	72	98.8- 99.3	30
97.6	6	97.8- 97.9	16	98.6- 98.9	48	99.4- 99.9	2
97.7	4	98.0- 98.1	27	99.0- 99.3	19	100.0-100.5	1
97.8	11	98.2- 98.3	30	99.4- 99.7	2		——
97.9	5	98.4- 98.5	42	99.8-100.1	1		205
98.0	20	98.6- 98.7	37		——		
98.1	7	98.8- 98.9	11		205		
98.2	15	99.0- 99.1	16				
98.3	15	99.2- 99.3	3				
98.4	29	99.4- 99.5	2				
98.5	13	99.6- 99.7	0				
98.6	26	99.8- 99.9	0				
98.7	11	100.0-100.1	1				
98.8	8		——				
98.9	3		205				
99.0	10						
99.1	6						
99.2	1						
99.3	2						
99.5	2						
100.0	1						
	——						
	205						
Pop. Mean (μ) 98.35°		98.41°		98.42°		98.39°	
Pop. S.D. (σ) 0.47°		0.47°		0.48°		0.48°	

[1]Measurements were rounded to 0.1° below, e.g., any measurement between 98.1° and 98.2° was considered by the investigator to be 98.1°. Ordinarily, rounding off is made to the *nearest* .1°. For purposes of simplicity, we shall treat the data as if rounded off to the nearest .1°.

Grouping of Data: The first column presents the data as originally rounded off. The distribution is presented in succeeding columns partially summarized, i.e., grouped by class intervals. How fine should class intervals be? Not so wide that the distribution is distorted or calculated parameters markedly changed. Not so narrow that summarization is not achieved nor inherent accuracy of measurement ignored. For example, the data in Table 9-1 suggest that 0.1 degree of temperature cannot be measured accurately — there is a "heaping" of individuals at "even" digits (0.2 degrees) *digit preference*. When grouped by 0.4 degrees, information about the distribution is still adequate. That is, the reduction of the data has not introduced any significant error.

Other distributions

Figure 9-1B shows a distribution which is

symmetrical but *not normal*. Several types of non-symmetrical, or skewed, distributions are shown in Figure 9-1C, D, and E. Figure 9-1C is positively skewed (has an elongated tail to the right, or positive, direction), while Figure 9-1D is skewed to the left (negative skewness). Figure C might describe a distribution of families by income.

The log normal (Figure 9-1E) is a distribution which is skewed when the raw data (x values) are plotted directly, but is transformed to a normal curve (Figure 9-1F) when the logarithms of the x values are plotted. These logarithms may be to the base 10, e (2.718) or any other value. Distances on an arithmetic scale represent *absolute* change; on a logarithmic scale, *percentage* or *relative* change. Certain types of biological data, such as tolerance to a drug, and heart rate, have a log normal distribution. In some cases, the distribution can be attributed to a limitation of the possible range or variation in one direction. A hypothetical example of log normal data is given in Table 9-4.

*Johns Hopkins University School of Hygiene and Public Health

FIGURE 9-2

MOUTH TEMPERATURE OF 205 HEALTHY YOUNG MEN
Percentage Distribution According to Class Intervals of 0.4° F

Histogram and superimposed Frequency polygon
Histogram — bar covers width of class interval; height represents relative frequency (percentage)
Frequency (line) polygon — plotted at *midpoint* of class interval (e.g., 97.2, 97.6 etc.)

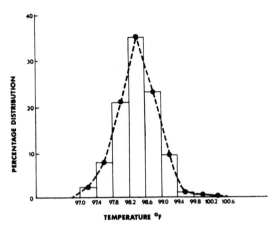

Note that in this instance all class intervals are the same (0.4°F). Where class intervals are not equal it is necesary to adjust the height of the bar for the length of the class interval so that area (height times length) equals frequency in the interval.

MEASURES OF CENTRAL TENDENCY

We can summarize our data succinctly by one or more measures of "central tendency" — mode, median, or mean (Figure 9-1):

The *mode* is the most frequent value (point of maximum concentration).

The *median* is the middle value of data ordered (arrayed) from the lowest to highest (50% of the population has a value as small or smaller and 50% a value as large or larger than the median). The median of an <u>even</u> number of observations is taken, arbitrarily, as the average of the two middle values, e.g., the median of the values 8, 8, 13, and 15 is 10.5.

The *mean* is the arithmetic average (μ). In algebraic notation the formula for the mean is written as $\dfrac{\Sigma x}{N}$ which says: add <u>all</u> the elements of the population $x_1 \ldots x_N$ and divide by the total number of elements, N. For example, the mean of 8, 8, 13, and 15 is $\dfrac{44}{4} = 11$. For grouped data, the formula for the mean is a *weighted* average

$$\mu = \frac{\Sigma \left[(\text{midpoint of class}) \times (\text{frequency of the class}) \right]}{\Sigma \text{ frequencies} = N}$$

The method of computing the mean for our population of temperatures of healthy young men is illustrated in Table 9-2 for ungrouped data and in Table 9-3 for grouped data.

The limits of class intervals and rounding off rules in measurement must be clearly indicated so that a correct midpoint can be assigned. The above example makes the assumption that the precision of the thermometer is such that it can be read to more than one decimal place.

In symmetrical distributions, the median and mean values coincide (Figure 9-1A). In highly skewed populations, the median is a more "representative" average because it is not affected as much as the mean is by extreme values in one direction. For example, in Figure 9-1C, where the tail is to the right, the mean is larger than the median because the mean is affected more by the few high values. In Figure 9-1D the mean is smaller than the median because of the extreme low values. In log normal distributions (Figures 9-1E, F and Table 9-4) such as dose response data, either the median or the *geometric mean* (the antilog of the mean of the logarithms) is more "representative" than the arithmetic mean.

On the other hand the mean is typically more useful than the median for statistics of inference, that is for estimating population parameters from sample values. Also, in combining different populations a combined mean can be obtained directly by weighting each mean by the number of items it represents (or size of the population). Medians cannot be combined directly. Instead the combined population must be reordered to find its midpoint or median.

MEASURES OF DISPERSION OR VARIABILITY

In addition to average values, the scatter of the population (variability) must be described. Do items tend to be alike (cluster together) or do they instead differ markedly from each other? Summary measures of the variability of individuals in a population are useful for describing the population distribution. As will be shown in Chapter 11, these measures are also needed for estimating the reliability of statistics based on samples from the population. It is important to note that the variability of individuals in a population is an <u>inherent</u> characteristic and cannot

TABLE 9-2

Calculation of Mean, Variance and
Standard Deviation for Ungrouped Data
Mouth Temperatures of 205 Healthy Young Men (0.1°F intervals)

Individual	Temperature (x)	Deviation from Mean $(x-\mu)$	Squared Deviation $(x-\mu)^2$
1	97.0	−1.35	1.8225
2	97.0	−1.35	1.8225
3	97.2	−1.15	1.3225
•	•	•	•
•	•	•	•
205	100.0	+1.65	2.7225
Total	20160.9°	0	45.1890

$$\text{Pop. Mean} = \mu = \frac{\Sigma x}{N} = \frac{20160.9}{205} = 98.35°$$

$$\text{Pop. Variance} = \sigma^2 = \frac{\Sigma (x-\mu)^2}{N} = \frac{45.19}{205} = .222$$

$$\text{Pop. Standard Deviation} = \sigma = \sqrt{\frac{\Sigma (x-\mu)^2}{N}} = \sqrt{.222} = .47°$$

TABLE 9-3

Calculation of Mean, Variance
and
Standard Deviation for Grouped Data
(Class Interval of 0.4° F)

Mouth Temperatures of 205 Healthy Young Men

Temperature (°F)	Mid-pt. x	Freq. f	*Weighted* Freq. xf	Deviation From Mean $(x-\mu)$	Squared Deviation $(x-\mu)^2$	*Weighted* Squared Deviation $(x-\mu)^2 f$
97.0 and under 97.4	97.2	4	388.8	−1.22	1.4884	5.9536
97.4 and under 97.8	97.6	16	1561.6	−0.82	.6724	10.7584
97.8 and under 98.2	98.0	43	4214.0	−0.42	.1764	7.5852
98.2 and under 98.6	98.4	72	7084.8	−0.02	.0400	0.0288
98.6 and under 99.0	?8.8	48	4742.4	+0.38	.1444	6.9312
99.0 and under 99.4	99.2	19	1884.8	+0.78	.6084	11.5596
99.4 and under 99.8	99.6	2	199.2	+1.18	1.3924	2.7848
99.8 and under 100.2	100.0	1	100.0	+1.58	2.4964	2.4964
Total		205	20175.6			48.0981

$$\text{Pop. Mean, } \mu = \frac{\Sigma x f}{\Sigma f = N} = \frac{20175.6}{205} = 98.42°$$

$$\text{Pop. Variance, } \sigma^2 = \frac{\Sigma (x-\mu)^2 f}{\Sigma f = N} = \frac{48.0981}{205} = .2346$$

Pop. Standard deviation, SD or $\sigma = \sqrt{.2346} = 0.48°$

NOTE: For all computations, such as mean or standard deviation, the *midpoint* of the interval represents the x value for every member in the class. The *frequency* (f), or number of individuals in the class, is the *"weighting"* factor.

be affected by the size of the population. (Similarly, the variability of individuals in a sample is not affected by the size of the sample.)

The most useful measure of variability is the *population standard deviation* (σ). Its square, the *population variance* (σ^2), is computed first. The variance is the <u>average</u> squared deviation around the mean and <u>can</u> be expressed algebraically by $\frac{\Sigma (x-\mu)^2}{N}$. This formula says: (1) obtain the deviation of each item from the mean, (2) square the deviation, (3) sum up all items in the population, and (4) divide by the total number of items (N) to obtain the <u>average</u> squared deviation. Examples of this <u>calculation</u> are illustrated in Table 9-2 for ungrouped data and in Table 9-3 for grouped data. A short-cut computational formula is shown in the footnote[1] and is illustrated in Problem 14-13.

The Standard Deviation (σ) is the <u>square root</u> of the variance, S.D. $= \sqrt{\text{variance}}$. Therefore, its algebraic form is $\sqrt{\frac{\Sigma (x-\mu)^2}{N}}$. Thus the variance of the distribution of mouth temperatures (in 0.4° class intervals) (Table 9-3) is .2346 and its square root, the standard deviation, is .48°.

The square root operation converts the measure of variability back to its original (unsquared) dimension. Why then are the deviations squared? Why not add the original deviations without regard to "+" or "−" sign to obtain a *mean absolute deviation?*[2]

Because measures based on squared deviations (i.e., variances) are very useful statistically: (1) When populations or samples are combined their variances can be <u>pooled</u> after appropriate weighting; for example, the comparison of treatment results from two investigators of breast cancer requires knowledge of the respective variances which are subsequently pooled. (2) Conversely, a variance can be <u>partitioned</u> into its components such as differences <u>between</u> treatment groups and differences <u>within</u> treatment groups (the topic of

TABLE 9-4
Example of a Logarithmic Transformation

Following are data (fictitious) which illustrate "distortion" of the arithmetic mean as a measure of central tendency when the distribution is highly skewed. These data represent thresholds of 13 experimental animals to a given drug, with values arrayed in order of magnitude.

Threshold of Animal (mg per kg body weight)	Logarithm of Threshold
4	0.6021
6	0.7782
8	0.9031
9	0.9542
9	0.9542
14	1.1461
15	1.1761
16	1.2041
18	1.2553
25	1.3979
28	1.4472
70	1.8451
160	2.2041
Total 382	15.8677

The arithmetic mean of these values is 382/13 = 29.4 mg/kg. Note that 11 of the 13 animals showed a smaller threshold than the mean while only 2 showed a bigger threshold. Since the logarithms of thresholds are often found to be distributed normally, or nearly so, a logarithmic "transformation" should be attempted. That is, we should deal with the logarithms of the values rather than with the values themselves.

The mean of the logarithms is 15.8677/13 = 1.2206. The antilog of this value is called the geometric mean and in this instance is equal to 16.6 mg/kg. Note how much more typical or representative this value is than the arithmetic mean. Note also that the median, which is affected much less by skewness than is the arithmetic mean, is equal to 15 mg/kg, ---- a value approximating the geometric mean but much smaller than the arithmetic mean. This reflects the tremendous reduction in skewness resulting from the logarithmic transformation. (From Menduke, H., class material.)

---

[1]The sum of squared deviations around the mean used in the numerator of the variance formula, $\Sigma (x-\mu)^2$, can be shown to equal $\Sigma x^2 - \frac{(\Sigma x)^2}{N}$. Therefore the population variance,

$$\sigma^2 = \frac{\Sigma (x-\mu)^2}{N} = \frac{1}{N}\left[\Sigma x^2 - \frac{(\Sigma x)^2}{N} \right] = \frac{\Sigma x^2}{N} - \left[\frac{\Sigma x}{N} \right]^2$$

These identities are the basis of short-cut computational formula.

[2]If they were added with "+" and "−" signs retained, they would add to zero, since deviations around a mean add up to zero.

Analysis of Variance and Design of Experiments.)

Another advantage is that if the population follows a normal distribution then we know from the mean (μ) and the square root of the variance, i.e., the standard deviation (σ), its precise probability areas. Even if a population is <u>not normally</u> distributed we know that at least $\frac{3}{4}$ of the measurements will lie between the mean (μ) and 2 σ's on either side, and 8/9 within 3 σ's on either side (Tchebycheff's inequality).

Finally, a measure of the reliability of sample statistics is given by the Standard Error, which, as will be shown in Chapter 11, is directly related to the Standard Deviation of the population.

The *coefficient* of *variation* (C.V.) is another useful term. It is used to compare the variability of two diverse populations with different units of measure, such as blood pressure and blood cell diameter. The formula C.V. $= \dfrac{\sigma}{\mu}$ x 100 expresses the size of the standard deviation in relation to the size of the mean. The multiplication by 100 converts this relative variation to a percentage. Since the dimensions in the numerator and denominator cancel, C.V. is dimensionless. Thus, whether we record children's height in inches or in centimeters, the C.V. will be the same. We can even compare the variability of blood sugar level (mg/100 ml.) with that of respiration (breaths/min.).

In the next chapter, we will discuss how one can use a *cumulative* frequency or percentage distribution in order to describe a population.

PROBLEM 9-1

Indicate *true or false* for each item in the statement below:

In a normally distributed population

(a) The mean and median are identical.

(b) The distribution is symmetrical.

(c) The mode differs from the mean.

(d) If you take any point on the **x** axis and add one Standard Deviation, 34% of the area will fall between these two points.

ANSWER 9-1

(a) *True*

(b) *True*

(c) *False*. Mode = mean = median in a normal distribution.

(d) *False*. It is *only* at the center of the dis-

tribution (μ) where one can encompass 34% of the observations by adding 1 Standard Deviation, i.e., ($\mu + 1$ S. D.)

PROBLEM 9-2

Comparison of Two Groups:

	Healthy Men	Men with Tuberculosis
Mean Temperature	98.4°	99.4°
Standard Deviation	0.5°	1.0°

Assuming that each group is normally distributed;

(a) What proportion of the healthy men have temperatures between 97.4° and 99.4°?

(b) What temperatures will include 68% of the healthy men? 95% of the healthy men?*

(c) What temperatures will include 68% of the tuberculous men? 95% of the tuberculous men?*

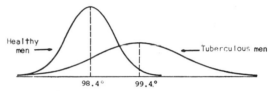

ANSWER 9-2

(a) By the z scale since $\mu = 98.4°$ and $\sigma = .5°$ we see that 97.4°-99.4° represents $\mu \pm 2\sigma$. Therefore it includes 95% of the observations.

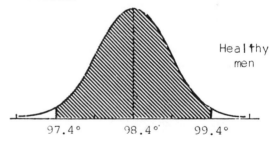

(b) 68% of the area under a normal curve is represented by $\mu \pm 1\sigma = 98.4° \pm 0.5° = 97.9°$ to 98.9°. Similarly, 95% is represented by $\mu \pm 2\sigma = 98.4° \pm 2(0.5)° = 97.4°$ to 99.4°.

(c) In a similar manner, for tuberculous men

68% = $\mu \pm 1\sigma = 99.4° \pm 1.0° = 98.4°$ to 100.4°

95% = $\mu \pm 2\sigma = 99.4° \pm 2(1.0)° = 97.4°$ to 101.4°

---

*Without further specification, we assume that the question refers to the area around the mean.

PROBLEM 9-3

The heights of a large population of men are found to follow fairly closely a normal distribution with a mean of 67 inches and a standard deviation of 2 inches.

What proportions of the population would you expect to find with a height:

(a) above 70 in.?

(b) below 65 in.?

(c) between 65 and 70 in.?

(d) What height is exceeded by 2.5% of the population?

ANSWER 9-3

This exercise demonstrates the usefulness of the normal curve.

(a) We translate to the z scale by

$$z = \frac{x - \mu}{\sigma}$$

μ is 67 in.

σ is 2 in.

Here x is 70 in.

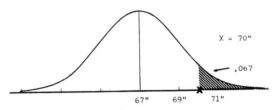

$$\therefore z = \frac{70'' - 67''}{2''} = \frac{3''}{2''} = 1.5 \text{ and}$$

P = .134. However, we are interested only in the area in the upper tail or

$$\frac{P}{2} = \frac{.134}{2} = .067$$

(b) Here x = 65 in.

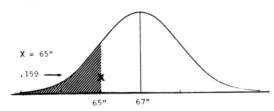

$$\therefore z = \frac{65'' - 67''}{2''} = \frac{-2''}{2''} = -1 \text{ and}$$

P = .317. Here we are interested only in the lower tail or

$$\frac{P}{2} = \frac{.317}{2} = .159$$

(c) The area between 65″ and 70″ is the sum of the area between 65″ and 67″ and between 67″ and 70″. It can be obtained in 2 ways:

(1) By adding the two 1-P areas (A + B = C):

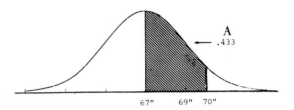

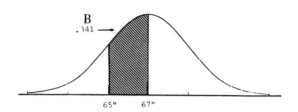

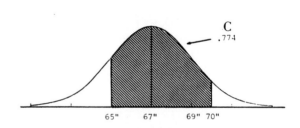

$$A \left[z = \frac{70'' - 67''}{2''} = \frac{3''}{2''} = 1.5. \right.$$

Here we need 1-P associated with this z value. 1-P = .867. Half of this is .433 $\Big]$.

$$+$$

$$B \left[z = \frac{65'' - 67''}{2''} = \frac{-2''}{2''} = -1 \right.$$

Therefore, 1-P = .683 and $\frac{1\text{-}P}{2} = .341 \Big]$.

C. Hence, the Total area = .433 + .341 = .744

(2) By adding the area in both tails beyond 65″ to 70″ and deducting this from the total curve area or 1: The area beyond 65″ to 70″ is the sum of the area in (a) and (b) or .067 + .159 = .226. Therefore, 1—.226 = .774

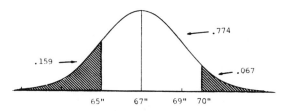

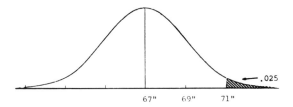

(d) The height *exceeded* by 2.5% of the population can be determined by solving for x

when $\dfrac{P}{2} = .025$. We know that a z of 1.96 is associated with a P of .05 or $\dfrac{P}{2}$ of .025

$$\therefore 1.96 \text{ (or 2)} = \frac{x-67''}{2''}$$

$$4'' = x-67'' \text{ and } \therefore x = 71''$$

PROBLEM 9-4

What does the mean or median alone, and together, tell about the distribution of a population?

ANSWER 9-4

The mean is the "weighted" center of the distribution comparable to the "fulcrum" in a balanced seesaw. The median divides the distribution in half so that 50% of the distribution lies above and 50% below this value. Neither parameter by itself tells you the shape of the distribution. The median and mean together, however, can tell you if the distribution is symmetrical or skewed.

— if symmetrical, mean = median
— if skewed to the right (tail on the right) the mean will be greater than the median.
— if skewed to the left (tail on the left) the mean will be less than the median.

PROBLEM 9-5

The standard deviation of a distribution of heights or weights does not depend on the mean value. *True or False?*

ANSWER 9-5

True. This may seem to contradict the standard deviation formula since S.D. is obtained by squaring individual deviations from the mean. However, the standard deviation of heights measures only how much the heights of individuals vary one from another. The mean is derived from the individuals. The mean does not give any information about the size of S.D. of heights. It is possible to have the same standard deviation with a large mean or with a small mean.

(However, it should be pointed out that for some distributions, such as the Poisson, the mean and variance are identical and therefore the standard deviation is determined by the mean.)

PROBLEM 9-6

Indicate *True* or *False* for each item in the statement below:

For grouped measurement data

(a) The frequency in each interval is used for the calculation of mean and standard deviation.

(b) When measurements are recorded to the nearest mm., the midpoints of the intervals 6-8 mm. and 9-11 mm. are 7 and 10 mm. respectively.

(c) The width of the interval in (b) is 2 mm.

ANSWER 9-6

(a) *True.* The frequency (f) is the "weighting" factor used in all calculations.

(b) *True.* The class limits are shown graphically below along with the midpoints x:

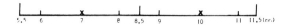

(c) *False.* The width of the class interval is 3 mm., i.e., 5.5 to 8.5 mm. Since measurements are rounded to the nearest mm., a measurement of exactly 8.5 would be rounded as 8 half the time and as 9 half the time.

PROBLEM 9-7

The data* below on daily log output of nicotinamide methochloride of several populations of rats represent an interesting genetic example:

Distributions of the logarithm of the daily output (in micrograms) of nicotinamide methochloride.

Log. output (μg.)[1]	Albino A	Hooded H	First cross F_1	Backcross $F_1 \times A$	Backcross $F_1 \times H$	Second Cross F_2
<1.50	2	—	—	—	—	1
1.50—	7	—	—	7	—	—
1.65—	9	—	--	2	—	1
1.80—	6	—	—	5	—	1
1.95—	17	—	—	18	1	5
2.10—	9	—	5	34	6	6
2.25—	—	—	19	47	24	6
2.40—	—	—	17	17	29	4
2.55—	—	1	10	10	25	2
2.70—	—	17	—	1	39	5
2.85—	—	23	—	1	43	3
3.00—	—	12	—	—	31	3
3.15—	—	4	—	1	4	2
3.30—	—	—	—	—	—	—
Total no. of rats	50	57	51	143	202	39
Mean	1.89	2.92	2.42	2.24	2.72	2.45
S.D.	0.22	0.14	0.14	0.26	0.27	0.43

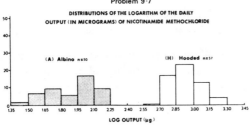

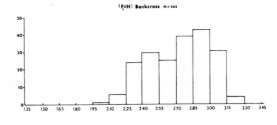

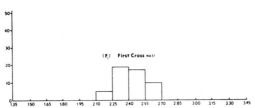

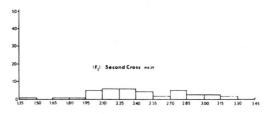

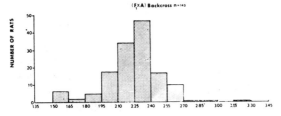

A (Albino) and H (Hooded) are two inbred strains of rats. The F_1 generation is obtained by crossing the two inbred strains. The two backcross generations, $F_1 \times A$ and $F_1 \times H$, are obtained by crossing the F_1 with each of the inbred strains. The F_2 generation is obtained by interbreeding the F_1.

*Source: London School of Hygiene and Tropical Medicine

[1]Lower limit of class

Histograms of the distributions are shown in the graph.

The means and standard deviations are given in the table. Note that:

(1) the F_1 and F_2 means are about midway between those of the two parent strains,

(2) the two backcross means F_1A and F_1H are about midway between the means for F_1 and parent (A and H),

(3) the S.D. for the F_1 generation is less than the average of the S.D.'s for the parent strains (this phenomenon is often observed),

(4) the S.D. for the F_2 generation is very much larger than for the parent or F_1 generations, owing to segregation of genes.

This is a typical picture of inheritance of a measurement controlled by a large number of genes.

Check your ability to calculate the mean and standard deviation for grouped data by verifying the values for First Cross F_1.

Before carrying out the calculations, answer the following questions:

(a) Is this a continuous or a discrete distribution? Why?

(b) What are the class limits? The class midpoint?

ANSWER 9-7

(a) Log output of nicotinamide methochloride represents *continuous* data. There is an infinite number of points along the scale. The output is *not* exactly 1 μg., 2 μg., etc as with number of teeth (*discrete* data).

(b) Only the lower class limit is shown. Therefore, the upper class limits and the midpoint would be:

Lower limit	Upper limit	Midpoint
1.50	— 1.6499	1.575
1.65	— 1.7999	1.725
1.80	— 1.9499	1.875

The midpoint may be obtained by adding the two lower limits (1.50 + 1.65) and dividing by 2 = 1.575. The calculation of the mean and Standard Deviation for First Cross (F_1) is shown:

Calculations of Mean and Standard Deviation
First Cross (F_1)
(Log Output in μg.)

Class interval	Midpoint	Frequency	Weighted Frequency	Deviation from mean	Squared Deviation	Weighted Squared Deviation
	(x)	(f)	(xf)	$(x-\mu)$	$(x-\mu)^2$	$(x-\mu)^2 f$
2.10-2.2499	2.175	5	10.875	.245	.060025	.300125
2.25-2.3999	2.325	19	44.175	.095	.009025	.171475
2.40-2.5499	2.475	17	42.075	—.055	.003025	.051425
2.55-2.6999	2.625	10	26.250	—.205	.042025	.420250
Total		51	123.375			.943275

$$\text{Mean} = \frac{\Sigma xf}{\Sigma f = N} = \frac{122.375}{51} = 2.40; \quad \text{Variance} = \frac{\Sigma (x-\mu)^2 f}{\Sigma f = N} = \frac{.943,275}{51} = .01849; \quad \text{S.D.} = \sqrt{.01849} \text{ or } .14$$

SUMMARY OF CHAPTER 9

In this chapter we have learned that a population of continuous data can have many different shapes:

—normal

—log normal

—other symmetrical and nonsymmetrical distributions

A large population of continuous data can be summarized by:

—grouping the data into classes

—measures of central tendency (mean, median, mode)

—measures of spread or variation

Of especial use is the Standard Deviation and its square, the Variance. These measure the inherent variability of individuals in the population.

CUMULATIVE GLOSSARY I: TERMS

Chapter 9

Skewed Distribution	A distribution with one elongated tail.
Positively Skewed	With elongated tail to the right (positive direction or large numbers).
Negatively Skewed	With elongated tail to the left (negative direction or small numbers).
Uniform (Rectangular) Distribution	A distribution with equal frequency for all x values.
Parametric Test	A test which assumes that the underlying population has the parameters or shape of a particular distribution.
Non-Parametric Test	A test which makes no assumption about the parameters or shape of the underlying population.
Transformation	Mathematical operation which changes the algebraic expression of a set of values.
Lognormal Distribution	A skewed distribution which can be transformed to a normal distribution by taking the logarithms of the x values.
Measure of Central Tendency	Average value.
Mean	The arithmetic average; see 'μ' in Glossary II.
Mode	The most frequent value (point of maximum concentration).
Median	The middle value of data ordered from lowest to highest.
Geometric mean	Antilog of the mean of logarithmic data.
Frequency (f)	Number of individuals with value x (or in the xth class interval). A weighting factor in calculations.
Variance	A measure of variability represented by the average squared deviation around the mean. See σ^2 in Glossary II.
Standard Deviation	A measure of dispersion obtained by taking the square root of the variance. See σ in Glossary II.
Coefficient of Variation	The size of the standard deviation relative to the size of the mean (in percentage). See C.V. in Glossary II.
Class interval	Arbitrary unit into which raw data are grouped.
Frequency Distribution	Arrangement of data indicating the frequency of specified x values.
Frequency Polygon	A many-sided figure. Formed by straight lines which connect the points representing the frequencies of the x values. In grouped data, the frequencies are plotted at the midpoints of the class intervals.
Histogram	A bar graph for grouped data. Assuming equal class intervals, the frequency of a class is represented by the height and the class interval by the width of the bar.

CUMULATIVE GLOSSARY II: SYMBOLS

Chapter 9

N   number of individuals in a population (*population* size)[*]

μ mu, the mean or arithmetic average of a population of individuals

$$\frac{\Sigma x}{N}$$

σ^2 sigma squared, the variance of a population

$$\frac{\Sigma(x-\mu)^2}{N}$$

σ sigma, the standard deviation of a population (or S.D.)

$$\sqrt{\frac{\Sigma(x-\mu)^2}{N}}$$

C.V.   Coefficient of Variation (in %)

$$\frac{\sigma}{\mu} \times 100$$

---

*Remember (from Chapter 2) that n= number of individuals in a sample (*sample* size).

10

Cumulative Frequency Distributions and Ordered Data

Cumulative Frequency Distribution • Application to Pharmacology • Other Measures Based on Ordered Data

In the previous chapter we discussed various types of continuous populations and some of the summary measures used to describe them. In this chapter we continue the general theme of descriptive statistics for populations using the *cumulative* frequency distribution and measures based on ordered data.

CUMULATIVE FREQUENCY DISTRIBUTION

The data are ordered by size as in the uncumulated frequency polygon and then cumulated successively. Table 10-1 illustrates this method for the data on temperatures of 205 healthy young men (Table 9-3). The cumulative number or cumulative per cent indicates that portion of the population which has a certain x value or less. The uses of the cumulative percentage distribution are discussed in the following paragraphs.

It is helpful to graph the data before proceeding further. Special care must be taken when grouped data are plotted. The cumulative percentages must correspond to the end of the class interval (Figure 10-1). Recall that with the uncumulated frequency polygon, frequencies or percentages are plotted at the midpoint of the class interval (Figure 9-2).

One use of the cumulative graph is for visual inspection; does it approximate a normal curve? If a population is normally distributed the cumulative curve characteristically will be *sigmoid* in shape; it will be an S-shaped curve, approaching linearity in the middle and curved at either end. The data can be plotted on a special type of paper called *probability paper,* which exaggerates the upper and lower ends of the scale (Figure 10-2) in such a manner that the cumulative normal curve is "straightened out". Thus any set of cumulative data which plots as a straight line on (arithmetic) probability paper must be normally distributed.

An important characteristic of the normal curve is that the mean (μ) and the median are identical. (This is true of all symmetrical distributions). The median is the x value below which 50% of the population values lie, and above which the other 50% are found. Therefore, if one reads from the cumulative graph the value on the x scale which corresponds to the 50% point on the y scale, it will provide an estimate of the mean if the population is approximately symmetrical.

Another characteristic of the normal distribution is that the mean (μ) $\pm$ 1 standard deviation will include 68% of the area under the curve. That is, 34% of the population will lie between (the mean) and (the mean *minus* one standard deviation) and 34% between (the mean) and (the mean *plus* one standard deviation). The cumulative graph, therefore, can be used to estimate the standard deviation for a normal distribution: read the x values corresponding to the 50% and 16% points. The difference between these x values represents 1 standard deviation. Similarly, read the x values corresponding to the 50% and 84% points. The difference between these two values provides another estimate of the standard deviation. If the data are approximately normally distributed, the distribution will be symmetrical and the two estimates of the standard deviation will be about the same. An average of the two will estimate the actual standard deviation computed as $\sqrt{\dfrac{\Sigma (x-\mu)^2}{N}}$ (See Chapter 9).

TABLE 10-1

Calculation of Quartile Values from Cumulative Percentage Distribution
Mouth Temperatures of 205 Healthy Young Men[1]
(Grouped in 0.4° F)

Midpoint of Class Interval	Class Interval				Frequency in %	Cumulative %
97.2° F	97.0° F to less than			97.4° F	1.95	1.95
97.6	97.4	"	"	" 97.8	7.80	9.75
98.0	97.8	"	"	" 98.2	20.97	30.72
98.4	98.2	"	"	" 98.6	35.12	65.84
98.8	98.6	"	"	" 99.0	23.41	89.25
99.2	99.0	"	"	" 99.4	9.27	98.52
99.6	99.4	"	"	" 99.8	.98	99.50
100.0	99.8	"	"	" 100.2	.49	99.99

(difference = percentage points remaining)

(beginning of interval)   (width of class interval)   (prorated portion of interval) (width of interval)

$$Q_1 \ (25\%) = 97.8° + \left[\frac{25\% - 9.75\%}{30.72\% - 9.75\%}\right] (.4)° = 97.8° + (.727) (.4)° = 98.09°$$
.29

(difference = relative frequency of class interval)

$$Q_2 \ (50\%) = 98.2° + \left[\frac{50\% - 30.72\%}{65.84\% - 30.72\%}\right] (.4)° = 98.2° + (.549) (.4)° = 98.42°$$
.22

$$Q_3 \ (75\%) = 98.6° + \left[\frac{75\% - 65.84\%}{89.25\% - 65.84\%}\right] (.4)° = 98.6° + (.391) (.4)° = 98.76°$$
.16

[1] See Table 9-3.

This is illustrated in Figure 10-1 for mouth temperatures. It can be seen from this graph that the distribution of mouth temperatures is approximately normal since the difference between the 84th and 50th percentiles is .48°, the same as the calculated standard deviation of .48°. The difference between the 50% and 16% values is approximately .50° which is not too disparate.

The standard deviation is a measure of the inherent variability of individuals in the population. The larger the standard deviation the greater will be the distance between the x values corresponding to the 50th and 84th (or 16th and 50th) percentage points. A more variable population has a cumulative curve with a slope that is less steep (Figure 10-3, curve B) than that of a less variable population (Figure 10-3, curve A). The steepness of the slope of the cumulative graph (especially the linear portion) is, therefore, a measure of the variability of the population.

APPLICATION TO PHARMACOLOGY

It is not possible to discuss in detail the statistics of pharmacology, such as the evaluation of drug potency and toxicity or bioassay. The material in the preceding paragraphs, however, provides a brief introduction to this topic since the cumulative normal curve has its most practical application here. An elementary understanding of this application is desirable.

It was mentioned in Chapter 9 that the distribution of a population of thresholds* to a drug is frequently log-normal. In other words, if the logarithms of the doses are plotted on an arithmetic scale (or if the doses are plotted on a logarithmic scale) then the thresholds will follow a normal distribution. If we give a series of graded doses to

*The *threshold* of an individual to a particular drug is the amount of that drug just necessary to produce a response in that individual.

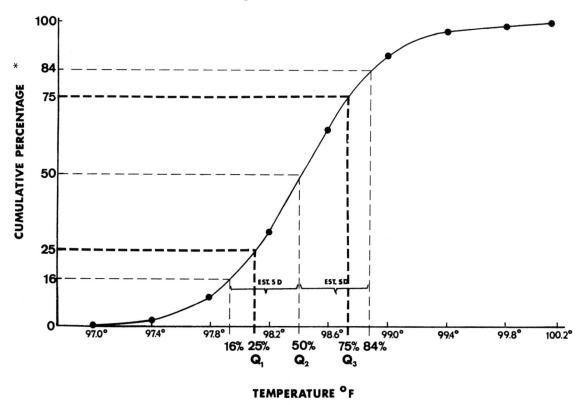

FIGURE 10-1

MOUTH TEMPERATURE OF 205 HEALTHY YOUNG MEN

Cumulative Percentage Distribution Class Intervals of 0.4°F

*Percentage with temperature less than stated value

ESTIMATED STANDARD DEVIATION

$$84\% = 98.88° \atop 50\% = 98.40°\} = .48°$$
$$50\% = 98.40° \atop 16\% = 97.90°\} = .50°$$

ESTIMATED QUARTILES:

$Q_1 = 25\% = 98.10°$
$Q_2 = 50\% = 98.40°$
$Q_3 = 75\% = 98.74°$

---

groups of subjects and plot the percentage responding to each dose we have in effect a "cumulative" curve of thresholds. This is called a *dose-response* curve.

The response may be *quantal* (all or none response of an animal — the curve represents an increasing percentage of the animals responding to a drug) or *graded* (the response is of increasing magnitude within an animal or tissue). We shall use a simple example of quantal response (qualitative) data for illustration (Figure 10-4).

From a dose-response curve one can readily determine the median effective dose, ED_{50}, e.g., that dose to which 50 percent of the popu-

lation will respond. If the curve represents the percentages of an experimental animal population for which specified doses are just lethal, then that dose at which 50% of the animals will die is referred to as the LD_{50} (Table 10-2 and Figure 10-4).

As pointed out before, the slope of the cumulative curve reflects the variability of the population. The steeper the slope, the smaller will be the standard deviation or difference between the 50% and 84% (or 16% and 50%) values. Therefore, two drugs can be compared as to (1) *potency* (if their slopes are parallel): the dose-response curve or ED_{50} for the less potent drug will be to

FIGURE 10-2

CUMULATIVE PERCENTAGE DISTRIBUTION
ON PROBABILITY PAPER
MOUTH TEMPERATURES OF
205 HEALTHY YOUNG MEN

Class Intervals of 0.4°F

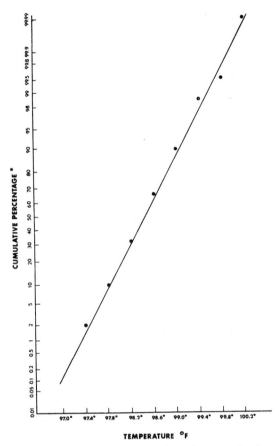

*Percentage with temperature less than stated value

the right of that for the more potent drug since a larger dose of the less potent drug is necessary to affect 50% of the population, and (2) *variability* of population response: this is reflected in the slope of the dose-response curve. Minor tranquilizers such as meprobamate have a relatively flat dose-response curve: many subjects can be tranquilized by relatively small doses while others require relatively large doses. It takes a comparatively large increase in dose to affect a relatively small additional segment of the population. For other drugs such as digitalis, the dose-response curve is much steeper, reflecting the fact that very small increments in dose will digitalize additional large segments of the population. Thus, it is quite easy to overdigitalize inadvertently. For further discussion of this topic, much abbreviated here,

the reader is referred to other texts.[1,2]

FIGURE 10-3
TWO HYPOTHETICAL CUMULATIVE
PERCENTAGE DISTRIBUTIONS WITH THE
SAME MEDIAN VALUE BUT DIFFERENT SLOPES

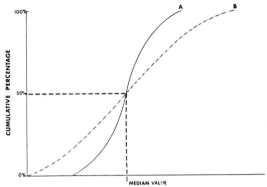

A = steeper slope, therefore smaller standard deviation

B = less steep slope, therefore larger standard deviation

TABLE 10-2
Cat Assay for Digitalis*

Dose mg per 10 kg of Cat	Log dose	No. dying in closed interval	Dying *below* specified dose No.	%
3.8—	.58—	1		
4.2—	.62—	5	1	.5
4.6—	.66—	4	6	2.8
5.0—	.70—	24	10	4.6
5.5—	.74—	30	34	15.7
6.0—	.78—	49	64	29.6
6.6—	.82—	49	113	52.3
7.2—	.86—	26	162	75.0
7.9—	.90—	21	188	87.0
8.7—	.94—	5	209	96.8
9.6—	.98—	2	214	99.1
10.5—	1.02—		216	100.0
		216		

From C. I. Bliss, J. A. Ph. A. 33: 225,1944

*It should be pointed out that digitalis is one of the few compounds where it is possible to obtain the threshold of each individual because of the immediacy of the response to the drug. Ordinarily, the best that can be done is to give a series of graded doses to groups of animals, i.e., group A gets .01 mg, group B gets .10 mg, etc. Data on the proportion responding within each group provide a cumulative threshold distribution since all animals responding at a particular dose have a threshold *below* or equal to that dose and all animals failing to respond have a threshold *above* that dose.

1. Goldstein, A.: *Biostatistics: An Introductory Text.* Macmillan Company, New York, 1964.
2. Finney, D. J.: *Probit Analysis, A Statistical Treatment of the Sigmoid Response Curve.* Cambridge, 1964, 2nd edition.

OTHER MEASURES BASED ON ORDERED DATA

A number of other measures characterize a population of items arrayed from the lowest to the highest values. The *range* is the <u>difference</u> between the highest and lowest values. It is often used as a measure of variation in place of the standard deviation. The range is limited, however, because it only measures the difference between the most extreme values and does not take into account any intermediate values of the distribution. Therefore it usually has a more variable sampling distribution than a measure based on the whole set of numbers in a sample. Another consideration is that the range of a sample will tend to increase as the sample size increases because extreme elements in the population will be included with greater likelihood.[1] This is not true of the sample standard deviation. As the sample size increases there are more terms in the numerator of the formula but there is simultaneously an increase in the number in the denominator $(n-1)$ (see Chapter 11).

Other measures based on ordered data include

---

[1]Advantageous use is made of this property of the sample range in estimating the S. D. of a normal population (See Chapter 11).

FIGURE 10-4

CAT ASSAY FOR DIGITALIS

LETHAL DOSE FOR INDIVIDUAL ANIMALS

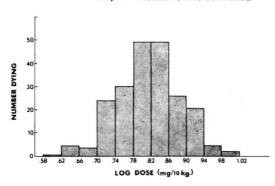

Graph A - NUMBER DYING IN INTERVAL

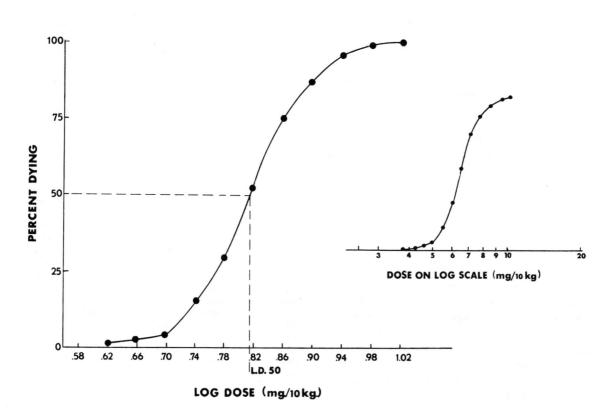

Graph B - PERCENT DYING BELOW SPECIFIED DOSE

percentiles, *deciles*, and *quartiles*. *Percentiles* are values that divide a distribution of ordered data into 100 equal parts; *deciles*, into 10 equal parts; and *quartiles*, into 4 equal parts (or quarters.) Quartile Q_1 is the 25th per cent value; Q_2, the 50th per cent; and Q_3, the 75th per cent value. Note that Q_2, the 50th percentile, is the middle value of ordered data and therefore the same as the median. These and other percentage values can be estimated graphically from the cumulative percentage curve (Figure 10-1) or by interpolation (Table 10-1).

The general procedure for calculating a quartile value (or any other percentage value) by interpolation is as follows:

To determine Q_1 (25th percentage value) we note from the cumulative percentage column of Table 10-1 that the 25th percentile falls somewhere in the third class interval. The lower limit of this class is 97.8° and the upper limit approaches 98.2°. If we look at Figure 10-1 we see that there is no question that we must pass at least 97.8° on the x scale to reach 25%, but *how much further* toward 98.2° must we travel?

Stated in terms of percentages, since the cumulative percentage point reached by the beginning of the third interval is 9.75% and that reached by the end of the interval is 30.72%, there are (30.72%—9.75%) or 20.97% percentage points falling within this interval. We cannot include the entire interval because this would bring our cumulative percentage to 30.72%. We must add only that portion of the interval that will bring us to 25%. The proportion of the interval needed is therefore:

$$\frac{25\% - 9.75\%}{30.72\% - 9.75\%} = \frac{15.25\%}{20.97\%} = .727$$

Thus, only .727 of the third interval is appropriately included to reach Q_1. This proportion must be multiplied by the width of the interval (0.4°) or (.727 × 0.4°) = .29°. Therefore .29° is the additional distance to be travelled along the x axis (Figure 10-1) to reach 25%. The correct answer is:

97.80° (the x value corresponding to the beginning of the third class interval)

+

.29° (the additional x distance needed to reach 25%)

98.09° (Q_1)

The calculations of Q_1, Q_2, and Q_3 are summarized in Table 10-1.

Quartile values are frequently used for describing skewed distributions. If a distribution is balanced (symmetrical) the distances between the quartiles on either side of the median are equal $(Q_3 - Q_2) = (Q_2 - Q_1)$; also, the median equals the mean. Thus for the data on temperatures of 205 healthy men (Table 10-1), Q_3, the 75th percentile value = 98.75°; Q_2, the median value (50th percentile) = 98.41°; and Q_1, the 25th percentile = 98.08°. The distribution is symmetrical since 98.75° minus 98.41° = .34° and, 98.41° minus 98.08° = .33°, approximately the same value. Also, the mean (98.42°) is approximately the same as the median (98.41°).

We have discussed briefly some population distributions of continuous data and the principal measures for summarizing these data. These "tools" allow us to reduce a mass of data to simple numerical quantities which are more readily "digested". With these "tools" we can see relationships about our data which might otherwise be missed. Also we can more readily compare different sets of data.

Relatively rarely, however, do we obtain data on an entire population. Measuring an entire population may be impossible, too costly, or inefficient. Instead, we rely upon samples to provide estimates of the characteristics or parameters of the respective populations. This will be discussed in Chapter 11.

PROBLEM 10-1

Indicate *True or False* for each item in the statement below:

When a distribution is non-symmetrical

(a) The variance is always smaller than in a normal distribution.

(b) It can always be converted to a log normal distribution.

(c) $Q_3 - Q_2$ will include 25 per cent of the population.

(d) A non-parametric test can still be applied.

ANSWER 10-1

(a) *False.*

(b) *False.* Only certain distributions have the characteristic that the log of x follows the normal distribution.

(c) *True.* Q_3 refers to the 75th percentile value and Q_2 to the 50th percentile value. Therefore, the difference between these two values will include 25 per cent of the observations.

(d) *True.* A non-parametric test does not require that the population be normally distributed.

PROBLEM 10-2

Distribution of cholesterol values in a random sample of 100 adult males

Cholesterol (mg %)	No.
100 and up to 200	15
200 and up to 300	40
300 and up to 400	35
400 and up to 500	10

(a) Label the y scale and draw a frequency polygon of the distribution on the graph below.

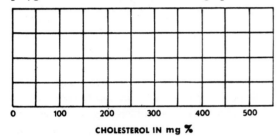

CHOLESTEROL IN mg %

(b) Label the y scale and draw a cumulative % curve on the graph below.

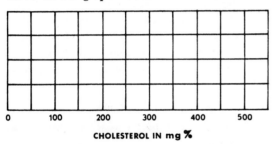

CHOLESTEROL IN mg %

(c) Estimate the standard deviation from the graph.

(d) Calculate Q_1 from the data.

ANSWER 10-2

Although the example refers to a sample, we can use the same descriptive methods as for a population.

(a) Frequency polygon

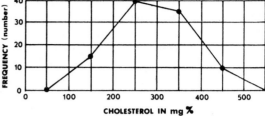

CHOLESTEROL IN mg %

Note that the frequencies are plotted at the midpoint of the class interval.

(b) Before graphing the cumulative percentage distribution, we successively add the frequencies to obtain the number with less than the stated value.

Cholesterol (mg %)	Cumulative frequency
Less than 200	15
" 300	55
" 400	90
" 500	100

Since the frequencies cumulate to 100, we can consider this as a percentage distribution.

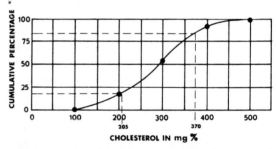

CHOLESTEROL IN mg %

*Percentage with cholesterol less than stated level. Note that the cumulative values are plotted at the end of the class interval.

(c) The dashed lines in graph (b) represent the estimated 84% and 16% values: 370 and 205 mg %. The difference, 370—205 represents 68% of the area. Stated in another way it represents the area falling between the mean ± 1 S. D. (or the area falling within 2 S. D.'s around the mean) of a normal curve. Therefore

$$\frac{370-205}{2} = \frac{165}{2} = \frac{82.5}{\text{mg \%}} = 1 \text{ S. D. (estimated standard deviation).}$$

(d) $Q_1 = 200 + \left\{\frac{(25\%-15\%)}{(55\%-15\%)}\right\} \times (100) = 200 + \frac{(10\%)}{(40\%)}(100)$

corresponds to beginning of second interval

proportion of interval to be included.

width of interval

$$= 200 + (\tfrac{1}{4})(100) = 225 \text{ mg \%}$$

PROBLEM 10-3

Cumulative (normal) Distribution of Systolic Blood Pressures for Populations A and B

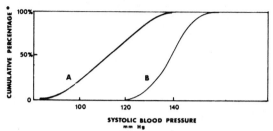

*Percentage with systolic blood pressure less than stated level

Answer (a) and (b) from the above chart: *True or False?*

(a) The mean systolic blood pressure is larger for B than A.

(b) The standard deviation of individual blood pressures is greater for B than A.

ANSWER 10-3

(a) *True.* The 50% value is approximately 140 mm Hg for B but only 110 mm Hg for A.

(b) *False.* The slope is steeper for B than for A. Therefore, the standard deviation (difference between 84% & 50% values on the x scale) will be less for B than A. Population A is more variable in systolic blood pressure.

PROBLEM 10-4

The following table gives the percentage distribution by weight of 9,651 white male infants delivered on the Obstetrical Service of the Johns Hopkins Hospital during a certain period:

Weight at Birth of White Males

Weight in Hectograms	Per cent of Infants
5< 9	0.05
9<13	0.40
13<17	1.02
17<21	1.41
21<25	2.95
25<29	9.29
29<33	23.21
33<37	28.26
37<41	21.25
41<45	7.98
45<49	3.21
49<53	0.76
53<57	0.18
57<61	0.02
61<65	0.01
	100.00

Mean (μ) = 34.9 hectograms (1 hectogram = 100 grams)

Variance (σ^2) = 39.85

(1) What are the limits of the first class interval? The second class interval? What is the midpoint of the first class interval? The second class interval?

(2) The distribution is plotted in Graph A in uncumulated form and in Graph B in cumulated form. Which of the two values — midpoint or class limit — is used for plotting Graph A? Graph B?

(3) Calculate the standard deviation and coefficient of variation.

(4) From Graph B estimate the first quartile, median, and third quartile. What do these data indicate about the distribution?

(5) Also estimate the mean and standard deviation from Graph B and compare these estimates with the calculated values.

(6) If we use the calculated mean and standard deviation we find from the frequency distribution that $\mu \pm 1$ S.D. includes approximately 75%, $\mu \pm 2$ S.D. includes 95% and $\mu \pm 3$ S.D. includes 98% of the values. What does this suggest about the nature of the distribution?

WEIGHT AT BIRTH OF WHITE MALES
(in hectograms)

Graph A UNCUMULATED PERCENTAGE DISTRIBUTION
(smoothed curve)

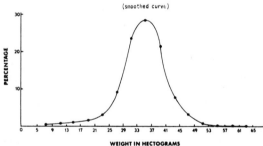

Graph B CUMULATED PERCENTAGE DISTRIBUTION

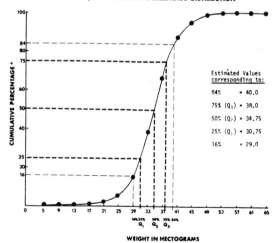

Estimated Values corresponding to:

84%	= 40.0
75% (Q_3)	= 38.0
50% (Q_2)	= 34.75
25% (Q_1)	= 30.75
16%	= 29.0

*Percentage with weight less than stated value.

ANSWER 10-4

(1) The limits of the first and second class intervals can be visualized on a linear scale.

The first class interval is 4 hectograms in width, from 5 to 9; the second is from 9 to 13. The midpoint is that value (x) which divides the class interval exactly in half: 7 for the first class interval and 11 for the second.

(2) The uncumulated (frequency) distribution is plotted at the <u>midpoint</u> of the interval. The cumulated distribution is plotted at the <u>end</u> of the interval (i.e., value corresponding to the class limit).

(3) The standard deviation (σ) is the square root of the variance (σ^2). Therefore $\sigma = \sqrt{39.85} = 6.31$ hectograms. The coefficient of variation relates the standard deviation to the size of the

$$\text{mean} = \frac{\sigma}{\mu} \times 100 = \frac{6.31}{34.9} \times 100 = 18\%.$$

(4) From Graph B we can estimate the value for the median or 50% or $Q_2 = 34.75$

First quartile, 25% or $Q_1 = 30.75$

$$\left.\begin{array}{l} \text{Therefore, } Q_2 = 34.75 \\ Q_1 = \underline{30.75} \\ 4.00 \end{array}\right\} Q_2 - Q_1$$

$$\left.\begin{array}{l} \text{Third quartile, } 75\% \text{ or } Q_3 = 38.00 \\ Q_2 = \underline{34.75} \\ 3.25 \text{ hect.} \end{array}\right\} Q_3 - Q_2$$

The distances between $Q_3 - Q_2$ and $Q_2 - Q_1$ are not too dissimilar, suggesting some symmetry (the normal distribution is symmetrical).

(5) The estimated mean is the median value or
$$Q_2 = 34.75$$

$$\left.\begin{array}{l} \text{Standard Deviation, } 84\% = 40.00 \\ \phantom{\text{Standard Deviation, }}50\% = \underline{34.75} \\ \phantom{\text{Standard Deviation, }50\% = }5.25 \end{array}\right\} 34\% \text{ of area}$$

$$\left.\begin{array}{l} \text{Also } 50\% 34.75 \\ \phantom{\text{Also }}16\% = \underline{29.00} \\ \phantom{\text{Also }16\% = }5.75 \text{ hectograms} \end{array}\right\} 34\% \text{ of area}$$

Again, the two graphical estimates of the standard deviation (5.25 and 5.75) are not too disparate. However, both estimates of the standard deviation are lower than the calculated standard deviation of 6.31. Therefore, the distribution of birth weights has somewhat <u>less</u> spread than the normal distribution.

The median (34.75) is fairly close to the calculated mean (34.9) as would be expected in a normal distribution.

(6) The distribution fairly resembles that of a normal curve since the corresponding values from the normal curve are 68%, 95% and 99.7%.

In conclusion, on the whole the fit to a normal curve is not bad. It is probable that the differences from a normal curve are not large enough to be of clinical importance. A significance test (such as Chi Square Goodness of Fit test) would be necessary to determine whether the discrepancy from normality is sufficient to be significant.

PROBLEM 10-5

The following table (taken from Price-Jones — "Red Blood Cell Diameters") * gives the distribution of diameters (in microns) of 500 red blood cells from a blood sample of a male age 45 with pernicious anemia before and after liver treatment.

Red Blood Cell Diameters of Male Age 45 with Pernicious Anemia, Before and After Liver Treatment in Microns

Mid-points of Class Interval[1]	Number of Cells	
	Before	After
5.25	1	
5.50	2	
5.75	1	1
6.00	5	1
6.25	4	6
6.50	2	5
6.75	4	12
7.00	8	37
7.25	18	107
7.50	18	125
7.75	18	101
8.00	40	57
8.25	49	28
8.50	57	11
8.75	68	5
9.00	74	2
9.25	52	2
9.50	29	
9.75	16	
10.00	13	
10.25	9	
10.50	6	
10.75	3	
11.00	2	
11.25	0	
11.50	1	
Total	500	500
Mean =	8.62	7.56
Standard Deviation =	0.91	0.46

[1]It might be preferable to group the data into larger class intervals because the distribution is not smooth.
*Price-Jones C.: Red Blood Cell Diameters, Oxford Medical Publications, London, 1933.

Graphs of the frequency distributions (uncumulated) are given (Graph A). Also a cumulative frequency distribution (after treatment) is provided below and graphed in percentage form (Graph B). [Note that the cumulative % distribution is plotted at the *end* of the class interval whereas the "uncumulated" frequency (or %) distribution is plotted at the *mid-point* of the class interval.]

after treatment?

(b) What is the source of variation exhibited by the measurement of diameter before and after treatment?

(c) Calculate the median and quartiles of the

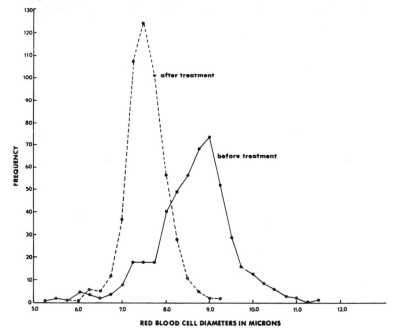

Graph A

FREQUENCY
DISTRIBUTION OF
RED BLOOD CELL
DIAMETER OF 500
CELLS OF MALE
AGE 45 WITH
PERNICIOUS ANEMIA
BEFORE AND AFTER
TREATMENT
(class interval of
.25 microns)

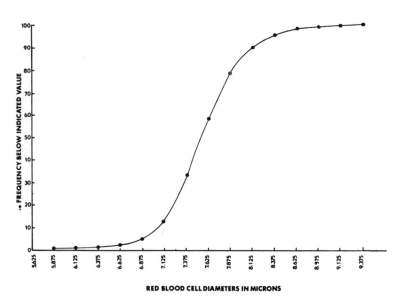

Graph B

CUMULATIVE
PERCENTAGE
DISTRIBUTION OF
RED BLOOD CELL
DIAMETERS AFTER
TREATMENT

(a) Compute the Coefficient of Variation (C.V.) for both groups. Is there more relative variability in red blood cell diameter before or

distribution of diameters <u>after treatment</u> from the cumulative percentage distribution. Compare these values with estimates obtained from the graph of the cumulative percentage distribution (Graph B).

(d) What does the comparison of the mean and median values suggest about the nature of the distribution? What does the comparison of the distance (Q_2-Q_1) and (Q_3-Q_2) tell us?

(e) Estimate the mean diameter (μ) and the standard deviation (σ) from Graph B. Compare these graphical estimates with the two computed values. What does this comparison suggest con-

cerning the nature of the distribution?

(f) From the actual distribution of diameters after treatment, what is the estimated probability (for this male) of encountering a red cell diameter greater than 7.875 microns? What is this probability if calculated from the normal curve?

DIAMETERS IN MICRONS AFTER TREATMENT

Class Interval	Frequency	Cumulative Frequency	%	Cumulative %
5.625 up to 5.875	1	1	.2	.2
5.875 " " 6.125	1	2	.2	.4
6.125 " " 6.375	6	8	1.2	1.6
6.375 " " 6.625	5	13	1.0	2.6
6.625 " " 6.875	12	25	2.4	5.0
6.875 " " 7.125	37	62	7.4	12.4
7.125 " " 7.375	107	169	21.4	33.8
7.375 " " 7.625	125	294	25.0	58.8
7.625 " " 7.875	101	395	20.2	79.0
7.875 " " 8.125	57	452	11.4	90.4
8.125 " " 8.375	28	480	5.6	96.0
8.375 " " 8.625	11	491	2.2	98.2
8.625 " " 8.875	5	496	1.0	99.2
8.875 " " 9.125	2	498	.4	99.6
9.125 " " 9.375	2	500	.4	100.0
	500		100.0	

ANSWER 10-5

(a) Coefficient of Variation (in %) = $\dfrac{\text{Standard Deviation} \quad (\sigma)}{\text{Mean} \qquad (\mu)} \times 100$

$$\text{Before} = \frac{0.91 \text{ micron}}{8.62 \text{ microns}} = 10.5\% \qquad \text{After} = \frac{0.46 \text{ micron}}{7.56 \text{ microns}} = 6.1\%$$

The Coefficient of Variation is larger before treatment than after. This indicates that there is more variability in blood cell diameter before treatment relative to the average size at that time.

(b) <u>Before treatment</u>: The source of variation is probably a combination of two factors: (1) red blood cells vary naturally to a certain extent, and (2) the disease itself may be partly responsible for the variation.

<u>After treatment</u>: Assuming that the cells once

formed have been unaffected by the treatment, variation is due solely to the nature of red blood cells (biologic variability). Both measurements may vary because of the limitations of the instrument used and the possibility of human error.

(c) The 25th, 50th and 75th percentile values calculated from the cumulative percentage data are given below. "Interpolation" or "proportioning" is necessary where the percentiles fall within a class interval (See Table 10-1)

$$Q_1 (25\%) = 7.125 + \left[\frac{63}{107}\right]^* \times (\text{width of interval} = .250) = 7.125 + .145 = 7.27 \text{ microns}$$

$$Q_2 (50\%) = 7.375 + \left[\frac{81}{125}\right] (.250) = 7.54 \text{ microns}$$

$$Q_3 (75\%) = 7.625 + \left[\frac{81}{101}\right] (.250) = 7.83 \text{ microns}$$

The corresponding values estimated from the graph (See Graph C) are: 7.250, 7.550 and 7.825 microns.

*or one could use $\dfrac{12.6\%}{21.4\%}$ This factor indicates the proportion of the interval needed to reach the 25th percentile.

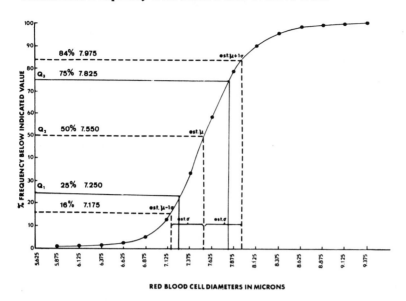

RED BLOOD CELL DIAMETERS IN MICRONS

Graph C

CUMULATIVE
PERCENTAGE
DISTRIBUTION OF
RED BLOOD CELL
DIAMETERS AFTER
TREATMENT

(d) The median (Q_2) is 7.54 microns while the mean is 7.56 microns; thus they are approximately equal. We know that in a normal distribution the mean and median are equal. We wish to investigate further and determine if the distribution of diameters is approximately normal. We note from the computed values that

$Q_2 - Q_1 = 7.54 - 7.27 = .27$; and
$Q_3 - Q_2 = 7.83 - 7.54 = .29$

Therefore, the curve is fairly symmetrical, another property of the normal distribution.

(e) As we have already seen, if the distribution is normal, the median (50th percentile) will estimate the mean. Also, one standard deviation on either side of the mean (or median) will include 34% of the area or frequency distribution, i.e., the difference between the 84th and 50th percentile values should equal the calculated standard deviation. Similarly, the difference between the 50th and 16th percentile values should equal the calculated standard deviation.

From the graph we obtain the following approximate values:

84% = 7.975	50% = 7.550
−50% = 7.550	−16% = 7.175
34% = .425	34% = .375

The average of these two estimates of σ is:
$\frac{.425 + .375}{2} = .40$. This compares with our given computed value for σ of .46. On the basis of the graph, **68% of the diameters fall between 7.175 and 7.975** whereas based on the computed values and properties of the normal curve, we

would expect 68% of them to fall between 7.10 and 8.02 (i.e., 7.56 ± .46). While not a perfect fit, these comparisons suggest that the distribution of diameters after treatment is approximately normal.

(f) From the cumulated % frequency distribution, we note that 79% of the diameters fall below 7.875 microns. Therefore, the probability of encountering a red blood cell larger than 7.875 is $1.00 - .79 = .21$.

Since the distribution is approximately normal, we can also calculate this probability from the areas of the standard normal curve where;

(observed value)   (center of normal curve)

$$z = \frac{x - \mu}{\sigma}$$

(standard deviation of curve)

$$= \frac{7.875 - 7.56}{.46} = \frac{.315}{.46} = .69$$

Thus, our x value (7.875) is approximately .69 σ distance from μ (7.56). P associated with a z of .69 is approximately .50. However, we are only interested in the area in <u>one</u> tail (the probability of *exceeding* x). Therefore, we must divide the P area by 2:

$$\frac{P}{2} = \frac{.50}{2} = .25$$

To conclude, if the distribution were exactly normal, the probability of encountering a red blood cell diameter larger than 7.875μ would be .25. From the actual distribution, however, this probability is only .21. Returning to Graph A, it can be seen that the area in the right tail of the curve is less than that in the left, accounting for the discrepancy from the normal expected value. Therefore, some deviation from normality is suggested. A Goodness of Fit Test is necessary, however, to determine if the deviation from a normal distribution is significant.

PROBLEM 10-6

In the assay of digitalis, a tincture of digitalis is infused at a slow and steady rate intravenously into an etherized cat until the cat dies. The experiment is stopped and the total dose injected (the "just fatal" dose) is read. The data following are log doses (± 0.5) for a standard tincture (tested on 10 cats) and an unknown (tested on 8 cats):

	STANDARD		UNKNOWN	
Cat #	1 .077	Cat #	11	.186
	2 .156		12	.316
	3 .163		13	.344
	4 .194		14	.348
	5 .221		15	.350
	6 .251		16	.389
	7 .256		17	.423
	8 .260		18	.476
	9 .289			
	10 .359			

For each drug, plot on probability paper the log dose against the percentage of animals killed by that dose or a smaller dose. How would you interpret the data if the curves for the two drugs were parallel straight lines?

ANSWER 10-6

We calculate the cumulative percentage distribution of the two groups (see below and graph).

PERCENTAGE OF ANIMALS KILLED FOR
LOG DOSES STANDARD TINCTURE
AND UNKNOWN
(on Probability Paper)

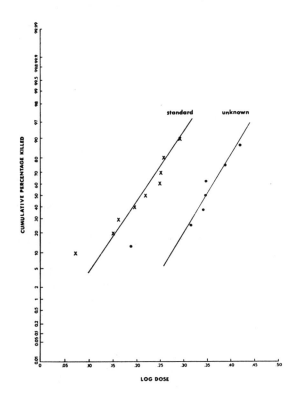

If the curves for the two drugs were parallel straight lines on probability paper it would indicate that the drugs had essentially the same variability in their effects on animals but that one was more potent than the other. In the graph plotted, the drug to the left (standard) is more potent since it takes less of that tincture to produce the same result as the unknown.

STANDARD

CAT #	LOG DOSE	CUMULATIVE %
1	.077	10
2	.156	20
3	.163	30
4	.194	40
5	.221	50
6	.251	60
7	.256	70
8	.260	80
9	.289	90
10	.359	100

10 OBSERVATIONS

UNKNOWN

CAT #	LOG DOSE	CUMULATIVE %
1	.186	12.5
2	.316	25.0
3	.344	37.5
4	.348	50.0
5	.350	62.5
6	.389	75.0
7	.423	87.5
8	.476	**100.0**

8 OBSERVATIONS

SUMMARY OF CHAPTER 10

In this chapter we have continued our analysis of a population of continuous data by ordering the data according to size.

Cumulative percentage graphs (% with stated value *or less*)

—facilitate comparison with a normal distribution

—when the distribution is normal, permit estimates of the mean and standard deviation

—are of particular use in the study of drug potency and toxicity

Quartiles provide an additional method of

—describing a population, particularly one that is skewed

—verifying the symmetry of the population

CUMULATIVE GLOSSARY I: TERMS

Chapter 10

Cumulative Distribution	A distribution of ordered data cumulated successively. The cumulative number (or per cent) indicates that portion of the population which has a certain x value or less.
Sigmoid Curve	S-shaped curve, approaching linearity in the middle and curved at either end, which is characteristic of the cumulative normal distribution.
Probability Paper	Paper which exaggerates the upper and lower ends of the cumulative normal curve in such a manner that it plots as a straight line.
Bioassay	The estimation of the potency and other characteristics of a drug or other material by studying the reaction in living matter.
Dose Response Curve	Curve indicating per cent response to a specified (log) dose or less. The curve may represent an increasing percentage of animals responding to a drug or an increasing magnitude of response within an individual animal or tissue.
Slope of a Line	Change in y value (ordinate) per unit change in the x value (abscissa).
Percentiles	Values that divide a distribution of ordered data into 100 equal parts.
Deciles	Values that divide a distribution of ordered data into 10 equal parts.
Quartiles	Values that divide a distribution of ordered data into 4 equal parts.
Interpolation	The process of obtaining intermediate terms, usually by the method of linear proportioning.

CUMULATIVE GLOSSARY II: SYMBOLS

Chapter 10

ED_{50}	median effective dose
LD_{50}	median lethal dose
Q_1	25th percentage value = first quartile
Q_2	50th percentage value (median) = second quartile
Q_3	75th percentage value = third quartile

11

Description of a Quantitative Sample; Comparison of a Sample Mean with an Expected Mean

*Distribution of a Single Random Sample; Sample Estimators •
Distribution of Sample Means • Significance Test on a Sample
Mean, Population Variance (σ^2) Known • Significance Test
on a Sample Mean, Population Variance (σ^2) Not Known;
t-Distribution*

In Chapters 9 and 10, *populations* of quantitative (continuous) data were described and a variety of summary measures (*parameters*) defined which can help to characterize such distributions. Thus we were concerned with what might be called *descriptive statistics*.

Usually, however, data are not available on an entire population. It may not be feasible or efficient to collect that much data. Instead, we obtain a sample from the population and attempt to draw inferences from the sample which apply to the entire population (*inferential statistics*). In order to use a sample in this way, we need to know two things: (1) the properties of the distribution of a single random sample drawn from the population and of an estimate or *statistic* from it (such as a sample mean) and (2) the properties of the distribution of very many such sample estimates which are called a *sampling distribution*. Let us consider first what a single sample and its estimate are like.

DISTRIBUTION OF A SINGLE RANDOM SAMPLE; SAMPLE ESTIMATORS

Does the distribution of a single sample drawn at random from a population tend to resemble the population distribution? The intuitive answer is, "Yes," a random sample does tend to resemble its parent population. A random sample from a log-normal population, for example, will tend to have a log-normal distribution (Figure 11-1). One can expect intuitively, also, that larger samples will tend to resemble more closely the parent population than smaller samples will. For example, in the extreme case where an entire (finite) population is included in a sample, the distribution of the sample and of the population will be identical.

Since a random sample tends to be a replica of the population, sample values serve as estimators of the corresponding population parameters. The *sample mean*, designated $\bar{x} = \dfrac{\Sigma x}{n}$, where n is the number of elements in the sample, is an *unbiased* estimate of the population or true mean, $\mu = \dfrac{\Sigma x}{N}$.* "Unbiased" refers to the fact that the average of all such sample estimates equals the population value.

To illustrate, the means of two random samples of size 5 from the population of oral temperatures of 205 healthy young men (Table 9-3) is shown in Table 11-1. (For purposes of simplicity, an adjustment to the variance formula required for sampling without replacement from a finite population will not be made.) Although these sample means are 98.52° and 98.36° respectively, the average of means of all possible random samples of size 5 from the population of temperatures

---

*The mathematical formulas for μ and $\bar{x}$ are

$$\mu = \frac{\sum\limits_{i=1}^{N} x_i}{N} \quad \text{and} \quad \bar{x} = \frac{\sum\limits_{i=1}^{N} a_i x_i}{\sum\limits_{i=1}^{N} a_i = n}$$

where x_i = each element in the population

$\sum\limits_{i=1}^{N} x_i$ = sum of the elements for $i = 1, 2, \ldots N$

a_i = 1 if the element is in the sample
a_i = 0 if the element is not in the sample

Similar mathematical notations are used for the variance terms σ^2 and s^2.

FIGURE 11-1

HYPOTHETICAL EXAMPLES OF DISTRIBUTIONS

NORMAL   **LOG NORMAL**

A. Parent Population of Individuals

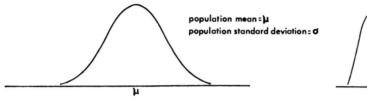

population mean = μ
population standard deviation = σ

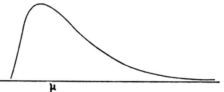

B. One Random Sample of Individuals from Population

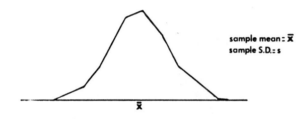

sample mean = x̄
sample S.D. = s

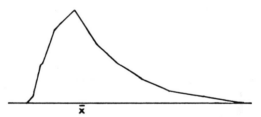

C. Sampling Distribution of Means (x̄) of Many Random Samples Like B.

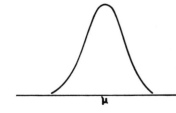

mean = μ
S.D. = $\sigma_{\bar{x}}$ or $\dfrac{\sigma}{\sqrt{n}}$ or $SE_{\bar{x}}$

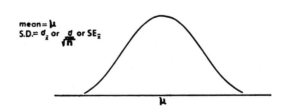

would be the population mean temperature $(\mu) =$ 98.42°. Table 11-2 shows the results of 20 such samples. The average of these sample means is 98.41°, which is very close to 98.42°, the population mean (μ).

Also, the *sample variance*, $s^2 = \dfrac{\Sigma\,(x-\bar{x})^2}{n-1}$, is an unbiased estimate of the population variance, $\sigma^2 = \dfrac{\Sigma\,(x-\mu)^2}{N}$. It is important to note that in this case the sample denominator is $n-1$ and not n. It can be shown that if the denominator were n, then the sample variance on the average

would **underestimate** the population variance. A rationale for the use of n—1 is as follows: although the sample variance is based on n squared deviations from the mean, only n—1 of them are independent because the mean itself is estimated from the data (i.e., there are n—1 degrees of freedom).

Thus, in our example in Table 11-1 the variance of Sample 1 is computed by obtaining the squared deviation of each of the 5 sample values from the sample mean, 98.52°, and summing them: $(98.6°-98.52°)^2 + \ldots + (98.7° - 98.52°)^2 = (.08)^2 + \ldots + (.18)^2 = 0.1480.$ The

TABLE 11-1

Oral Temperatures

I. <u>POPULATION</u> of 205 men (0.4°F) *

Population Mean	$= \mu = \Sigma x/N$	$= 98.42^c$
Population Variance	$= \sigma^2 = \dfrac{\Sigma\,(x-\mu)^2}{N} =$	0.23
Population Standard Deviation	$= \sigma = \sqrt{\dfrac{\Sigma\,(x-\mu)^2}{N}} =$	$0.48°$
Exact SE$_{\bar{x}}$ (for n = 5) or $\sigma_{\bar{x}}$	$= \dfrac{\sigma}{\sqrt{n}} = \dfrac{0.48°}{\sqrt{5}} =$	$0.21°$

II. Example of two random <u>SAMPLES</u>, each of size 5, from this population

		Sample 1	Sample 2
		98.6°	98.6°
		98.2°	98.8°
		98.6°	98.0°
		98.5°	98.7°
		98.7°	97.7°
Sample Total	$= \Sigma x$	492.6°	491.8°
Sample Mean	$= \bar{x} = \Sigma x/n$	98.52°	98.36°
Sample Sum of Squares	$= \Sigma\,(x-\bar{x})^2$	0.1480	0.9320
Sample Variance	$= s^2 = \dfrac{\Sigma\,(x-\bar{x})^2}{n-1}$	0.0370	0.2330
Sample S. D.	$= s = \sqrt{\dfrac{\Sigma\,(x-\bar{x})^2}{n-1}}$	0.1923°	0.4827°
Est. SE$_{\bar{x}}$	$= \dfrac{s}{\sqrt{n}}$	0.0860°	0.2158°

*Since it is doubtful that measurements can be made accurately to 0.1°F we shall use the data grouped by 0.4°F (Table 9-3) for our "population" values.

sum of squares is then divided by $n-1 = 5-1 = 4$, to obtain the sample variance, $s^2 = .0370.$[1] The average of the variances of all possible random samples calculated in this fashion will be the population variance $(\sigma^2) = 0.23$.

The *sample standard deviation* $s = \sqrt{\dfrac{\Sigma (x-\bar{x})^2}{n-1}}$ is the square root of the sample variance. It is an estimate of the population standard deviation, $\sigma = \sqrt{\dfrac{\Sigma (x-\mu)^2}{N}}$. The sample standard deviation in our example is:- $s = \sqrt{0.0370} = 0.19°$. The average of the standard deviations of all possible random samples of size 5 will estimate the true standard deviation of the population, $\sigma = 0.48°$ (Tables 11-1 and 11-2).

It is useful to compute the *sample range* (the difference between the highest and lowest sample values) if the sample is from a <u>normally distributed population</u>. The reason is that it provides another sample estimate of the standard deviation of the population. We use the formula:

estimated S.D. of a normal population $=$

$$\frac{\text{Sample Range}}{K}$$

where K is a constant determined by the sample size (see Table 11-3). This gives us a rough check of the standard deviation calculated by the formula: $s = \sqrt{\dfrac{\Sigma (x-\bar{x})^2}{n-1}}$.

As an example, in our Sample 1 of size 5 from the normally distributed population of 205 oral temperatures of healthy young men, the sample range is $98.7° - 98.2° = 0.5°$, and K (for $n = 5$) is 2.3 (from Table 11-3). The estimated standard deviation, therefore, by this method is $\dfrac{0.5°}{2.3} = 0.22°$, which is in the same "ball park" as the previously calculated S.D. of 0.19°. For Sample 2, the range is $98.8° - 97.7° = 1.1°$, K is again 2.3, and the estimated S.D. is $\dfrac{1.1°}{2.3} = 0.48°$, which agrees with the calculated S.D. of 0.48°. Therefore this is a useful check on our calculations.

---

[1]A short-cut formula for s^2 which also avoids rounding errors is:

$$s^2 = \frac{\Sigma x^2 - \dfrac{(\Sigma x)^2}{n}}{n-1}$$

See Problem 14-13.

In addition to mean, variance, and standard deviation, other population parameters such as the mode, median (Q_2), and the quartiles (Q_1) and (Q_3) can be estimated from corresponding sample values.

TABLE 11-2*
Oral Temperatures of Healthy Men —
Samples of size $n = 5$

Samples of size 5	Sample Mean	Sample Standard Deviation	Estimated Standard Error of the Mean
	$\bar{x}$	s	Est. $SE\bar{x} = \dfrac{s}{\sqrt{n}}$
	°F	°F	°F
1	98.41	.48	.21
2	98.57	.19	.08
3	98.43	.47	.21
4	98.29	.27	.12
5	98.47	.61	.27
6	98.49	.43	.19
7	98.71	.86	.38
8	98.55	.25	.11
9	98.69	.65	.29
10	98.27	.27	.12
11	98.19	.39	.17
12	98.33	.64	.29
13	98.05	.37	.17
14	98.45	.56	.25
15	98.33	.48	.21
16	98.43	.61	.27
17	98.09	.27	.12
18	98.63	.69	.31
19	98.33	.17	.08
20	98.33	.37	.17
Mean of Samples	98.41	.44	.20

*Source: Johns Hopkins University School of Hygiene and Public Health.

TABLE 11-3
Estimate of σ by Range Method
(Normal Populations)

To check calculation of standard deviation, determine sample range. This will provide an estimate of σ (for normal populations), as follows:

$$\text{Est. } \sigma = \frac{\text{Range}}{K}$$

Size of Sample (n)	K	Size of Sample (n)	K
5	2.3	50	4.5
10	3.1	100	5.0
15	3.5	200	5.5
20	3.7	300	5.8
30	4.1	500	6.1

DISTRIBUTION OF SAMPLE MEANS

We stated that the average of means of all possible random samples is equal to the true or population mean. But how good (i.e., *reliable*) is one sample mean as an estimate of the true mean? This depends in part on how variable sample means are. In a given sampling situation, do the sample means cluster around the population mean, or are they spread far apart? The closer a sample mean is to the population mean, the more reliable (the better estimate) it is.

Let us consider the properties of the distribution of sample means based on many samples of a specified size (n).[1] Note the similarities of these properties to those of the distribution of sample proportions (Chapter 4):

1. As the sample size (n) increases, the shape of the distribution of sample means ($\bar{x}$) from a large number of random samples of that size approaches the normal distribution (this is the *Central Limit Theorem*). Figure 11-2 shows a hypothetical population that is certainly not normal. Yet the distribution of means of 1000 samples of size 4 from that population is almost normal. This property, that as $n \rightarrow \infty$ the distribution of sample means approaches the normal distribution, is true for samples from a quantitative population of **any** shape.[2] We showed in Chapter 4 that even for samples from a binomial population, as the sample size (n) increases, the distribution of sample proportions (called the binomial distribution) is approximated by the normal distribution.

2. The center of the distribution of sample means is the population mean (μ).

3. A measure of the dispersion of sample means around the population mean is the standard deviation of that distribution of sample means (Figure 11-1C). This standard deviation is called the Stan-

FIGURE 11-2

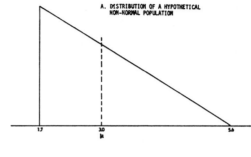

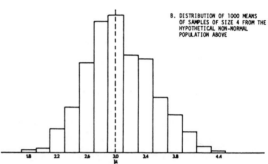

From Cornfield, J.: Mimeographed lecture material, Johns Hopkins University School of Hygiene and Public Health, based on data from Schewhart, D.: Economic Control of Quality of Manufactured Product (page 183), D. Van Nostrand Co., Princeton, N. J., 1931.

distribution of sample means ($\bar{x}$) from the standard deviation of the distribution of the individuals (x) in the original population, we shall use the symbol $\sigma_{\bar{x}}$ for the former, and σ_x or just σ for the latter.

$SE_{\bar{x}}$ or $\sigma_{\bar{x}}$ is obtained by dividing the standard deviation of the population by the square root of the number of items in the sample. Thus, in the example in Table 11-1 of oral temperatures, the *exact* $SE_{\bar{x}}$ for *every* random sample of size 5 is:

dard Error of the Mean and is denoted by $SE_{\bar{x}}$ (just as we designated the standard deviation of the distribution of sample proportions as the Standard Error of the Proportion, $SE_{\hat{p}}$). To distinguish symbolically the standard deviation of the

$$SE_{\bar{x}} = \sigma_{\bar{x}} = \frac{\sigma}{\sqrt{n}} = \frac{\text{Population S.D.}}{\sqrt{\text{size of sample or n}}} = \frac{0.48°}{\sqrt{5}} = .21°$$

Note that the standard deviation of the sampling distribution of means must be smaller than the S.D. of individuals in the population, since S.D. (or σ) divided by the square root of the sample size determines $SE_{\bar{x}}$.

Thus there are *two* factors which affect the reliability of the sample mean (i.e., the size of the Standard Error of the Mean): (1) *the variability of the original population* (σ) — it can be seen

[1] Note that it is **not** the number of samples that is important here but the number of elements in each sample (n). Also, it is understood that for any one sampling distribution all samples are of the **same** size and from the same population.

[2] The Central Limit Theorem has only two assumptions: (a) that the samples are random, and (b) that the parent distribution has a finite variance, a property which is true of all distributions of interest to us.

that if there were no variability whatsoever in the population and all items were identical (i.e., $\sigma = 0$), then any *one* item would always correctly estimate the population mean; (2) *the size of the sample* (n) — it is obvious that as the size of the sample increases and n approaches N, the sample is more likely to include elements from all parts of the population and, therefore, provide a better estimate of its parameters.

SIGNIFICANCE TEST ON A SAMPLE MEAN, POPULATION VARIANCE (σ^2) KNOWN

We can now use the above properties of the distribution of sample means to compare a sample mean with an expected or known mean. Since means of large samples from any shaped population follow a normal distribution, we use the standard normal deviate or z test (Chapter 4) to answer the question: is this sample mean likely to have arisen from a specified population with mean μ and differ from μ by chance alone? Remember the generalized form of the z test (Chapter 4) is:

$$z = \frac{\overset{\text{observed value}}{\overbrace{\text{X}}} - \mu \leftarrow \text{center of normal curve}}{\sigma \leftarrow \text{standard deviation of normal curve}}$$

Here, in specific terms, (1) the center of the normal curve of sample means is μ, (2) the observed value is the observed sample mean $\bar{x}$, and (3) the specific standard deviation of this normal curve (sampling distribution) is the

Standard Error of the Mean: $SE_{\bar{x}} = \sigma_{\bar{x}} = \dfrac{\sigma}{\sqrt{n}}$.

Therefore, the specific standard normal deviate, z, for a sampling distribution of means, when the population variance (σ^2) or standard deviation (σ) is known, is $z = \dfrac{\bar{x} - \mu}{SE_{\bar{x}}} = \dfrac{\bar{x} - \mu}{\sigma/\sqrt{n}}$. It is thus possible to locate an observed sample mean $\bar{x}$ on the theoretical distribution of sample means and determine its distance from the expected or population mean in Standard Error or z units.

Let us apply these concepts to test whether the mean, 98.52°, of Sample 1 in Table 11-1 is significantly different from the population mean, 98.42°.

$$z \text{ is } \frac{\bar{x} - \mu}{\sigma/\sqrt{n}} = \frac{98.52° - 98.42°}{0.48°/\sqrt{5}} = \frac{.10°}{.21°} = .46.$$

From the values of the normal table (more complete than the values in Table 4-1) we note that a z of .46 is associated with a P of .68. That is,

when random samples of size 5 are taken from this population, a sample mean as far away from the population mean as that observed or further will occur by chance alone more than 2/3 of the time (68 in 100 trials). As this is a very frequent chance occurrence the Null Hypothesis cannot be rejected. (Since in this case we *know* that the data are a random sample from the specified population, we also *know* that no error was made in this decision process, see Chapter 8).

SIGNIFICANCE TEST ON A SAMPLE MEAN, POPULATION VARIANCE (σ^2) NOT KNOWN; *t*-DISTRIBUTION

Suppose, in the more usual situation, we do not know that the population variance (σ^2) is 0.23, and therefore σ is 0.48°, and must estimate these values from the sample variance (s^2) (Tables 11-1 and 11-2). We then replace σ by s in the Standard Error formula to obtain an *estimated* $SE_{\bar{x}}$.* In doing this we are replacing also the variate $z = \dfrac{\bar{x} - \mu}{\sigma/\sqrt{n}}$ which follows a normal distribution (standard normal deviate) with the variate $t = \dfrac{\bar{x} - \mu}{s/\sqrt{n}}$ which follows the *t*-distribution (Table 11-4). As with z, the tabled values consider only the magnitude of t.

---

*Although in this instance we replace σ by s we can refer to (σ^2) as the unknown parameter since the Standard Deviation (σ) is the square root of the variance (σ^2).

TABLE 11-4*

Short Table of *t* Corresponding to Selected Values of P

df			P			
	.50	.20	.10	.05	.02	.01
3	.76	1.64	2.35	3.18	4.54	5.84
4	.74	1.53	2.13	2.78	3.75	4.60
5	.73	1.48	2.02	2.57	3.36	4.03
10	.70	1.37	1.81	2.23	2.76	3.17
15	.69	1.34	1.75	2.13	2.60	2.95
20	.69	1.32	1.72	2.09	2.53	2.84
30	.68	1.31	1.70	2.04	2.46	2.75
∞	.67	1.28	1.64	1.96	2.33	2.58

P = Probability of attaining or exceeding t, through chance alone, if the Null Hypothesis is true.

df = Degrees of Freedom

---

*Abridged from Table III of Fisher & Yates, Statistical Tables for Biological, Agricultural and Medical Research (Sixth Edition) published by Oliver and Boyd, Edinburgh, and by permission of the authors and publishers. See also Appendix, Table D.

The *t*-distribution is symmetrical and shaped like the normal (z distribution) but, for small samples, has more area in the tails, i.e., a relatively greater spread (Figure 11-3). An explanation for the greater spread of *t*, is that the variability of z, the standard normal deviate, reflects only a variation due to the sampling of x̄ around μ while the *t*-variate incorporates also the variation of s around σ. The *t*-distribution is an important distribution in medical statistics; its underlying assumptions are discussed in the next chapter.

FIGURE 11-3

t-DISTRIBUTION COMPARED WITH NORMAL DISTRIBUTION

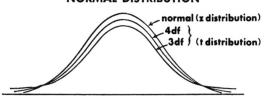

An important property of the *t*-distribution is that its shape, like that of the Chi Square distribution, depends upon the number of degrees of freedom (df) which enter into the statistic (Table 11-4). In the *t*-distribution, however, df refers to the number of independent differences or (n—1) items that contribute to the sample variance estimate (s²). Remember that it is n—1 that is used as the denominator in calculating s². One df is "lost" because the sample data are used to estimate the mean.

With large samples (n more than 30) the *t*-distribution approaches the normal distribution (t → z) and the z variate can be used instead of *t*. For small samples, however, the *t*-distribution must be used since it is quite different from the normal.

Let us return to Sample 1 in Table 11-1 to illustrate the use of the *t*-test. If we do not know the population variance (σ²), we must use the sample variance estimate (s²) instead for the formula for SE_x̄ to determine the critical ratio. Our test then is

$$ t = \frac{\bar{X}-\mu}{s/\sqrt{n}} = \frac{98.52°-98.42°}{0.19°/\sqrt{5}} = \frac{.10°}{.085°} = 1.18; $$

df = n—1 = 5—1 or 4. From Table 11-4, we see that this *t* value for 4 df is associated with a P of approximately .20, and again, the Null Hypothesis is accepted.

Note that because of the greater area in the tails, for the P = .05 level *t* for 4 df is 2.78 instead of the familiar 1.96 for z. Thus, a mean of a small sample (n of 30 or less) must be *further away from the center* of the *t*- than the z (normal) distribution to be significant (i.e., 2.78 instead of only 1.96 Standard Errors distance from μ).

In this chapter, we have illustrated that: (1) A random sample can be a miniature of the population; as a result, sample statistics serve as estimates of population parameters. (2) Means of samples from any shaped population will follow a normal distribution if the sample size is sufficiently large. This is an important property for significance tests on the mean. (3) The standard deviation of the curve of sample means is called the Standard Error of the Mean. Its formula $\frac{\sigma}{\sqrt{n}}$ involves the square root of the population variance (i.e., the population standard deviation σ). (4) If the population variance σ² (or standard deviation σ) is known, the normal deviate test can be used to compare an observed sample mean with an expected (population) mean. (5) If the population standard deviation is not known and the sample standard deviation (s) must be used in its place to estimate the Standard Error of the Mean, the *t*-distribution with n—1 degrees of freedom is used instead of the normal distribution. This is an important modification where n is small (30 or less).

In the next chapter we will begin the discussion of the comparison of *two* sample means.

PROBLEM 11-1

Below are given measurements on the colonic temperature of 6 rats:

Colonic Temperature of 6 Rats
(Degrees Centigrade)

| 38.0° |
| 38.2° |
| 38.1° |
| 38.0° |
| 38.4° |
| 38.5° |

(a) Calculate the mean, median, range, and standard deviation.

(b) Assume that the sample was drawn at random from a normal population. Estimate the population standard deviation from the range. (The K value for n = 6 is 2.3.)

ANSWER 11-1

(a) Our sample values are:

Mean $= \bar{x} = 38.2°$ (Note that for sample values like this, one need only add the last digit $(.0 + .2 + .1 + .0 + .4 + .5 = 1.2°)$ and divide by 6 to obtain 0.2° which is added on to 38°.

Median is the $\frac{n+1}{2}$ value of the ordered data: 38.0°, 38.0°, 38.1°, 38.2°, 38.4°, 38.5°. Thus, it falls midway between 38.1° and 38.2° or 38.15°.

Range $= 38.5° - 38.0° = 0.5°$.

Standard Deviation $= s = \sqrt{\dfrac{\Sigma\,(x-\bar{x})^2}{n-1}}$

Again, working only with the last digit, we obtain $\Sigma\,(x-\bar{x})^2$ or the sum of squared deviations from the mean:

$$(.0-.2)^2 + (.2-.2)^2 + (.1-.2)^2 + (.0-.2)^2 + (.4-.2)^2 + (.5-.2)^2$$
$$= (-.2)^2 + (0)^2 + (-.1)^2 + (-.2)^2 + (.2)^2 + (.3)^2$$
$$= .04 + .01 + .04 + .04 + .09 = .22°$$

$$s^2 = \frac{\Sigma\,(x-\bar{x})^2}{n-1} = \frac{.22}{5} = 0.044$$

$$s = \sqrt{.044} = .21°$$

(b) Estimated $\sigma = \dfrac{Range}{K} = \dfrac{0.5°}{2.3} = .22°$

This agrees fairly well with the calculated Standard Deviation (s) of .21°.

PROBLEM 11-2

The following data are taken from Salk, J. E., Poliomyelitis Vaccine in the Fall of 1955, Am. J. of Pub. Health, 46: 1-14, 1956.

Type I Antibody Levels After One Dose of Poliomyelitis Vaccine in 17 Persons Who Prior to Vaccination Gave Immune Responses to Types II and III Vaccine.

2048	64
1024	32
512	16
512	16
512	8
256	8
256	4
256	4
64	

(a) Convert the antibody levels to logarithms to the base 2. (Hint: What exponent or power will raise 2 to the number 4? to the number 8?, etc.)

(b) What effect does the logarithmic transformation have on this series of measures?

(c) For these logarithms compute the mean, median, standard deviation, and mean ± 2 standard deviations. What value is there in knowing the mean ± 2 S.D.?

(d) Determine the geometric mean by reconverting to original measure.

ANSWER 11-2*

(a) Antibody Levels	Log (base 2)	Antibody Levels	Log (base 2)
2048	11	64	6
1024	10	32	5
512	9	16	4
512	9	16	4
512	9	8	3
256	8	8	3
256	8	4	2
256	8	4	2
64	6		

(b) After the logarithmic transformation, the curve more closely approximates a normal distribution. (The original curve is so skewed that it cannot be plotted readily on an arithmetic scale.)

(c) Log values:

Mean $\bar{x} = \dfrac{\Sigma x}{n} = \dfrac{107}{17} = 6.29$

Median $= 6$

---

*A *logarithm* is that power or *exponent* (x) to which a *base* (b) must be raised so that b^x equals a particular value. For example if 10 is the base, the log of 100 is 2 because $10^2 = 100$ (i.e., the exponent is 2). Similarly, the log of 1000 to the base 10 is 3 because $10^3 = 1000$. Any number can serve as the *base*. If we ask: What is the log of 36 to the base 6, the answer is 2, for if $6^x = 36$, the exponent x must be 2. The numbers used most often as the base are (a) 10 (logs associated with the base 10 are called *common logarithms*) and (b) 2.71828 . . . which by convention is designated as e (logs associated with the base e are called *natural logarithms*).

Variance, $s^2 = \dfrac{\Sigma\,(x-\bar{x})^2}{n-1} = \dfrac{137.53}{16} = 8.60$

Standard Deviation, $s = \sqrt{\dfrac{\Sigma\,(x-\bar{x})^2}{n-1}} = \sqrt{8.60} = 2.93$

Mean $\pm$ 2 S.D. $= 6.29 \pm 2(2.93)$

$\qquad\qquad\quad = 6.29 \pm 5.86$

$\qquad\qquad\quad = 0.43$ to 12.15

Since the log values are approximately normally distributed, we know that 95% of them will fall between 0.43 and 12.15 (mean $\pm$ 2 S. D.)

(d) The geometric mean is the antilog of the mean. Antilog (to the base 2) of 6.29 is 78.

PROBLEM 11-3

No matter what the distribution of the parent population, means of sufficiently large random samples will tend to follow a normal distribution. *True or False?*

ANSWER 11-3

True.[1] This is the Central Limit Theorem which underlies statistical inference. Examples have been given for binomial and other non-normal populations.

PROBLEM 11-4

The Standard Error of the Mean indicates the variability among means of random samples of the same size from a population. In contrast, the Standard Deviation of the population indicates the variability among individuals in that population. *True or False?* Explain your answer.

ANSWER 11-4

True. The Standard Deviation of individuals in a population measures how alike or unlike the individuals are, i.e., their "spread". The Standard Error is a term specifically applied to the Standard Deviation of the distribution of a sample statistic, e.g., the chance distribution of means of samples of size 10 from a population. The Standard Error of this distribution indicates how much sample means differ from each other. In turn this depends upon the size of the sample (n) and the Standard Deviation (σ) of the individuals in the population since $SE_{\bar{x}} = \sigma_{\bar{x}} = \dfrac{\sigma}{\sqrt{n}}$

PROBLEM 11-5

Compare the Standard Error of the Mean ($SE_{\bar{x}}$) for a sample of size 9 with that for size 36, from the same universe.

ANSWER 11-5

The formula for the Standard Error of the Mean is $\dfrac{\sigma}{\sqrt{n}}$. Therefore, the Standard Error of the Mean for a sample of size 9 will be *twice* that for a sample of size 36:

$$\left. \begin{array}{l} \text{If } n = 9,\ SE_{\bar{x}} = \dfrac{\sigma}{\sqrt{9}} = \dfrac{\sigma}{3} \\[2mm] \text{If } n = 36,\ SE_{\bar{x}} = \dfrac{\sigma}{\sqrt{36}} = \dfrac{\sigma}{6} \end{array} \right\} \text{ and } \dfrac{\sigma}{3} = 2 \times \dfrac{\sigma}{6}$$

PROBLEM 11-6

The standard deviation of the distribution of sample means for a certain measure can be larger than the standard deviation of the population of individuals with respect to that measure. *True or False?*

ANSWER 11-6

False. The standard deviation of the chance distribution of sample means is represented by the Standard Error of the Mean ($SE_{\bar{x}}$). Its formula is $\dfrac{\sigma}{\sqrt{n}}$. Therefore, it is equal to the standard deviation (σ) of the individuals in a population *divided* by the $\sqrt{\text{sample size (n)}}$. For this reason $SE_{\bar{x}}$ can *never* be larger than the standard deviation of the population but only smaller (if the sample is larger than 1).

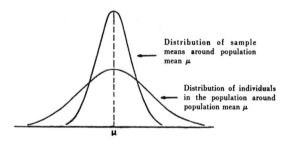

Distribution of sample means around population mean μ

Distribution of individuals in the population around population mean μ

PROBLEM 11-7

(a) What two factors determine the size of the Standard Error of the Mean ($SE_{\bar{x}}$)?

(b) Illustrate how the shape of the normal curve of sample means varies according to size

---

[1]The only exceptions are certain mathematical distributions that do not have a finite variance and about which we need not be concerned.

of $SE_{\bar{x}}$. Why is it often advantageous to take a large sample?

ANSWER 11-7

(a) The size of $SE_{\bar{x}}$, the Standard Error of the Mean, is determined by (1) the population standard deviation (σ) and (2) the sample size (n):

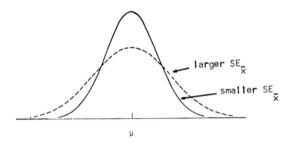

$$SE_{\bar{x}} = \frac{\sigma}{\sqrt{n}} \text{ where } \sigma = \sqrt{\frac{\Sigma\,(x-\mu)^2}{N}}$$

(b) Two curves with different size Standard Errors of the Mean are shown below:

It is often advantageous to take a large sample because one is then more likely to obtain a sample mean close to the population mean. This is reflected in the size of the Standard Error of the Mean ($SE_{\bar{x}}$) (the Standard Deviation of the distribution of sample means) which is smaller where n is larger.

PROBLEM 11-8

Indicate *True or False* for all items in the statement below. Give reasons for your answer.

The Standard Error of the Mean for samples from continuous data depends on

(a) The value of the Standard Deviation of individuals.

(b) The sample size.

(c) The number of samples taken.

(d) The value of the population mean.

ANSWER 11-8

(a) *True.* The degree to which the individuals in a population differ from each other (σ or Standard Deviation) is one factor determining the size of the Standard Error of the Mean.

(b) *True.* The size of the sample also enters into the $SE_{\bar{x}}$ formula which is $\frac{SD}{\sqrt{n}}$. The larger the sample, the smaller is $SE_{\bar{x}}$.

(c) *False.* The number of samples taken in no

way affects the Standard Error of the Mean. Rather it is the *number of elements* (n) of the sample (i.e., sample size) which determines how *precise* the sample mean is as an estimate of the population mean.

(d) *False.* The value of the population mean does not affect the Standard Error of the mean. This is related to the fact that in most quantitative distributions the mean does not influence the Standard Deviation of the individuals in the population (see Problem 9-5).

PROBLEM 11-9

The graph below by Keys, Ancel: The Age Trend of Serum Concentrations of Cholesterol and of S_f 10-20 ("G") Substances in Adults, reproduced with permission from J. Gerontology, 7:201, April, 1952, shows by age the mean serum cholesterol level of healthy men. Lines are drawn representing the mean ± 1 Standard Deviation and the mean ± 1 Standard Error.

(a) How do you interpret these lines?

(b) Why are the lines for the Standard Error closer to the mean than the lines for the Standard Deviation?

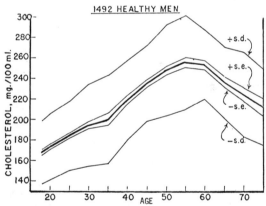

Mean serum total cholesterol and age in adult Americans, together with the lines for $\pm$ the standard deviation and $\pm$ the standard error.

ANSWER 11-9

(a) The sample Standard Deviation indicates how variable the cholesterol level is among *individuals* in each sample (healthy adult men at <u>each</u> age). If each sample is normally distributed, the sample mean ± 1 S. D. includes 68% of the sample observations (individuals) of that age. It would appear from the graph that the cholesterol levels of sample men aged 60 are less variable than those of men aged 55 since the S. D. lines at age 60 are closer together.

The lines pertaining to the Standard Error tell us how *precise* the sample means are at each age. 68% of all sample means at each age can be expected to fall within the limits of the sample mean $\pm$ 1 $SE_{\bar{x}}$ (assuming more than 30 men in the sample at each age or a true $SE_{\bar{x}}$.)

(b) The lines for the Standard Error are closer to the mean because the S.E. is a smaller value than the S.D. The Formula for $SE_{\bar{x}}$ is $\dfrac{S\ D}{\sqrt{n}}$. Thus, the Standard Error of the Mean is equal to the Standard Deviation of individuals divided by the square root of the sample size. In contrast to the Standard Deviation of individuals, $SE_{\bar{x}}$ is affected by sample size.

As seen from the graph, the $SE_{\bar{x}}$ is larger at age 70 than at younger ages. Since the Standard Deviation has not increased markedly in size, the increase in $SE_{\bar{x}}$ must be due to the smaller number of men in the sample at age 70 than at other ages.

PROBLEM 11-10

(a) Why are the median (Q_2) and the Q_1 and Q_3 values useful in describing a skewed distribution?

(b) Why is the mean more useful than the median in describing a population that is not skewed? Hint: Standard Error of Mean $= \sigma/\sqrt{n}$; Standard Error of Median $= 1.253\ (\sigma/\sqrt{n})$.

(c) Why is the range less useful than the standard deviation as a measure of dispersion?

ANSWER 11-10

(a) A comparison of the distance between Q_1 and Q_2 (the 25th and 50th percentiles) and Q_2 and Q_3 (the 50th and 75th percentiles) will give a general picture of the skewness and shape of the distribution. If the curve is symmetrical, these distances (Q_2-Q_1) and (Q_3-Q_2) will be identical (Chapter 10).

(b) A sample mean is a more reliable estimate of the population mean than the sample median is of its population parameter (population median). Note that the Standard Error of the Mean is smaller than the Standard Error of the Median (by a factor of 1.253).

Also one can combine the mean of several samples by appropriate weighting. The median has

to be calculated anew as more samples are added.

(c) The range is not very useful in scientific work because it takes account of the two most extreme values only and so wastes a lot of information. Another main problem is that it is very much affected by sample size. The range of the distribution of a single sample of size 10 would be much more likely to include extreme values and therefore be larger than the range for a sample of size 2.

In contrast, as sample size increases, the sample standard deviation will come closer to the population standard deviation (i.e., be more reliable) but it will not systematically increase (or decrease). The reason is that it is the square root of the variance which is the average squared deviation from the mean. Of course, the larger the sample, the more squared deviations from the mean are computed. At the same time, however, the magnitude of the divisor $(n - 1)$ increases in the variance calculation. For example, if there are ten times as many squared deviations included in the numerator, the denominator will be correspondingly larger:

$$s^2 = \frac{(10)\ \Sigma\ (x-\bar{x})^2}{(10n - 1)},\ \text{and 10 will tend to cancel out.}$$

PROBLEM 11-11

A random sample of 100 children of a certain age in an "underdeveloped" country have an average height of 44.0" and a standard deviation of heights of 1.4".

(a) Is the sample mean value significantly different from the mean value of 45.5" found for a very large series of children of this age in "developed" countries of similar racial background where the standard deviation in height is 1.5"?

(b) How would you answer this question if the standard deviation of heights in developed countries were not known?

ANSWER 11-11

(a) Here we are comparing a sample mean value of 44.0" with a *population* mean value of 45.5". The latter can be considered a population value or parameter since it is based on a "very large series of cases". We must determine P, the probability of drawing from this population a sample with a mean as different from the population mean (or more extreme) by chance alone.

Since we know the population variance (1.5")

we can determine P from a normal distribution of sample means. The test of the Null Hypothesis using the normal curve is always $z = \frac{x - \mu}{\sigma}$. Here x represents the observed sample mean value ($\bar{x}$), μ is the population or expected mean and σ is the standard deviation of the distribution of means of samples of size 100 drawn from this population. Therefore it is the Standard Error of the Mean, $SE_{\bar{x}}$ or $\sigma_{\bar{x}}$. Thus, we can rewrite z as $\frac{\bar{x} - \mu}{SE_{\bar{x}}}$, where

$$SE_{\bar{x}} = \frac{\sigma}{\sqrt{n}} = \frac{\text{population standard deviation}}{\sqrt{\text{sample size}}} = \frac{1.5''}{\sqrt{100}} = .15''$$

Thus $z = \frac{44.0'' - 45.5''}{.15''} = \frac{-1.5''}{.15''} = -10$

z tells us that the sample mean is 10 Standard Errors away from the expected mean on the chance distribution of sample means (under the Null Hypothesis). The P value is $\ll .0001$; very rarely would such an outcome arise by chance alone. It is, therefore, highly significant.

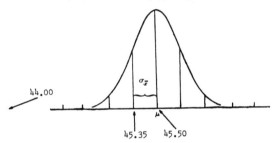

(b) If the population standard deviation (σ) of the "developed" countries is not known, we have no choice but to use as our best estimate of σ the sample standard deviation, s, of 1.4''. We then calculate an estimated $SE_{\bar{x}}$. The formula is:

$$\text{est. } SE_{\bar{x}} = \frac{s}{\sqrt{n}} = \frac{\text{sample standard deviation}}{\sqrt{\text{sample size}}} = \frac{1.4''}{\sqrt{100}} = .14''$$

In this case the critical ratio is $t = \frac{\bar{x} - \mu}{s/\sqrt{n}}$ df $= n-1 = 100-1 = 99$

$$t_{99df} = \frac{44.0'' - 45.5''}{.14''} = \frac{1.5''}{.14''} = 11 \qquad \text{P is} <<< .0001$$

Note that the t distribution for samples of n > 30 is similar to the z or normal distribution. The difference again is highly significant.

PROBLEM 11-12

Why for small samples is the critical value corresponding to a P of .05 greater in the t-distribution than in the normal distribution?

ANSWER 11-12

The t- distribution for small samples (df 30 or less) has greater area in the tails. Therefore, the observed t ratio must be larger than z in order to include a P of only .05 beyond it. That is, the sample result must be <u>more</u> standard error units away from the center of the curve to achieve the same level of significance.

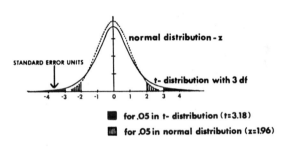

■ for .05 in t- distribution (t=3.18)
▦ for .05 in normal distribution (z=1.96)

PROBLEM 11-13

The table below from McGuire, J., et al., Arch. Int. Med., Feb. 1939: Relation of Cardiac Output To Congestive Heart Failure, pp. 290-297, shows measurements of cardiac output on 16 apparently normal subjects (liters per square meter of body surface per minute).

Cardiac Output in 16 Healthy Subjects

Individual Number	Cardiac Output (x)
1	2.59
2	1.84
3	1.93
4	2.39
5	1.96
6	2.14
7	2.02
8	2.32
9	1.80
10	1.90
11	2.18
12	2.21
13	1.70
14	1.96
15	2.35
16	2.33
Total	33.62

$$\bar{X} = 2.10 \text{ liters/sq.m./min.}$$

$$s = \sqrt{\frac{1.024}{15}} = 0.26 \text{ liters/sq.m./min.}$$

(1) Does the observed mean value differ significantly from the so-called "normal value" of 2.21 liters/sq.m./min. as given by Grollman in the Cardiac Output of Man in Health and Disease, Charles C Thomas, Springfield, Illinois, 1932, for presumably a large series of cases?

(2) Is the mean value of 2.10 significantly *less* than the so-called "normal value"?

ANSWER 11-13

(1) Given:

$\mu = 2.21$ liters/sq.m./min. (population mean)
$\bar{X} = 2.10$ liters/sq.m./min. (sample mean)
$s = .26$ liters/sq.m./min. (sample standard deviation)

We calculate est. $SE_{\bar{X}}$ and form the critical t ratio:

$$\text{est. } SE_{\bar{X}} = \frac{s}{\sqrt{n}} = \frac{.26}{\sqrt{16}} = .065 \text{ liters/sq.m./min.}$$

$$\text{observed } t = \frac{\bar{X}-\mu}{\text{est } SE_{\bar{X}}} = \frac{2.10-2.21}{.065} = \frac{-.11}{.065} = -1.69$$

$$df = n-1 = 16-1 = 15$$

$$t_{15df\,(.05)} \text{ is } |2.13|.$$

Since our observed t is only -1.69, P $>$ .05 and the difference is not significant.

(2) This involves the same critical ratio as before, observed $t = -1.69$. But now the question is whether the sample mean value is significantly *less* than the so-called normal value. Therefore, a one-tailed test is appropriate. To have .05 in one tail, P must be .10 in order that $\frac{P}{2} = .05$. The critical t value, $t_{15df(.10)} = -1.75$. This critical value is *further* from μ than our observed t value of -1.69. Therefore the sample mean is not significantly *less* than the so-called normal value.

SUMMARY OF CHAPTER 11

A random sample from a continuous population (or any other population) tends to be a replica of that population. Therefore, sample statistics (summary data based on samples) can estimate population parameters:

- - $\bar{X}$ estimates μ
- - s estimates σ

The distribution of sample means from *any* population of interest will follow the normal curve if n is sufficiently large.

The center of this sampling distribution is the population mean (μ).

The standard deviation of this sampling distribution is the Standard Error of the Mean $(SE_{\bar{X}}) = \sigma_{\bar{X}} = \frac{\sigma}{\sqrt{n}}$. Therefore,

$\cdots$ a sample mean can be compared with a population mean by the z test $= \frac{\bar{X}-\mu}{\sigma/\sqrt{n}}$

- - if σ is not known, s is substituted and we use the *t*-test $= \frac{\bar{X}-\mu}{s/\sqrt{n}}$ especially for small samples (n of 30 or less).

CUMULATIVE GLOSSARY I: TERMS

Chapter 11

Descriptive Statistics   Methods used to describe or summarize a set of data which do not involve generalization to a larger set of data.

Inferential Statistics   Methods used to summarize a relatively small set of data (e.g., a sample) in order to make generalizations concerning a much larger set of possible data (e.g., a population).

Unbiased Estimate	A sample estimate which has the property that the average of all possible sample estimates obtained in the specified manner equals exactly the population parameter.

Sum of Squares   Sum of squared deviations around the population mean, $\Sigma\,(x-\mu)^2$, or sample mean, $\Sigma\,(x-\bar{x})^2$. The numerator of the variance term.

t-Distribution   A distribution of the variate $t = \dfrac{\bar{X}-\mu}{s/\sqrt{n}}$. Note that s has replaced σ in the critical ratio (i.e., compare with $z = \dfrac{\bar{X}-\mu}{\sigma/\sqrt{n}}$). Shape of the distribution depends on the number of degrees of freedom: it approaches the normal distribution as df $\longrightarrow \infty$. Use to test small samples (df 30 or less) where the population variance is unknown.

Central Limit Theorem   The distribution of means of random samples from a non-normal population approaches the normal distribution as the sample size (n) becomes sufficiently large (e.g., see *t-Distribution* above).

CUMULATIVE GLOSSARY II: SYMBOLS

Chapter 11

$\bar{x}$ Sample mean $= \dfrac{\Sigma\,x}{n}$. Unbiased estimate of population mean, μ.

s^2 Sample variance $= \dfrac{\Sigma\,(x-\bar{x})^2}{n-1}$. Unbiased estimate of population variance, σ^2.

s Sample standard deviation $= \sqrt{\dfrac{\Sigma\,(x-\bar{x})^2}{n-1}}$. An estimate of the population standard deviation, σ.

K Constant, whose value depends on size of sample, used in the formula $\dfrac{\text{Sample Range}}{K}$ to estimate the standard deviation of a normal population.

t Variate or critical ratio $\dfrac{\bar{X}-\mu}{s/\sqrt{n}}$. See Glossary I.

$\sigma_{\bar{x}}$ (SE$_{\bar{x}}$)   Standard deviation of the distribution of sample means, hence the Standard Error of the Mean. Equal to the population standard deviation divided by the square root of the sample size $= \dfrac{\sigma}{\sqrt{n}}$. Estimated by $\dfrac{s}{\sqrt{n}}$.

CUMULATIVE REVIEW III
(Chapters 1-11)

These notes review our discusion thus far on the description of continuous (quantitative) populations and on inferences based on samples from such populations. Comparisons between quantitative and qualitative data are also highlighted.

DESCRIPTIVE STATISTICS
FOR A CONTINUOUS POPULATION OR SAMPLE

1. Measures of central tendency = mean (μ or $\bar{x}$), mode, median (Q_2). The median is a better measure than the mean if the population is skewed.

2. Standard Deviation = most useful measure of variability = σ or s.

3. Relative Variability = Coefficient of Variation in % = $\dfrac{\sigma}{\mu} \times 100$, or, $\dfrac{s}{\bar{x}} \times 100$.

4. Measures based on ordered data: Q_1, Q_2 (median), Q_3.

5. The sample range can be used to estimate the Standard Deviation of a normal population: $\dfrac{\text{Range}}{\text{K}}$ = est. Population Standard Deviation (σ) where K depends on sample size.

6. If the distribution is balanced (symmetrical), then: a) $Q_2 - Q_1 = Q_3 - Q_2$
  b) Median = Mean

CUMULATIVE FREQUENCY DISTRIBUTION

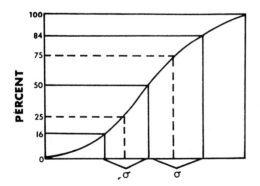

values corresponding to: 84−50 = 34% = σ or s
  50−16 = 34% = σ or s

7. In addition, if the distribution is normal, then the Standard Deviation calculated as

$$\sigma = \sqrt{\dfrac{\Sigma\,(x-\mu)^2}{N}}, \text{ or } s = \sqrt{\dfrac{\Sigma\,(x-\bar{x})^2}{n-1}}$$

will include 34% of the distribution on either side of the mean.

8. Examples of Distributions:
  a) symmetrical, normal
  b) symmetrical, non-normal
  c) nonsymmetrical
  d) log normal

The next page illustrates, for both qualitative and quantitative data, three types of distributions which must be clearly distinguished. These are: (1) the population; (2) a sample from the population; and (3) the distribution of a sample statistic such as the means of many random samples of size n taken from the population and called a *sampling distribution.*

The standard deviation of the first two curves is a measure of the variability of individuals in the population (or sample). The standard deviation of the third curve is a measure of the variability or error of the sampling statistic and is appropriately called a Standard Error.

The size of the standard deviation of individuals (σ) is an inherent property of the population. It tells us how much individuals differ from each other. It cannot be affected by the number of individuals in the population. The Standard Error of a sampling statistic, on the other hand, depends on (1) the variability of the individuals in the population (σ), and (2) the size of the sample (n) on which the estimate is based.

As can be seen in these illustrations, there are many similarities between quantitative and qualitative data. A principal difference is that binomial data have only one independent parameter (p) while quantitative data typically have two independent parameters (μ and σ). Stated in another way, the variability of most quantitative populations does not depend on the mean value.

In Chapter 12, we will discuss a fourth type of distribution: a sampling distribution of *differences* between sample means.

ANALOGIES BETWEEN INFERENCE
FOR QUALITATIVE AND QUANTITATIVE DATA

DISTRIBUTION OF A BINOMIAL POPULATION

Note that if we know p, we also know pq

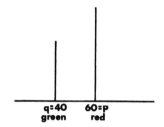

q=40   60=p
green   red

Population Mean (proportion) = p

Population Variance = pq

Population S. D. = $\sqrt{pq}$

DISTRIBUTION OF ONE SAMPLE OF n= 25 FROM ABOVE POPULATION

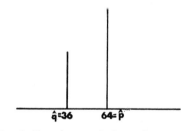

$\hat{q}$=36   64=$\hat{p}$

Sample Mean (proportion) = $\hat{p}$

Sample Variance = $\hat{p}\,\hat{q}$

Sample S. D. = $\sqrt{\hat{p}\,\hat{q}}$

DISTRIBUTION OF ONE MILLION SAMPLE PROPORTIONS ($\hat{p}$) WHERE n=25 FROM ABOVE POPULATION

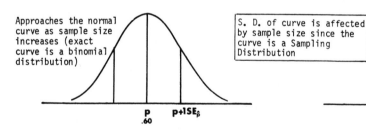

Approaches the normal curve as sample size increases (exact curve is a binomial distribution)

S. D. of curve is affected by sample size since the curve is a Sampling Distribution

P   p+1SE$_{\hat{p}}$
.60

Mean of curve = true p of population

Variance of curve = $\dfrac{pq}{n}$ = $\dfrac{\text{population variance}}{\text{size of sample}}$

S. D. = SE$_{\hat{p}}$= $\dfrac{\sqrt{pq}}{\sqrt{n}}$ = $\dfrac{\sqrt{pq}}{\sqrt{n}}$ = $\dfrac{\text{population S. D.}}{\sqrt{\text{size of sample}}}$

(Standard Error of Proportion)

DISTRIBUTION OF A CONTINUOUS POPULATION

If it is a normal distribution $\mu \pm 1\sigma$ will include 68% of the values

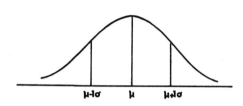

μ-1σ μ μ+1σ

Population Mean = μ = $\dfrac{\Sigma x}{N}$

Population Variance = σ^2 = $\dfrac{\Sigma(x-\mu)^2}{N}$

Population S. D. = $\sigma = \sqrt{\dfrac{\Sigma(x-\mu)^2}{N}}$

DISTRIBUTION OF ONE SAMPLE OF n= 25 FROM ABOVE POPULATION

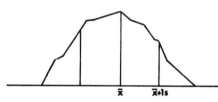

$\bar{x}$ $\bar{x}$+1s

Sample Mean = $\bar{x}$ = $\dfrac{\Sigma x}{n}$

Sample Variance = s^2 = $\dfrac{\Sigma(x-\bar{x})^2}{n-1}$

Sample S. D. = s = $\sqrt{\dfrac{\Sigma(x-\bar{x})^2}{n-1}}$

DISTRIBUTION OF ONE MILLION SAMPLE MEANS ($\bar{x}$) WHERE n=25 FROM ABOVE POPULATION

Approaches the normal curve as sample size increases

μ μ+1SE$_{\bar{x}}$

Mean of curve = true μ of population

Variance of curve = $\dfrac{\sigma^2}{n}$ = $\dfrac{\text{population variance}}{\text{size of sample}}$

S. D. = SE$_{\bar{x}}$ = $\sigma_{\bar{x}}$ = $\dfrac{\sigma}{\sqrt{n}}$ = $\dfrac{\text{population S. D.}}{\sqrt{\text{size of sample}}}$

(Standard Error of Mean)

12

Difference Between
Two Independent Sample Means

*Significance Test on Difference Between Two Independent Sample
Means, Population Variance (σ^2) Known • Significance Test on
Difference Between Two Independent Sample Means, Population
Variance (σ^2) Not Known: $n_1 = n_2$ (Samples of Same Size);
$n_1 \neq n_2$ (Samples of Different Size) • Assumptions of the t-Test*

In the last chapter we discussed distributions of
sample means around a population mean (1)
where the population variance σ^2 is known, and
(2) where σ^2 is not known.

(1) In the first case since the population
variance σ^2 is known, the exact $SE_{\bar{x}}$ value can be
determined. Furthermore the variate $z = \dfrac{\bar{X} - \mu}{\sigma/\sqrt{n}}$
will follow the normal distribution. Therefore,
areas of the normal table can be used to do a
test on a sample mean. That is we locate a sample
mean on the standard normal distribution of random sample means in order to determine P, the
probability of a deviation from the expected mean
as large or larger *if* the Null Hypothesis is true.

(2) Where the population variance (σ^2) is not
known, the sample variance (s^2) is used in
estimating $SE_{\bar{x}}$. That is s replaces σ in the $SE_{\bar{x}}$
formula. As a result, the z variate of the normal
distribution is replaced by the variate $t = \dfrac{\bar{X} - \mu}{s/\sqrt{n}}$
The t-distribution (n 30 or less) has more area
in the tails than the normal. Therefore, a sample
mean to be associated with an area, P, of only .05
in the tails must be further from the expected
mean. Compare $t_{4df} = 2.78$ with $z = 1.96$.

This chapter extends our theory of sampling
distributions to *differences* between two *independent* sample means. Two samples are independent when the items or values of one sample
are not related to or affected by those of the
other. If two samples represent two entirely
different populations, e.g., healthy men and tuberculous men, or are otherwise unpaired, they are
independent. On the other hand if one sample
includes littermates of individuals in the other
sample, or if they represent "before" and "after"
measurements on the same individuals, they are
not independent.

SIGNIFICANCE TEST ON A DIFFERENCE
BETWEEN TWO INDEPENDENT SAMPLE MEANS,
POPULATION VARIANCE (σ^2) KNOWN

Just as the distribution of sample means is
analogous to the distribution of sample proportions
(Cumulative Review III), distributions of differences between independent sample means and
sample proportions are comparable: (1) the
center of the distribution of a million differences
between means of two random samples of sizes n_1
and n_2 is zero, the true difference (see Figure
12-1); (2) the standard deviation of the sampling
distribution is $\sigma_{\bar{x}_1 - \bar{x}_2}$, also called the Standard
Error of the Difference $= SE_{\bar{x}_1 - \bar{x}_2}$. This term
can be computed from the two sample Standard
Errors of the Mean ($SE_{\bar{x}}$) in squared form or
directly from the population variance (σ^2). The
various alternative formulas are shown below:

$$SE_{\bar{x}_1 - \bar{x}_2} = \sqrt{(SE_{\bar{x}_1})^2 + (SE_{\bar{x}_2})^2}$$

$$= \sqrt{\frac{\sigma^2}{n_1} + \frac{\sigma^2}{n_2}} = \sqrt{\sigma^2 \left(\frac{1}{n_1} + \frac{1}{n_2} \right)}$$

Note that the same (known) population variance (σ^2) enters into the $SE_{\bar{x}}$ term for each sample, that the sizes of the samples affect the Standard Error and that the formula is analogous to that

for $SE_{\hat{p}_1 - \hat{p}_2} = \sqrt{\hat{p}\hat{q} \left(\frac{1}{n_1} + \frac{1}{n_2} \right)}$

(See Chapter 5).

FIGURE 12-1

DISTRIBUTION OF CHANCE DIFFERENCES

BETWEEN TWO SAMPLE MEANS

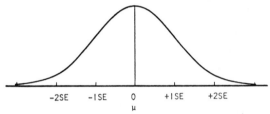

$SE_{\bar{x}_1 - \bar{x}_2} = \sigma_{\bar{x}_1 - \bar{x}_2} =$ Standard Deviation of Distribution of Differences or Standard Error of the Difference

For illustration, we use data from Chapter 11 on two random samples, each of size 5, from a population of 205 temperatures of healthy young men. The two sample means are 98.52° and 98.36°. Is the difference between the two means significant? Recall that for this population the standard deviation σ is known to be 0.48° and each $n = 5$. Therefore, each $SE_{\bar{x}}$ is equal to

$$\frac{\sigma}{\sqrt{n}} = \frac{0.48°}{\sqrt{5}} = 0.21°.$$

Since the population variance is known, the Critical Ratio or test statistic for the difference between the two sample means is z, the Standard Normal deviate, whose general form is:

$$z = \frac{\overset{\text{observed value}}{\overset{\downarrow}{\bar{x}} - \mu \longleftarrow \text{center of normal curve}}}{\sigma \longleftarrow \text{standard deviation of normal curve}}$$

In this instance, x is the observed difference $(\bar{x}_1 - \bar{x}_2)$, μ is 0 under the Null Hypothesis that $\mu_1 - \mu_2 = 0$ (there is no difference) and σ is $\sigma_{\bar{x}_1 - \bar{x}_2}$ or $SE_{\bar{x}_1 - \bar{x}_2}$.

Therefore, the Critical Ratio is $z = \dfrac{(\bar{x}_1 - \bar{x}_2) - 0}{SE_{\bar{x}_1 - \bar{x}_2}}$

Since the population variance σ^2 is known, the

formula for $SE_{\bar{x}_1 - \bar{x}_2}$ is:

$$\sqrt{\sigma^2 \left(\frac{1}{n_1} + \frac{1}{n_2} \right)} \text{ or } \sqrt{(SE_{\bar{x}_1})^2 + (SE_{\bar{x}_2})^2}$$

Using the latter formula we obtain

$$SE_{\bar{x}_1 - \bar{x}_2} = \sqrt{(0.21°)^2 + (0.21°)^2} = .30°$$

Alternatively, computing $SE_{\bar{x}_1 - \bar{x}_2}$ from

$$\sqrt{\sigma^2 \left(\frac{1}{n_1} + \frac{1}{n_2} \right)}$$

we obtain

$$\sqrt{(0.48°)^2 \left(\frac{1}{5} + \frac{1}{5} \right)}$$

$$= \sqrt{(.23) \ (.2 + .2)} = .30°$$

Therefore

$$z = \frac{(98.52° - 98.36°) - 0}{.30°} = \frac{.16°}{.30°} = .53$$

The P associated with a z of .53 is approximately .30 (Normal table). Therefore, the difference between the sample means is not significant. (The difference could frequently arise by chance alone when the Null Hypothesis is true.) Again, since we know that these are two random samples from the same population, we know that no error (Type I) was made (Chapter 8).

SIGNIFICANCE TEST ON A DIFFERENCE
BETWEEN TWO INDEPENDENT SAMPLE MEANS,
POPULATION VARIANCE (σ^2) NOT KNOWN

Much more commonly the population variance is not known and must be estimated from the sample variances (s_1^2 and s_2^2). Note that we now have two samples which contribute to the estimate of the population variance. In order to make this estimate and to use the t-test we shall assume no true difference between population variances. (See end of chapter, Assumptions of the t-test.)[1]

It is best to consider two different situations: where the two samples are of the same size and where they are of different sizes. In both cases we shall first concern ourselves with estimating the Standard Error of the Difference ($SE_{\bar{x}_1 - \bar{x}_2}$).

$n_1 = n_2$. If the samples are of the same size, s_1^2 and s_2^2 contribute equally to the overall estimate (called s^2_{pooled}) of the population variance. Therefore this pooled estimate, s_p^2, can be computed as a simple average of s_1^2 and s_2^2 $\left(\text{i.e., } s_p^2 = \frac{s_1^2 + s_2^2}{2} \right)$. We then substitute s_p^2

---

[1]Where σ_1^2 and σ_2^2 are not equal, a weighted t-test may be used as described in Snedecor, G., and Cochran, W., Statistical Methods, 6th ed., pp. 114-116, Iowa State Press, 1967.

for σ^2 in the estimated $SE_{\bar{x}_1 - \bar{x}_2}$ formula.

Thus, est. $SE_{\bar{x}_1 - \bar{x}_2} = \sqrt{s_p^2\left(\dfrac{1}{n_1} + \dfrac{1}{n_2}\right)}$

Equivalently, we can calculate for each sample an estimated Standard Error of the Mean, using s in place of σ (est. $SE_{\bar{x}} = \dfrac{s}{\sqrt{n}}$). We then add these est. $SE_{\bar{x}}$ terms in squared form and take the square root to obtain est. $SE_{\bar{x}_1 - \bar{x}_2}$. The formula for $SE_{\bar{x}_1 - \bar{x}_2}$ and its alternative form by this method is therefore:

est. $SE_{\bar{x}_1 - \bar{x}_2} = \sqrt{(\text{est. } SE_{\bar{x}_1})^2 + (\text{est. } SE_{\bar{x}_2})^2}$

$= \sqrt{\dfrac{s_1^2}{n_1} + \dfrac{s_2^2}{n^2}}$

To illustrate, we use Samples 1 and 2 from Table 11-1:

	Sample 1	Sample 2
Size of sample (n)	5	5
Sample mean ($\bar{x}$)	98.52°	98.36°
Sample variance (s^2)	0.0370	0.2330
Sample S.D. (s)	0.1923	0.4827
Est. $SE_{\bar{x}}\left(\dfrac{s}{\sqrt{n}}\right)$	$\dfrac{0.1923}{\sqrt{5}} = .0860$	$\dfrac{0.4827}{\sqrt{5}}$

$= 0.2158$

Since $n_1 = n_2$, a pooled variance estimate s_p^2 can be obtained by averaging (s_1^2) and (s_2^2):

$s_p^2 = \dfrac{(.0370) + (.2330)}{2} = .135$

Substituting this for σ^2 we estimate

$SE_{\bar{x}_1 - \bar{x}_2} = \sqrt{s_p^2\left(\dfrac{1}{n_1} + \dfrac{1}{n_2}\right)}$

$= \sqrt{.135\left(\dfrac{1}{5} + \dfrac{1}{5}\right)} = .23°$

Equivalently using the estimated $SE_{\bar{x}}$ values we obtain:

est. $SE_{\bar{x}_1 - \bar{x}_2} = \sqrt{(\text{est. } SE_{\bar{x}_1})^2 + (\text{est. } SE_{\bar{x}_2})^2}$

$= \sqrt{(.0860)^2 + (.2158)^2} = .23°$

$n_1 \neq n_2$. If the samples are not of the same size ($n_1 \neq n_2$) they do not contribute equally to the overall estimate of the population variance. Therefore, a pooled variance estimate (s^2_{pooled} or s_p^2) must be obtained by *weighting* each sample variance estimate by the $n-1$ degrees of freedom that enter into its computation (remember that the formula for $s^2 = \dfrac{\Sigma(x - \bar{x})^2}{n-1}$), and then dividing

by the sum of the weights. Therefore,

$s_p^2 = \dfrac{(n_1 - 1)\, s_1^2 + (n_2 - 1)\, s_2^2}{(n_1 - 1) + (n_2 - 1)}$

Thus s_p^2 is a weighted average of the two estimated variances *. Note its similarity to the estimate of the overall population proportions, p' and $\hat{q}$, a weighted average of the sample proportions, $\hat{p}_1$ and $\hat{p}_2$ (or $\hat{q}_1$ and $\hat{q}_2$).

After s_p^2 is computed it is substituted for σ^2 in the usual $SE_{\bar{x}_1 - \bar{x}_2}$ formula:

est. $SE_{\bar{x}_1 - \bar{x}_2} = \sqrt{s_p^2\left(\dfrac{1}{n_1} + \dfrac{1}{n_2}\right)} = \sqrt{\dfrac{s_p^2}{n_1} + \dfrac{s_p^2}{n_2}}$

Note that it can be shown that if $n_1 = n_2$, the above formula reduces as before to

est. $SE_{\bar{x}_1 - \bar{x}_2} = \sqrt{(\text{est. } SE_{\bar{x}_1})^2 + (\text{est. } SE_{\bar{x}_2})^2}$

As an example of this computation, let us again use two sample means of mouth temperatures. However, this time we use a mean based on a sample of size 5 and one based on a sample of size 6.

	Sample 1	Sample 2
Size of sample (n)	5	6
Sample mean ($\bar{x}$)	98.52°	98.60°
Sample sum of squares $\Sigma(x - \bar{x})^2$	0.1480	1.4775
Sample variance (s^2)	0.0370	0.2955

If we make the assumption that the population variances are the same (see below assumptions of the t-test) we can proceed as follows:

s^2_{pooled} or $(s_p^2) = \dfrac{(n_1 - 1)\, s_1^2 + (n_2 - 1)\, s_2^2}{(n_1 - 1) + (n_2 - 1)}$

$= \dfrac{(4)\,(.0370) + (5)\,(.2955)}{(4) + (5)}$

$= \dfrac{(.1480) + (1.4775)}{(4) + (5)} = .1806$

Thus, for our example,

est. $SE_{\bar{x}_1 - \bar{x}_2} = \sqrt{s_p^2\left(\dfrac{1}{n_1} + \dfrac{1}{n_2}\right)}$

$= \sqrt{(.1806)\left(\dfrac{1}{5} + \dfrac{1}{6}\right)} = .26°$

---

*s_p^2 can also be computed by "pooling" the two sample "sums of squares" or numerators of the individual variance terms and then dividing by the pooled denominators.

$s_p^2 = \dfrac{\Sigma(x - \bar{x}_1)^2 + \Sigma(x - \bar{x}_2)^2}{(n_1 - 1) + (n_2 - 1)} = \dfrac{.1480 + 1.4775}{(4) + (5)} = .1806$

The next step for both cases $(n_1 = n_2)$ and $(n_1 \neq n_2)$, once $SE_{\bar{X}_1-\bar{X}_2}$ is computed, is to complete our significance test on the difference between the sample means. Since an estimate based on the sample variances is substituted for the population variance in the Standard Error formula the t-variate is used rather than z.

The Critical Ratio is $t = \dfrac{(\bar{X}_1-\bar{X}_2) - 0}{SE_{\bar{X}_1-\bar{X}_2}}$

The number of degrees of freedom for t is the __total__ number of independent differences from which the __combined__ variance estimate (s_p^2) is made:

$$df = (n_1-1) + (n_2-1), \text{ or } (n_1+n_2-2)$$

Thus for our example where $n_1 = n_2$:

$$t = \frac{(\bar{X}_1-\bar{X}_2) - 0}{SE_{\bar{X}_1-\bar{X}_2}} = \frac{(98.52° - 98.36°) - 0°}{.23°} = \frac{0.16°}{.23°} = .69$$

$$df = (n_1 - 1) + (n_2 - 1) = 4 + 4 = 8; \quad P \sim .50$$

And for the example where $n_1 \neq n_2$:

$$t = \frac{(\bar{X}_1-\bar{X}_2) - 0}{SE_{\bar{X}_1-\bar{X}_2}} = \frac{(98.52° - 98.60°) - 0°}{.26°} = \frac{-.08°}{.26°} = -.31$$

$$df = (n_1 - 1) + (n_2 - 1) = 4 + 5 = 9; \quad P \sim .75$$

In both examples, since P is greater than .05, the Null Hypothesis is accepted. Note that if df is greater than 30, the z or Normal Deviate Test can be used instead of the t-test.

Table 12-1 summarizes the various significance tests on samples of mouth temperature illustrated in this chapter and in Chapter 11.

TABLE 12-1

Examples of Significance Tests for Continuous Data (Mouth Temperature Data)

I. To Compare *One* Sample Mean With An *Expected* Mean

A. σ^2 Known

$$z = \frac{\bar{X}-\mu}{SE_{\bar{X}}} = \frac{\bar{X}-\mu}{\sigma/\sqrt{n}}$$

$$= \frac{98.52° - 98.42°}{.48°/\sqrt{5}} = \frac{.10°}{.21°}$$

$$z = .46, P \sim .35$$

B. σ^2 Not Known

$$t = \frac{\bar{X}-\mu}{\text{est } SE_{\bar{X}}} = \frac{\bar{X}-\mu}{s/\sqrt{n}}$$

$$= \frac{98.52° - 98.42°}{.19°/\sqrt{5}} = \frac{.10°}{.085°}$$

$$t_{4df} = 1.18, P \sim .20$$

II. To Compare *Two* Independent Sample Means With *Each Other*

A. σ^2 Known

$$z = \frac{(\bar{X}_1-\bar{X}_2) - 0}{SE_{\bar{X}_1-\bar{X}_2}} = \frac{(\bar{X}_1-\bar{X}_2) - 0}{\sqrt{\sigma^2\left(\frac{1}{n_1} + \frac{1}{n_2}\right)}}$$

$$= \frac{(98.52° - 98.36°) - 0}{\sqrt{(.48°)^2\left(\frac{1}{5} + \frac{1}{5}\right)}} = \frac{.16°}{.30°}$$

$$z = .53, P \sim .38$$

B. σ^2 Not Known

$n_1 = n_2$

$$t = \frac{(\bar{X}_1-\bar{X}_2) - 0}{\text{est. } SE_{\bar{X}_1-\bar{X}_2}} = \frac{(\bar{X}_1-\bar{X}_2) - 0}{\sqrt{(SE_{\bar{X}_1})^2 + (SE_{\bar{X}_2})^2}}$$

$$= \frac{(98.52° - 98.36°) - 0}{\sqrt{(.0860°)^2 + (.2158°)^2}} = \frac{.16°}{.23°}$$

$$t_{8df} = .69, P \sim .50$$

$n_1 \neq n_2$

$$t = \frac{(\bar{X}_1-\bar{X}_2) - 0}{\text{est. } SE_{\bar{X}_1-\bar{X}_2}} = \frac{(\bar{X}_1-\bar{X}_2) - 0}{\sqrt{s_p^2\left(\frac{1}{n_1} + \frac{1}{n_2}\right)}}$$

$$= \frac{(98.52° - 98.60°) - 0}{\sqrt{(.1806)\left(\frac{1}{5} + \frac{1}{6}\right)}} = \frac{-.08°}{.26°}$$

$$t_{9df} = -.31, P \sim .75$$

ASSUMPTIONS OF THE t-TEST

In conducting the t-test, two assumptions were required:

(1) We assume that the underlying population data are __normally distributed__.[1] This assumption can be tested by (a) a Chi Square Goodness of Fit Test (Chapter 7) or (b) roughly by graphic inspection of the cumulative frequency distribu-

[1] If data are not normally distributed, use either a normalizing transformation or a non-parametric procedure.

tion. The difference between the 84th and 50th percentiles and between the 50th and 16th percentiles, since each includes 34% of the area on either side of the mean, should equal the S. D. of the population if it is normally distributed (Chapter 10).

(2) Where the test is between two sample means we assume that the <u>population variances are really the same (homogeneity of variances)</u>, i.e., $\sigma_1^2 = \sigma_2^2 = \sigma^2$. An "F" test of equality of variances (is s_1^2 significantly different from s_2^2?) can be carried out to test this assumption. The reader is referred to more advanced texts for information on the F-test. See also Chapter 15.

PROBLEM 12-1

$P = .01$ means that the probability is one in a hundred that the observed difference is due to chance. *True or False?*

ANSWER 12-1

False. This is a "tricky" question: The majority of students incorrectly answer *true*. First note that P should refer to a difference as extreme as that observed *or more extreme* (this phrase is missing). Secondly, note that the words *if the Null Hypothesis is true* are missing. If the Null Hypothesis is true, then, $P = .01$ represents the probability that a difference as extreme as that observed or more extreme will occur just by sampling variation. If the Null Hypothesis *is not true*, the probability of a chance difference as extreme as that observed or more extreme cannot be readily determined. (See Chapter 8.)

Stated in another way: P and 1-P refer to the probability of chance differences under the Null Hypothesis. It is not appropriate to interpret these terms as referring to the likelihood that the Null Hypothesis assumption is or is not correct.

PROBLEM 12-2

The t ratio, $\dfrac{(\bar{X}_1 - \bar{X}_2) - 0}{SE_{\bar{X}_1 - \bar{X}_2}}$ for a difference between two independent sample means is 2.01. The two samples are of sizes 8 and 10 respectively. Is the difference significant at the .05 level?

ANSWER 12-2

No. The degrees of freedom are $(n_1 - 1) + (n_2 - 1) = (8-1) + (10-1) = 16$. The critical t value for 16 df at the .05 level of significance is approximately 2.13. Since the observed t value is only 2.01, P is $> .05$ and the difference is not significant.

PROBLEM 12-3

The weight gain in two comparable groups of children fed on special diets is given below. Is there a significant difference in mean weight gain between the two groups?

Weight Gain in Children

	Group A	Group B
n	36	36
$\bar{x}$	50 gms	70 gms
s	18 gms	24 gms

ANSWER 12-3

The test statistic is $t = \dfrac{(\bar{X}_1 - \bar{X}_2) - 0}{SE_{\bar{X}_1 - \bar{X}_2}}$. This ratio enables us to locate the observed difference on the chance distribution of sample differences under the Null Hypothesis. Thus, the probability of such an event (or one more extreme) by chance alone can be determined.

Since $n_1 = n_2$, the simplest procedure is to calculate the Standard Error of the Difference $(SE_{\bar{X}_1 - \bar{X}_2})$ from the respective values for the Standard Error of the Mean (est. $SE_{\bar{x}}$).

$$SE_{\bar{X}_1 - \bar{X}_2} = \sqrt{(SE_{\bar{X}_1})^2 + (SE_{\bar{X}_2})^2}$$

Thus:

$$SE_{\bar{X}_1} = \frac{s_1}{\sqrt{n_1}} = \frac{18 \text{ gms}}{\sqrt{36}} = \frac{18}{6} = 3 \text{ gms}$$

$$SE_{\bar{X}_2} = \frac{s_2}{\sqrt{n_2}} = \frac{24 \text{ gms}}{\sqrt{36}} = \frac{24}{6} = 4 \text{ gms}$$

$$SE_{\bar{X}_1 - \bar{X}_2} = \sqrt{(3)^2 + (4)^2} = \sqrt{9 + 16} = 5 \text{ gms}$$

$$\text{Obs } t = \frac{50 \text{ gms} - 70 \text{ gms}}{5 \text{ gms}} = \frac{-20}{5} = -4$$

$$df = (n_1 - 1) + (n_2 - 1) = 35 + 35 = 70$$

Since df > 30 this is equivalent to the z or normal distribution:

$$t_{.05(70 \text{ df})} = 1.96$$

$\therefore$ P $< .05$; difference is significant

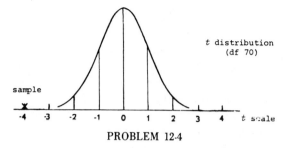

PROBLEM 12-4

Comparison of Two Samples:		Healthy men	Men with Tuberculosis
Size of sample	(n)	100	100
Mean temperature	($\bar{x}$)	98.4°	99.4°
Standard deviation	(s)	0.5°	1.0°

Is there a statistically significant difference between the two average temperatures? Explain your answer by appropriate calculations. Assume the population variances are the same.

ANSWER 12-4

Difference between two sample means is $\bar{x}_1 - \bar{x}_2 = 1.0°$. The Critical Ratio is

$$t = \frac{(\bar{x}_1 - \bar{x}_2) - 0}{SE_{\bar{x}_1 - \bar{x}_2}}$$

Since $n_1 = n_2$, $SE_{\bar{x}_1 - \bar{x}_2} = \sqrt{(SE_{\bar{x}_1})^2 + (SE_{\bar{x}_2})^2}$

$$SE_{\bar{x}_1} = \frac{s_1}{\sqrt{n_1}} = \frac{0.5°}{\sqrt{100}} = .05°$$

$$SE_{\bar{x}_2} = \frac{s_2}{\sqrt{n_2}} = \frac{1.0°}{\sqrt{100}} = .10°$$

$$\therefore SE_{\bar{x}_1 - \bar{x}_2} = \sqrt{(.05°)^2 + (.10°)^2} = \sqrt{.0025 + .01} = \sqrt{.0125} = \sim .11°$$

$$t = \frac{1.0° - 0}{.11°} = 9$$

This is considerably larger than $t_{.05, 198df}$ (or z) $= 1.96$ $P << .05$

Therefore, the difference is significant.

PROBLEM 12-5

In computing the Standard Error of the Difference between two independent sample means, one way to get an estimate of σ^2 is to obtain a pooled sample variance estimate s_p^2.

If $n_1 = 10$ and $s_1^2 = 5$
$n_2 = 5$ and $s_2^2 = 8$

What is s_p^2? What is $SE_{\bar{x}_1 - \bar{x}_2}$? (Data in gms).

ANSWER 12-5

$s_p^2 = $ the weighted average of the two sample

variances, Thus,

$$s_p^2 = \frac{(n_1-1) \ s_1^2 + (n_2-1) \ s_2^2}{(n_1-1) + (n_2-1)} = \frac{(10-1) \ (5) + (5-1) \ (8)}{(10-1) + (5-1)}$$

$$= \frac{45 + 32}{13} = \frac{77}{13} = 6 \text{ (approximately)}$$

$$SE_{\bar{x}_1 - \bar{x}_2} = \sqrt{s_p^2 \left(\frac{1}{n_1} + \frac{1}{n_2}\right)} = \sqrt{6 \left(\frac{1}{10} + \frac{1}{5}\right)}$$

$$= \sqrt{6 \ (.1 + .2)} = \sqrt{1.8} = 1.34 \text{ gms}$$

PROBLEM 12-6

The weight of an organ (in gm) determined after a certain procedure is listed below for 5 female and 6 male rats. Is there a significant difference in mean weight between females and males?

Female	Male
8.3	8.8
8.5	8.7
8.2	9.2
8.1	8.6
8.4	8.5
	9.0

ANSWER 12-6

We proceed systematically to calculate the sample means, sample variances and the Standard Error of the Difference in order to obtain the t value.

	Female		
	x	$(x-\bar{x})$	$(x-\bar{x})^2$
	8.3	0	0
	8.5	.2	.04
	8.2	−.1	.01
	8.1	−.2	.04
	8.4	.1	.01
$\Sigma x =$	41.5 gms	0*	.10
$\frac{\Sigma x}{n} =$	$8.3 = \bar{x}_1$	$s_1^2 = \frac{.10}{4} = .025$	

	Male		
	x	$(x-\bar{x})$	$(x-\bar{x})^2$
	8.8	0	0
	8.7	−.1	.01
	9.2	.4	.16
	8.6	−.2	.04
	8.5	−.3	.09
	9.0	.2	.04
$\Sigma x =$	52.8 gms	0*	.34
$\frac{\Sigma x}{n} =$	$8.8 = \bar{x}_2$	$s_2^2 = \frac{.34}{5} = .068$	

*The sum of the deviations from the mean should always add to 0.

We can summarize these statistics as follows:

Data in gms	Female	Male
No $= n$	5	6
Total $= \Sigma x$	41.5	52.8
$\bar{x} = \Sigma x/n$	8.3	8.8
$s^2 = \dfrac{\Sigma(x-\bar{x})^2}{n-1}$	.025	.068

We now proceed to calculate $SE_{\bar{x}_1 - \bar{x}_2}$. Since $n_1 \neq n_2$, we must use a formula for $SE_{\bar{x}_1 - \bar{x}_2}$ which involves $s^2{}_{pooled}$:

$$SE_{\bar{x}_1 - \bar{x}_2} = \sqrt{s^2{}_{pooled}\left(\frac{1}{n_1} + \frac{1}{n_2}\right)} \text{ where}$$

$s^2{}_{pooled}$ is the weighted average of the two sample variances

$$= \frac{(n_1-1)\; s_1{}^2 + (n_2-1)\; s_2{}^2}{(n_1-1) + (n_2-1)}$$

$$s^2{}_{pooled} = \frac{4(.025) + 5(.068)}{4 + 5} = \frac{.10 + .34}{9} = \frac{.44}{9} = .05$$

(Note that this is equivalent to pooling the two "sums of squares", $\Sigma(x-\bar{x}_1)^2$ and $\Sigma(x-\bar{x}_2)^2$, or .10 and .34, respectively, and dividing by the pooled df.)

Then, $SE_{\bar{x}_1 - \bar{x}_2} = \sqrt{(.05)\left(\dfrac{1}{5} + \dfrac{1}{6}\right)}$

$$= \sqrt{(.05)\;(.20 + .17)} = \sqrt{.0185} = .14$$

obs. $t = \dfrac{(8.3 - 8.8)}{.14} = \dfrac{-.50}{.14} = -3.6$

$df = (n_1-1) + (n_2-1) = 9 \text{ df}$

$t_{.05\; 9df}{}^* = 2.23$ (*approximately the same as 10 df)

Difference is significant since observed t of -3.6 is larger than $t_{.05.9df}$ of 2.23 in magnitude.

PROBLEM 12-7

Choose the correct item.

(a) The larger the number of degrees of freedom entering into the pooled variance estimate, the (smaller, larger) is the size of the t-ratio required at the .05 level of significance.

(b) The larger the observed t-ratio for a given number of df (e.g. $t_{obs.} = 3.00$ instead of 2.00 for 30 df), the (smaller, larger) is the significance level or P value.

ANSWER 12-7

(a) Smaller. As the sample size (and therefore the degrees of freedom) increases, the t-distribution approaches the normal. As it does so, the area in the tails is reduced (see Figure 11-3). Therefore, for a t at a given distance from the center (0), P will become less and less. Correspondingly the t at which P $= .05$ becomes smaller (closer to the center 0) approaching 1.96 at df > 30. See also Problem 11-12.

(b) Smaller. As with the z ratio, the larger the t-ratio, the further is the observed difference from the center (zero) of the curve of chance differences under the Null Hypothesis. Therefore, P, the probability of its occurrence or of an event more extreme by chance alone is smaller.

PROBLEM 12-8

What are the two assumptions made when the ordinary t-test on the difference between two independent sample means is carried out?

ANSWER 12-8

1. The samples are drawn from a normal population.
2. The population variances are really equal (homogeneous); the sample variances differ only by chance.

PROBLEM 12-9

The t-test can be applied validly to a comparison of more than two sample means. *True or False?*

ANSWER 12-9

False. The t-test is valid for a comparison of two samples only. A comparison of more than two samples requires the Analysis of Variance technique. (See Chapter 15.)

SUMMARY OF CHAPTER 12

The distribution of differences between random samples from the same population is a **normal curve**
—the center of the curve is the true difference, 0
The Standard Deviation of the curve $(\sigma_{\bar{x}_1 - \bar{x}_2})$ is the Standard Error of the Difference, $SE_{\bar{x}_1 - \bar{x}_2}$
The formula for $SE_{\bar{x}_1 - \bar{x}_2}$ for independent means varies:
—when σ^2 (population variance) is known:

$$\sqrt{(SE_{\bar{x}_1})^2 + (SE_{\bar{x}_2})^2} = \sqrt{\frac{\sigma^2}{n_1} + \frac{\sigma^2}{n_2}}$$

—when σ^2 is not known

and $n_1 = n_2$: $\sqrt{(\text{est. } SE_{\bar{X}_1})^2 + (\text{est. } SE_{\bar{X}_2})^2} = \sqrt{\dfrac{s_1^2}{n_1} + \dfrac{s_2^2}{n_2}}$

and $n_1 \neq n_2$: $\sqrt{s_p^2\left(\dfrac{1}{n_1} + \dfrac{1}{n_2}\right)}$ where $s_p^2 = \dfrac{(n_1-1)s_1^2 + (n_2-1)s_2^2}{(n_1-1) + (n_2-1)}$

The test between two means is:

—if σ^2 is known: $\dfrac{(\bar{X}_1 - \bar{X}_2) - 0}{SE_{\bar{X}_1 - \bar{X}_2}} = z$

—if σ^2 is not known: $\dfrac{(\bar{X}_1 - \bar{X}_2) - 0}{\text{est } SE_{\bar{X}_1 - \bar{X}_2}} = t$ with $(n_1 + n_2 - 2)$ df.

CUMULATIVE GLOSSARY I: TERMS
Chapter 12

Pooled Variance	Estimate of the population variance (σ^2) obtained by <u>pooling</u> the sample variance estimates (s^2). Each s^2 value is weighted by the $n-1$ terms which enter into its calculation. Also see Glossary II.
Standard Error of the Difference	Standard deviation of the distribution of chance differences between two sample means $(\bar{X}_1 - \bar{X}_2)$. Hence the Standard Error of the Difference. Formula varies depending upon (a) whether the population variance (σ^2) is known and (b) whether the sample sizes are equal or unequal. See Glossary II.
F Test	A test of the equality of two variances. For the test we use the F ratio $(F = s_1^2/s_2^2)$ which is compared with the F distribution (i.e., the distribution of the ratio of two independent sample estimates of a population variance). (See Chapter 15.)
Independent Samples	Samples whose values are independent of each other because they represent measurements on entirely different individuals or are otherwise unpaired or unrelated.
Non-Independent (Correlated) Samples	Samples whose values are correlated with each other because they represent measurements on the same or related individuals and hence are not independent.

CUMULATIVE GLOSSARY II: SYMBOLS

s^2_{pooled} — Pooled variance. Formula is $= \dfrac{(n_1-1)\,s_1^2 + (n_2-1)\,s_2^2}{(n_1-1) + (n_2-1)}$. See Glossary I.

$\sigma_{\bar{X}_1 - \bar{X}_2}$ } $(SE_{\bar{X}_1 - \bar{X}_2})$ } — Standard Error of the Difference between two sample means.
Formula for independent means —

when σ^2 (population variance) is known: $\sqrt{(SE_{\bar{X}_1})^2 + (SE_{\bar{X}_2})^2} = \sqrt{\dfrac{\sigma^2}{n_1} + \dfrac{\sigma^2}{n_2}}$

when σ^2 is not known

and $n_1 = n_2$: $\sqrt{(\text{est. } SE_{\bar{X}_1})^2 + (\text{est. } SE_{\bar{X}_2})^2} = \sqrt{\dfrac{s_1^2}{n_1} + \dfrac{s_2^2}{n_2}}$

and $n_1 \neq n_2$: $\sqrt{s_p^2\left(\dfrac{1}{n_1} + \dfrac{1}{n_2}\right)}$ where $s_p^2 = \dfrac{(n_1-1)\,s_1^2 + (n_2-1)\,s_2^2}{(n_1-1) + (n_2-1)}$

Also see Glossary I.

13

Difference
Between Correlated Sample Means
(Paired Data)

Comparison of Paired Data by the Usual t-Test (Adjusted) •
Comparison of Paired Data by the t-Test, Difference Method •
Comparison of Paired Data by the Sign Test •
Review of Principles for Testing Paired Data

In Chapter 12, we discussed significance tests on the difference between sample means where the data in the two samples were independent of each other. In this chapter, we will evaluate differences between means where the two samples are <u>not</u> independent of each other but are correlated, i.e., where the samples either refer to the same individuals or to "relatives," or are otherwise "paired" or matched.

Pairing is often done experimentally to reduce the variability between two sample groups. The purpose is to make them *homogeneous* with respect to all factors except the one tested, e.g., difference in treatment. It is often possible thereby to find a significant difference with a smaller sample size.

TABLE 13-1

| Individual | Temperatures on <u>Same</u> Individuals | |
	Fingers (x)	Toes (y)
1	31.0°	24.5°
2	29.5°	23.4°
3	28.5°	23.6°
4	34.6°	33.6°
5	35.0°	32.8°
6	35.0°	32.5°
Sample mean	32.27°	28.40°
Sample S.D.	2.96°	5.03°
Est. $SE_{mean} = \dfrac{S.D.}{\sqrt{n}}$	1.21°	2.05°

Source of data: Johns Hopkins University School of Hygiene and Public Health.

COMPARISON OF PAIRED DATA BY THE USUAL *t*-TEST (ADJUSTED)

Table 13-1 shows data on finger and toe temperatures for 6 individuals. Is there a significant difference between mean temperature of fingers and of toes? Note that if we carry out the *t*-test in the usual manner (as for independent samples) the difference between the means is not significant:

Since $n_1 = n_2$,

$$SE_{\bar{x}-\bar{y}} = \sqrt{(SE_{\bar{x}})^2 + (SE_{\bar{y}})^2}$$

Therefore,

$$t = \frac{(\bar{x} - \bar{y}) - 0}{\sqrt{(SE_{\bar{x}})^2 + (SE_{\bar{y}})^2}} = \frac{32.27 - 28.40}{\sqrt{(1.21)^2 + (2.05)^2}}$$

$$= \frac{3.87°}{2.38°} = 1.63$$

$$df = (n_x - 1) + (n_y - 1) = 10 \qquad P \sim .20$$

Inspection of the data indicates that the two distributions of temperatures for fingers and toes overlap.[1] For <u>each</u> individual, however, the temperature for fingers is <u>higher</u> than that for toes. This suggests that a significant difference may exist which is not evident by the test method used.

It can be shown that the above usual Standard Error formula (the denominator for the *t*-test) <u>overstates</u> the sampling variance for paired data whenever there is direct or posi-

[1] For example, finger temperatures range from 28.5° to 35.0°, toe temperatures from 23.4° to 33.6°.

144

tive correlation between the pairs. The correct $SE_{\bar{x}-\bar{y}}$ formula for paired data should be:

$$SE_{\bar{x}-\bar{y}} \text{ (paired data)}$$
$$= \sqrt{(SE_{\bar{x}})^2 + (SE_{\bar{y}})^2 - 2r(SE_{\bar{x}})(SE_{\bar{y}})}$$

where r is the *sample product moment correlation coefficient*. r indicates the strength of the association between x and y. It´ varies from -1 to $+1$. Its formula[1] is

$$r = \frac{\Sigma(x - \bar{x})(y - \bar{y})/(n-1)}{\sqrt{\left(\dfrac{\Sigma(x - \bar{x})^2}{n-1}\right)\left(\dfrac{\Sigma(y - \bar{y})^2}{n-1}\right)}}$$

$$= \frac{\text{Covariance } xy}{\sqrt{(\text{Variance } x)(\text{Variance } y)}}$$

Note that the numerator of r is the *covariance* of x and y. "Covariance" involves the multiplication of each x deviation from its mean ($\bar{x}$) with the corresponding y deviation from its mean ($\bar{y}$). That is, for each x, y pair, the product $(x - \bar{x})(y - \bar{y})$ is obtained and then summed over all pairs. In contrast, "variance" refers to the multiplication of each x deviation from the mean ($\bar{x}$) with itself, i.e., $(x - \bar{x})(x - \bar{x}) = (x - \bar{x})^2$.

The whole term $2r(SE_{\bar{x}})(SE_{\bar{y}})$ will be positive if x and y are positively correlated with each other (i.e., when r is between 0 and $+1$). That is, when x is high, y tends to be high, and conversely, when x is low, y tends to be low. When this positive term is *subtracted* from $[(SE_{\bar{x}})^2 + (SE_{\bar{y}})^2]$, it *reduces* the Standard Error of the Difference. Thus,

$$SE_{\bar{x}-\bar{y}} \text{ (paired data)}$$
$$= \sqrt{(SE_{\bar{x}})^2 + (SE_{\bar{y}})^2 - 2r(SE_{\bar{x}})(SE_{\bar{y}})}$$

For our data, $r = +.970$. Therefore,

$$2r(SE_{\bar{x}})(SE_{\bar{y}}) = 2(.970)(1.21)(2.05) = 4.802$$
$$\therefore SE_{\bar{x}-\bar{y}} = \sqrt{(1.21)^2 + (2.05)^2 - 4.802} = .93°$$

Note that is considerably less than the Standard Error of 2.38° obtained previously. The critical *t* ratio,

$$t = \frac{3.87°}{.93°} = 4.2$$

is now larger (4.2 instead of 1.63) because the Standard Error value is smaller.

This illustrates the reason for pairing when two sets of data are positively correlated. If two samples are <u>positively</u> correlated (that is, if r is between 0 and $+1$) with respect to a factor studied, the Standard Error of the Difference will be reduced. On the other hand, if they are <u>negatively</u> correlated (if r is between -1 and 0) the S.E. will be increased, and in this case pairing is disadvantageous. If the two samples are uncorrelated or independent, r will be equal to 0 and the whole term $[2r(SE_{\bar{x}})(SE_{\bar{y}})]$ will drop out. In that case we are left with our familiar formula for the Standard Error of the Difference between two independent or uncorrelated sample means:

$$SE_{\bar{x}_1-\bar{x}_2} = \sqrt{(SE_{\bar{x}_1})^2 + (SE_{\bar{x}_2})^2}$$

COMPARISON OF PAIRED DATA BY THE *t*-TEST, DIFFERENCE METHOD

The previous method adjusted the Standard Error of the Difference to reflect the correlation between the values in the two samples. The computation of the correlation coefficient, however, can be laborious without a computer. It is usually simpler to use a modified *t*-test, the "Difference Method." This is an important test and is shown step by step in Table 13-2 (see page 146).

(1) Compute the difference (d) between each x and y pair (be sure to enter + and − signs). The difference (d) is considered as a "new" variate from a population of differences (Fig. 13-1) (see page 147).

(2) Compute the *mean of the sample differences*, $\bar{d} = +3.87°$. Note that it is the same as the *difference between sample means*, $\bar{x} - \bar{y} = 32.27° - 28.40° = +3.87°$.

(3) Compute the deviation of each difference, d, from the sample mean difference $\bar{d}$, i.e., compute each $(d - \bar{d})$. Make sure that these deviations add to zero.

(4) Compute the square of the deviations, and sum these squared deviations.

---

[1] A short-cut computational formula for r which also avoids rounding errors is derived as follows:

$$r = \frac{\Sigma(x - \bar{x})(y - \bar{y})/(n-1)}{\sqrt{\Sigma(x - \bar{x})^2 \Sigma(y - \bar{y})^2}/(n-1)} = \frac{\Sigma(x - \bar{x})(y - \bar{y})}{\sqrt{\Sigma(x - \bar{x})^2 \Sigma(y - \bar{y})^2}}$$

$$= \frac{\Sigma xy - \dfrac{\Sigma x \, \Sigma y}{n}}{\sqrt{\left[\Sigma x^2 - \dfrac{(\Sigma x)^2}{n}\right]\left[\Sigma y^2 - \dfrac{(\Sigma y)^2}{n}\right]}}$$

TABLE 13-2. *Calculation of t-Ratio by Difference Method:*
Temperatures on Same Individuals

			Steps		
			(1)	(3)	(4)
Individual	Fingers (x)	Toes (y)	Difference $(x - y = d)$	$(d - \bar{d})$	$(d - \bar{d})^2$
1	31.0°	24.5°	+6.5°	+2.63°	6.917
2	29.5	23.4	+6.1	+2.23	4.973
3	28.5	23.6	+4.9	+1.03	1.061
4	34.6	33.6	+1.0	−2.87	8.237
5	35.0	32.8	+2.2	−1.67	2.789
6	35.0	32.5	+2.5	−1.37	1.877
Total	193.6	170.4	$+23.2 = \Sigma d$	~0	$25.854 = \Sigma(d - \bar{d})^2$
Means	32.27	28.40	$+3.87 = \bar{d}$		

Step (2) $\bar{d} = \dfrac{\Sigma d}{\text{No. of pairs}} = \dfrac{+23.2}{6} = 3.87°$

(5) $s_{\bar{d}}^2 = \dfrac{\Sigma(d - \bar{d})^2}{\text{No. of pairs} - 1} = \dfrac{25.854}{5} = 5.17$

(6) $s_d = \sqrt{\dfrac{\Sigma(d - \bar{d})^2}{\text{No. of pairs} - 1}} = \sqrt{5.170} = 2.27°$

(7) Check: $\dfrac{\text{Sample range}}{\text{K (based on number of pairs)}} = \dfrac{6.5° - 1.0°}{2.3} = \dfrac{5.5°}{2.3} = 2.4°$

(8) Est. $SE_{\bar{d}} = \dfrac{s_d}{\sqrt{\text{No. of pairs}}} = \dfrac{2.27°}{\sqrt{6}} = .93°$

(9) Obs. $t = \dfrac{\bar{d} - 0}{\text{Est. } SE_{\bar{d}}} = \dfrac{3.87° - 0}{.93°} = 4.2$

$df = \text{Number of pairs} - 1 = 6 - 1 = 5$

$P = < .05$; difference is significant

(5) The sample variance is then

$$s_{\bar{d}}^2 = \frac{\Sigma(d - \bar{d})^2}{\text{No. of pairs} - 1} = 5.17$$

Note that the denominator of this variance estimate is the number of pairs minus 1.

(6) Compute the sample standard deviation of differences by obtaining the square root of the sample variance

$$s_d = \sqrt{\frac{\Sigma(d - \bar{d})^2}{\text{No. of pairs} - 1}} = 2.27°$$

(7) Check this calculation by:

$$\frac{\text{Sample range}}{K} = \frac{5.5°}{2.3}$$

$$= 2.4° \quad \text{(roughly checks)}$$

(8) Obtain the estimated Standard Error of the Mean Difference ($SE_{\bar{d}}$) by dividing the sample standard deviation of differences by the square root of the number of pairs:

$$\frac{s_d}{\sqrt{\text{No. of pairs}}} = \frac{2.27°}{\sqrt{6}} = .93°$$

Note that this S.E. value is identical with that obtained by the formula for $SE_{\bar{x}-\bar{y}}$ when the formula is adjusted for paired data by using the correlation coefficient (r). In other words, $SE_{\bar{d}} = SE_{\bar{x}-\bar{y}}$ (paired data).

(9) The Null Hypothesis is that the true mean difference $\mu_d = 0$ and that $\bar{d}$ differs from 0 only by chance. Therefore, the critical ratio is:

$$\text{Observed } t = \frac{\bar{d} - 0}{SE_{\bar{d}}} = \frac{3.87° - 0}{0.93°} = 4.2$$

Again note that a t of 4.2 is identical with the result obtained by the previous method, which uses the correlation coefficient. The number of degrees of freedom for both methods is the number of independent values contributing to the variance estimate: (Number of pairs − 1) = 5. Thus obs. $t_{5df} = 4.2, P < .05$.

FIGURE 13-1

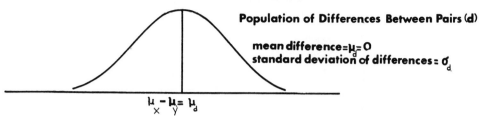

Population of Differences Between Pairs (d)

mean difference $= \mu_d = 0$
standard deviation of differences $= \sigma_d$

$\mu_x - \mu_y = \mu_d$

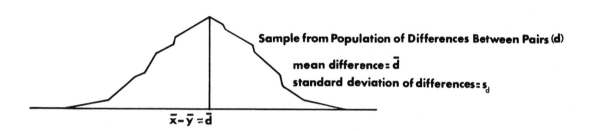

Sample from Population of Differences Between Pairs (d)

mean difference $= \bar{d}$
standard deviation of differences $= s_d$

$\bar{x} - \bar{y} = \bar{d}$

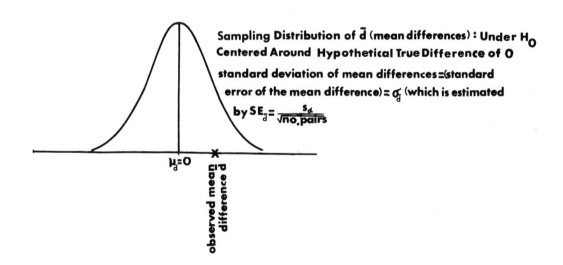

**Sampling Distribution of $\bar{d}$ (mean differences): Under H_0
Centered Around Hypothetical True Difference of 0**

standard deviation of mean differences = (standard
error of the mean difference) $= \sigma_{\bar{d}}$ (which is estimated

by $SE_{\bar{d}} = \dfrac{s_d}{\sqrt{\text{no. pairs}}}$

$\mu_d = 0$

observed mean
difference $\bar{d}$

The difference between mean finger and toe temperatures is, therefore, significant.

COMPARISON OF PAIRED DATA BY THE SIGN TEST

The *t*-test, you will recall, is based on the assumption that the population is normally distributed (i.e., that its parameters satisfy the criteria of a normal distribution). A test that is both "distribution-free" (non-para-

metric) and somewhat easier to compute is the *sign test*. The reasoning is as follows: If there is no true difference between the population of x values and the population of y values, we would expect as many pairs where the x values are higher than the y values (+ differences) as we would the reverse, i.e., x values lower than y values (− differences), and thus a distribution of x − y values symmetrically distributed around a true difference of 0. Therefore, for any pair of sample values

FIGURE 13-2

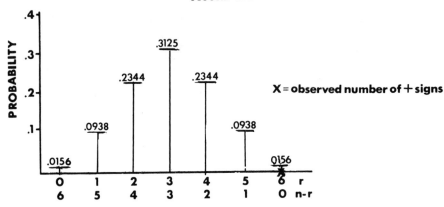

PROBABILITY (BINOMIAL) DISTRIBUTION
where p = 0.5, n = 6

there is a 50% chance that the difference has a + sign and a 50% chance it has a − sign. Hence, from the binomial formula

$$\frac{n!}{r!(n-r)!}\, p^r q^{n-r}$$

where p = .5 and q = .5, we can calculate the probability of obtaining a sample proportion with + (or −) sign as extreme or more extreme than that observed (Fig. 13-2). In

TABLE 13-3. *Sign Test for Temperatures on Same Individuals*

We use the binomial formula

$$\frac{n!}{r!(n-r)!}\, p^r q^{n-r}$$

where n = 6
    p = .5 (probability of a + sign)
    q = .5 (probability of a − sign)
    We note from Table 13-2 that all differences, d, have a + sign.

Let r = No. of observed + signs = 6
(n − r) = No. of observed − signs = 0

For a two-tailed test we want the P value associated with 6 + signs, or 0 + signs (both tails):

Prob (r = 6) + Prob (r = 0)

$$= \text{Prob }(6) = \frac{6!}{6!0!}\,(.5)^6(.5)^0 = (.5)^6 = \frac{1}{64}$$

and

$$\text{Prob }(0) = \frac{6!}{0!6!}\,(.5)^0(.5)^6 = (.5)^6 = \frac{1}{64}$$

$$\therefore P = \frac{2}{64} = .03$$

Since P < .05, the difference is significant.

this example, n = 6 and r, the number of + signs observed (finger temperature greater than toe temperature), is also 6. The calculations are shown in Table 13-3. P = .03, and therefore the difference is again significant. Note that, if there is a "tie" or zero difference between members of a pair, the pair is not counted when evaluating the result by the sign test.

If the assumption of normality is valid, however, the sign test will not be as *powerful* as the *t*-test in detecting a true difference between means. This is because the sign test considers the sign only and not the magnitude of the difference between pairs.[1] Therefore, if the population is normally distributed, for a test on the difference between means, the *t*-test is more likely than the sign test to lead to rejection of the null hypothesis when untrue.

Another limitation of the sign test is that the binomial with p = .5 cannot yield significant results for very small sample sizes. Therefore, for a two-tailed test at the .05 level, the number of non-tied pairs should be greater than 5. Countering this disadvantage is that if the number of pairs is very large, as with other binomial tests where (n × p) and (n × q) are equal to or larger than 5, the Normal

---

[1] Another non-parametric substitute for the *t*-test for paired samples is the Wilcoxon signed rank test. This test uses somewhat more information than the sign test since it is based on the relative sizes of the differences in addition to their signs.

Deviate test (with p = .5) can replace the sign test (see Problem 13-8).

REVIEW OF PRINCIPLES FOR TESTING PAIRED DATA

The physician must be able to distinguish readily between samples which are *independent*, such as temperatures of tuberculous men and of healthy men, and samples which are *not independent*, such as measurements on cases and matched controls or measurements on the same individual. If the samples are not independent, they may be positively correlated, i.e., both members of the pair tend to vary in the same direction with respect to a relevant characteristic such as temperature reading, reaction time, etc. This homogeneity of pairs reduces the variance estimate entering into the Standard Error formula. As a result, a difference may be found significant with smaller samples.

The *t*-test for independent sample means should not be used for paired means where there is a strong positive correlation between pairs with respect to the parameter being measured (as, in our example, when the temperature is high in the fingers it tends also to be high in the toes). Instead, the most appropriate test is a *t*-test which considers the sign and magnitude of the difference between each pair as the variate. The non-parametric sign test which considers only the sign of the difference may be used when the number of pairs (excluding those which are tied) is more than 5. Under conditions of normality, however, a result may be insignificant with the sign test but significant with the *t*-test.

We have considered thus far various significance tests on differences between means and proportions. We have left unanswered the important question of what true differences, other than the hypothetical difference of zero, the observed difference may be consistent with, and what true differences the observed difference is not consistent with.

If we make a significance test relative to all possible true values for the difference we would identify a range of values relative to which the observed difference is consistent at the probability level employed. The method for defining this *range, within which the true difference is likely to lie*, will be presented in Chapter 14. Similarly, we will indicate how to obtain such an interval estimate for the true mean (or true proportion).

PROBLEMS

Problem 13-1

Indicate whether each of the following sets of samples are (a) independent (b) not independent of each other and, therefore, whether the two sample means are likely to be uncorrelated or correlated.

(1) Weight gain of two random samples of children fed Formulas A and B respectively.

(2) A sample composed of one animal from each of 10 litters, and another sample composed of a second animal from each of the 10 litters, fed two experimental diets, respectively.

(3) The temperatures of samples of healthy men and of tuberculous men.

(4) Childhood rearing patterns in children from a psychiatric clinic and in children matched to same age, sex, and socioeconomic status chosen from the general population.

(5) Blood pressure measurements on a random sample of adult male patients with Disease A and on a sample of male siblings of these patients.

(6) Measurements on vital capacity of 25 emphysema patients before and after treatment.

Answer

(1) Independent.
(2) Not independent.
(3) Independent.
(4) Not independent (not as clear-cut as the others).
(5) Not independent.
(6) Not independent.

Problem 13-2

The coefficient of correlation (r) varies from −1 to +1. *True or False?*

Answer

True. r ranges from −1 (perfect negative linear correlation) to 0 (no correlation) to +1 (perfect positive correlation):

−1	0	+1

Range of r

Problem 13-3

If sample means are positively correlated, the Standard Error of the Difference will be smaller than if they are not correlated. *True or False?*

Answer

True. If sample means are positively correlated, r is some + value between 0 and +1. Therefore, the term $2r(SE_{\bar{x}})(SE_{\bar{y}})$ will be positive also. Because of the minus sign which precedes it in the S.E. formula, it will be subtracted from the variance term

$$SE_{\bar{x}-\bar{y}} = \sqrt{(SE_{\bar{x}})^2 + (SE_{\bar{y}})^2 - 2r(SE_{\bar{x}})(SE_{\bar{y}})}$$

As a result, the Standard Error of the Difference will be smaller than if the correlation coefficient r were 0.

This is the reason pairing is done in experiments when a positive correlation is expected. With a reduced Standard Error, the Critical Ratio will be larger. Therefore, a true difference is more likely to be found significant.

Problem 13-4

Given the following information:

No. of pairs: 100
Mean difference before and after treatment $(\bar{d}) = 30$ mm Hg
Standard Deviation of Differences $(s_d) = 100$ mm Hg

is there a significant mean paired difference before and after treatment?

Answer

The *t*-test for paired data is:

$$\text{Obs. } t = \frac{\bar{d} - 0}{SE_{\bar{d}}}$$

We determine Est. $SE_{\bar{d}}$ from

$$\frac{s_d}{\sqrt{\text{No. of pairs}}} = \frac{100}{\sqrt{100}} = 10 \text{ mm Hg}$$

$$\text{Obs. } t = \frac{30 - 0}{10} = 3$$

$$df = \text{No. of pairs} - 1 = 99$$

$$t_{.05,99df} = 1.96 \text{ (equivalent to z)}$$

Since the observed *t* value (3) is greater than the critical *t* (1.96), the difference is significant.

Problem 13-5

A non-parametric test makes no assumption about the type of distribution from which the data were taken. *True or False?*

Answer

True. A non-parametric test, such as the sign test, does not require that the parent population be normally distributed (this *is* a requirement of the *t*-test).

Problem 13-6

Measurements on the transverse diameter of an organ (in centimeters) were made on 5 animals before and after a therapeutic procedure.

Individual no.	After Rx	Before Rx
	x_2	x_1
1	17.0	16.2
2	14.7	14.5
3	9.5	9.7
4	13.2	13.1
5	14.7	14.6
Total (Σx)	69.1 cm	68.1 cm
Mean ($\bar{x}$)	13.82 cm	13.62 cm

Is there a significant difference in mean diameter before and after therapy?

Answer

Note that we are dealing with a series of two measurements on the *same* individuals. Therefore, the sample means are *not independent* of each other but may be correlated. The appropriate test for comparing the two means, therefore, is the *t*-test for paired data. This test is carried out below.

Individual	x_2 After	x_1 Before	$x_2 - x_1$ d	$(d - \bar{d})$	$(d - \bar{d})^2$
1	17.0	16.2	.8	.6	.36
2	14.7	14.5	.2	0	0
3	9.5	9.7	−.2	−.4	.16
4	13.2	13.1	.1	−.1	.01
5	14.7	14.6	.1	−.1	.01
Total	69.1	68.1	1.0	0	.54
Mean	13.82	13.62	$\bar{d} = .20$	Check	

We check our calculations as we proceed:

(a) The sum of the differences, $(\Sigma d = 1.0)$, is equal to the difference between the totals of the two samples $(69.1 - 68.1)$.

(b) The mean difference $\bar{d} = .20$ cm is equal to the difference between the means:

$$(\bar{x}_1 - \bar{x}_2) = (13.82 - 13.62)$$

(c) The sum of the deviations of the differences from the mean difference, $\Sigma(d - \bar{d})$, is equal to 0 as expected.

Sample Variance of Differences:

$$s_{\bar{d}}^2 = \frac{\Sigma(d - \bar{d})^2}{\text{No. of pairs} - 1} = \frac{.54}{4} = .135$$

Sample S.D. of Differences:

$$s_d = \sqrt{\frac{\Sigma(d - \bar{d})^2}{\text{No. of pairs} - 1}} = \sqrt{.135}$$
$$= .367 \text{ cm}$$

$$\text{Est. SE}_{\bar{d}} = \frac{s_d}{\sqrt{\text{No. of pairs}}} = \frac{.367}{\sqrt{5}} = .16$$

$$\text{df} = \text{No. of pairs} - 1 = 4$$

$$\text{Obs. } t_{4\text{df}} = \frac{\bar{d} - 0}{\text{SE}_{\bar{d}}} = \frac{.20}{.16} = 1.25$$

$$t_{.05,4\text{df}} = 2.78$$

$\therefore$ Difference is not significant. The null hypothesis is not rejected, since it could have given rise to the observed difference (or one more extreme) with a probability in excess of 5%.

The observed difference of 0.2 cm is not statistically significant nor is it likely to be clinically significant. That observed difference, however, may be consistent with a larger true difference, which could have clinical implication. The subject of setting limits on the true value of a parameter, rather than just testing a specific hypothetical value, will be taken up in Chapter 14.

Note that, since there are only five pairs, the sign test cannot be used. The sign test requires 6 or more pairs for the 0.05 level of significance using a two-tailed test.

Problem 13-7

In a comparison of 6 pairs of observations on the same individuals, 5 of the differences have a + sign and 1 has a − sign.

(a) Test for a significant difference between the means by the sign test.

(b) Can you conclude that the *t*-test also would give a non-significant result?

Answer

(a) We use the binomial formula for the sign test

$$\frac{n!}{r!(n-r)!} \, p^r q^{n-r}$$

where $n = 6$, $p = \frac{1}{2}$, $q = \frac{1}{2}$. We sum the probabilities of $r = 5$, $r = 6$ (outcomes as extreme or more extreme) and the probabilities of outcomes in the other direction or tail, i.e., $r = 1$, $r = 0$:

$$\text{Prob } (r = 5) = \frac{6!}{5!1!} \left(\frac{1}{2}\right)^5 \left(\frac{1}{2}\right)^1$$
$$= 6 \left(\frac{1}{2}\right)^6 = \frac{6}{64}$$
$$\text{Prob } (r = 6) = \frac{6!}{6!0!} \left(\frac{1}{2}\right)^6 \left(\frac{1}{2}\right)^0$$
$$= \left(\frac{1}{2}\right)^6 = \frac{1}{64}$$

$$\text{Sum} = \frac{7}{64}$$

Since $p = \frac{1}{2}$, the binomial distribution of chance outcomes is symmetrical. Therefore, the sum of Prob $(r = 1)$ + Prob $(r = 0)$ will also be 7/64.

$$\frac{7}{64} + \frac{7}{64} = \frac{14}{64} = .22 = P$$
$$P = .22 > .05$$

According to the sign test, therefore, the difference is *not* significant.

(b) *No.* The sign test considers only the direction of the difference and not the magnitude of the differences. Under conditions of normality it is possible that the sign test can give non-significant results although the *t*-test for paired data (which does take into account the magnitude of the differences) gives significant results. Therefore, if the sign test is not significant, it is advisable to then carry out the paired *t*-test.

Problem 13-8

Abramson et al. (Blood Flow in Extremities Affected by Anterior Poliomyelitis, Arch. Intern. Med. 71:391–402, 1943) report the following data on blood flow in 22 individuals who had had anterior poliomyelitis with unilateral involvement of an extremity:

(cc/min/100 cc of limb volume)

Individual	Normal limb	Affected limb
1	3.0	3.0
2	4.1	4.6
3	5.1	3.8
4	5.1	6.2
5	3.6	3.6
6	3.9	4.8
7	1.7	2.4
8	2.3	1.9
9	1.9	1.2
10	3.0	2.5
11	3.2	2.6
12	3.7	1.3
13	2.0	1.6
14	2.4	3.4
15	1.7	1.3
16	1.2	0.8
17	2.9	1.4
18	3.6	2.7
19	3.7	0.9
20	4.0	2.0
21	1.3	0.7
22	7.0	2.2

(a) Determine whether there is a significant difference in the average blood flow of the two limbs.

(b) Is it possible to come to any conclusion concerning the difference in the average blood flow by merely noting the consistency with which the normal limb has the higher flow?

Answer

(a) Table 13-4 is the work table to calculate $\bar{d}$ and s_d.

TABLE 13-4

Individual	Normal limb, x_1	Affected limb, x_2	Difference (d), $x_1 - x_2$	$(d - \bar{d})$	$(d - \bar{d})^2$
1	3.0	3.0	0 (tie)	−0.7	0.49
2	4.1	4.6	−0.5	−1.2	1.44
3	5.1	3.8	+1.3	+0.6	0.36
4	5.1	6.2	−1.1	−1.8	3.24
.5	3.6	3.6	0 (tie)	−0.7	0.49
6	3.9	4.8	−0.9	−1.6	2.56
7	1.7	2.4	−0.7	−1.4	1.96
8	2.3	1.9	+0.4	−0.3	0.09
9	1.9	1.2	+0.7	0	0
10	3.0	2.5	+0.5	−0.2	0.04
11	3.2	2.6	+0.6	−0.1	0.01
12	3.7	1.3	+2.4	+1.7	2.89
13	2.0	1.6	+0.4	−0.3	0.09
14	2.4	3.4	−1.0	−1.7	2.89
15	1.7	1.3	+0.4	−0.3	0.09
16	1.2	0.8	+0.4	−0.3	0.09
17	2.9	1.4	+1.5	+0.8	0.64

TABLE 13-4 (Cont.)

Individual	Normal limb, x_1	Affected limb, x_2	Difference (d), $x_1 - x_2$	$(d - \bar{d})$	$(d - \bar{d})^2$
18	3.6	2.7	+0.9	+0.2	0.04
19	3.7	0.9	+2.8	+2.1	4.41
20	4.0	2.0	+2.0	+1.3	1.69
21	1.3	0.7	+0.6	−0.1	0.01
22	7.0	2.2	+4.8	+4.1	16.81
Total	70.4	54.9	+15.5	~0	40.33
Mean	3.2	2.5	+ 0.7		

$$s_d = \sqrt{\frac{\Sigma(d - \bar{d})^2}{\text{No. of pairs} - 1}} = \sqrt{\frac{40.33}{21}}$$
$$= 1.39$$

$$SE_{\bar{d}} = \frac{s_d}{\sqrt{\text{No. of pairs}}} = \frac{1.39}{\sqrt{22}} = .30$$

$$\text{Obs. } t = \frac{\bar{d} - 0}{SE_{\bar{d}}} = \frac{.70}{.30} = 2.33$$

$$\text{df} = \text{No. of pairs} - 1 = 21$$

Critical $t_{.05, 21df} = 2.08 \qquad 2.33 > 2.08$

Therefore, difference is significant.

(b) To answer the second question we can simply apply the sign test, which uses the binomial formula:

$$\frac{n!}{r!(n - r)!} p^r q^{n-r}$$

where $p = .5$, $q = .5$. Note that n is only 20 instead of 22 pairs since we must exclude the two ties (or two zero differences).

Let r, the observed outcome, be 15 + signs. The probability of this occurrence or one less likely for a two-tailed test, is:

$$P = \left[\frac{20!}{15!5!}(.5)^{15}(.5)^5 + \cdots \right.$$
$$\left. \frac{20!}{20!0!}(.5)^{20}(.5)^0\right]$$
$$+ \left[\frac{20}{5!15!}(.5)^5(.5)^{15} + \cdots \right.$$
$$\left. \frac{20!}{0!20!}(.5)^0(.5)^{20}\right]$$
$$\text{Sum} = .042 < .05$$

$\therefore$ Difference is significant.

The number of untied pairs is fairly large (20). Also $(n \times p) = (20 \times .5) = 10$, which is larger than 5. Therefore, we can use the normal approximation to the binomial distribution, i.e., the Normal Deviate test:

$$z = \frac{\hat{p} - p}{SE_{\hat{p}}}$$

where

$$SE_{\hat{p}} = \sqrt{\frac{pq}{n}} = \sqrt{\frac{(.5)(.5)}{20}} = .11$$

We observe

$$\hat{p} = \frac{15}{20} = .75 = \text{sample proportion of } + \text{ signs}$$

$$\therefore z = \frac{.75 - .50}{.11} = 2.2$$

Since this z value is larger than 1.96, the difference is significant at the .05 level.

For n of ≥ 10 untied pairs, we can also use McNemar's test[1]:

$$\chi^2_{1df} = \frac{(\text{No. of positive pairs} - \text{No. of negative pairs})^2}{(\text{No. of positive pairs}) + (\text{No. of negative pairs})}$$

$$= \frac{(15-5)^2}{15+5} = 5.0 > 3.84 \text{ for } \chi^2_{.05}$$

Note: $\chi^2_{1df} = z^2$ or $5.0 \sim (2.2)^2$; the results are the same as the z test.

In this illustration, since the sign test (or its approximation) is significant, it is not necessary to do a *t*-test for paired data (contrast this with Problem 13-7).

SUMMARY OF CHAPTER 13

Paired data

—are not independent but are usually positively correlated. If they are positively correlated, the Standard Error of the Difference

$$SE_{\bar{x}_1 - \bar{x}_2}$$

is reduced by a term involving r, the correlation coefficient.

The t-test (for paired data)

This is simplified by working with the *difference* (d) between pairs. Thus:
  —the mean difference $= \bar{d} = \Sigma d / \text{No. of pairs}$.
  —the Standard Deviation of Differences $=$

$$s_d = \sqrt{\frac{\Sigma(d - \bar{d})^2}{\text{No. of pairs} - 1}}$$

  —the estimated Standard Error of the Difference $=$

$$\text{Est. SE}_{\bar{d}} = \frac{s_d}{\sqrt{\text{No. of pairs}}}$$

  —the *t*-test is then

$$t = \frac{\bar{d} - 0}{\text{Est. SE}_{\bar{d}}}$$

The sign test

  —is a nonparametric test.
  —is a quicker but less powerful test than the paired *t*-test when the data are normally distributed.
  —can be used when the number of untied pairs is 6 or more.
  —assumes p $= .5$ and evaluates the number of $+$ and $-$ sign differences by:

  The Binomial formula—if n is small
  The Normal Deviate approximation—if n is large

---

[1] In this test, to correct χ^2 for continuity, we subtract 1 from the numerator before squaring, i.e.:

$$\chi^2_c = \frac{(|15 - 5| - 1)^2}{15 + 5} = 4.05 > 3.84$$

CUMULATIVE GLOSSARY I: TERMS

Chapter 13

Paired Data

A set of observations where for each x value there is a corresponding (or matched) y value.

Covariance

For each x, y pair of data, the x deviation from the mean of all x's (i.e., $x - \bar{x}$) is multiplied by the y deviation from the mean of all y's (i.e., $y - \bar{y}$). These products are then summed for all pairs. Thus,

$$\text{The covariance of a sample} = \frac{\Sigma(x - \bar{x})(y - \bar{y})}{n - 1}$$

[Contrast this with the <u>variance</u> term for x (or y):

$$\frac{\Sigma(x - \bar{x})^2}{n - 1} \quad \text{or} \quad \frac{\Sigma(y - \bar{y})^2}{n - 1}\bigg]$$

Correlation Coefficient

A number, r, which indicates the strength of association (degree of *linear* relationship) between two variables. r varies between -1 (perfect negative correlation) and $+1$ (perfect positive correlation). See r in Glossary II: Symbols.

t-Test for Paired Data (Difference Method)

A *t*-test which treats the *difference*, d, between a pair of data (i.e., $x - y$) as the variable.

Non-Parametric Test

A test which makes no assumptions regarding the parameters of a distribution (distribution-free test), e.g., the sign test.

Sign Test

A non-parametric test based on the number of positive and negative differences between pairs. Under the null hypothesis, the number of $+$ and $-$ signs should be binomially distributed with $p = .5$.

McNemar's Test

A test for non-independent (correlated) proportions.

CUMULATIVE GLOSSARY II: SYMBOLS

Chapter 13

r

Correlation coefficient (also called Pearson's r or product moment coefficient)

$$= \frac{\Sigma(x - \bar{x})(y - \bar{y})/(n - 1)}{\sqrt{\Sigma(x - \bar{x})^2 \Sigma(y - \bar{y})^2}/(n - 1)}$$

$$= \frac{\text{Covariance of x and y}}{(\text{Standard Deviation of x})(\text{Standard Deviation of y})}$$

Note that r is the *sample* correlation coefficient which estimates ρ (rho), the *population* correlation coefficient.

d

Difference between each pair of data $(x - y)$.

μ_d

True mean of the population of differences between pairs:

$$\mu_d = \mu_x - \mu_y$$

$\bar{d}$

Mean of the sample of differences between pairs (sample mean difference)(estimate of μ_d):

$$\bar{d} = \bar{x} - \bar{y}$$

s_d^2

Variance of the sample of differences between pairs (estimate of σ_d^2):

$$s_d^2 = \frac{\Sigma(d - \bar{d})^2}{\text{No. of pairs} - 1}$$

s_d

Standard deviation of the sample of differences between pairs (estimate of σ_d):

$$s_d = \sqrt{\frac{\Sigma(d - \bar{d})^2}{\text{No. of pairs} - 1}}$$

Est. $SE_{\bar{d}}$

Estimated standard error of the mean difference between pairs (estimate of $\sigma_{\bar{d}}$):

$$\text{Est. } SE_{\bar{d}} = \frac{s_d}{\sqrt{\text{No. of pairs}}}$$

CUMULATIVE REVIEW IV
(Chapters 9–13)

SIGNIFICANCE TESTS FOR CONTINUOUS DATA

Population Variance (σ^2) Known   *Population Variance (σ^2) Not Known*

I. To compare *ONE* sample mean with an *EXPECTED* mean

$$z = \frac{\bar{x} - \mu}{SE_{\bar{x}}} = \frac{\bar{x} - \mu}{\sigma/\sqrt{n}}$$

Use normal distribution.

$$t = \frac{\bar{x} - \mu}{\text{Est. } SE_{\bar{x}}} = \frac{\bar{x} - \mu}{s/\sqrt{n}}$$

Since s is obtained from the sample, use *t* distribution, with $n - 1$ df.

II. To compare *TWO* sample means with *EACH OTHER FOR INDEPENDENT SAMPLES*

$$z = \frac{(\bar{x}_1 - \bar{x}_2) - 0}{SE_{\bar{x}_1 - \bar{x}_2}}$$

$$= \frac{(\bar{x}_1 - \bar{x}_2) - 0}{\sqrt{\sigma^2 \left(\frac{1}{n_1} + \frac{1}{n_2}\right)}}$$

$$= \frac{(\bar{x}_1 - \bar{x}_2) - 0}{\sqrt{\frac{\sigma^2}{n_1} + \frac{\sigma^2}{n_2}}}$$

Use normal distribution.

$$t = \frac{(\bar{x}_1 - \bar{x}_2) - 0}{\text{Est. } SE_{\bar{x}_1 - \bar{x}_2}}$$

$$= \frac{(\bar{x}_1 - \bar{x}_2) - 0}{\sqrt{s_p^2 \left(\frac{1}{n_1} + \frac{1}{n_2}\right)}} = \frac{(\bar{x}_1 - \bar{x}_2) - 0}{\sqrt{\frac{s_p^2}{n_1} + \frac{s_p^2}{n_2}}}$$

where s_p^2 represents the weighted (pooled) variance of the two sample variances computed as:

$$s_p^2 = \frac{(n_1 - 1)s_1^2 + (n_2 - 1)s_2^2}{(n_1 - 1) + (n_2 - 1)}$$

Note: If $n_1 = n_2$, then Est. $SE_{\bar{x}_1 - \bar{x}_2}$ is simplified to

$$\sqrt{(\text{Est. } SE_{\bar{x}_1})^2 + (\text{Est. } SE_{\bar{x}_2})^2}$$

Since s_p^2 is obtained from the samples, use t distribution with $n_1 + n_2 - 2$ df.

III. To compare *TWO* sample means with *EACH OTHER FOR PAIRED SAMPLES*

$$z = \frac{\bar{d} - 0}{SE_{\bar{d}}}$$

$$= \frac{\bar{d} - 0}{\sigma_d / \sqrt{\text{No. of pairs}}}$$

Use normal distribution.

$$t = \frac{\bar{d} - 0}{\text{Est. } SE_{\bar{d}}}$$

$$= \frac{\bar{d} - 0}{s_d / \sqrt{\text{No. of pairs}}}$$

Since s_d^2 is obtained from the samples, use t distribution with (number of pairs $- 1$) df.

14
Confidence Intervals for True Parameters

General Theory and Method for Interval Estimation •
Confidence Interval on a True Proportion (Qualitative Data) •
Confidence Interval on a True Mean (Quantitative Data) •
Confidence Interval on a True Difference Between Two Proportions
(Qualitative Data) •
Confidence Interval on a True Difference Between Two Independent
Means (Quantitative Data) •
Confidence Interval on a True Difference Between Paired Means
(Quantitative Data) •
Summary of Principles on Confidence Interval Estimation

We have been concerned with the question: Could this sample have come from a population with a certain true mean, the sample mean differing from the true mean only by chance? To answer this question, the null hypothesis

$$H_0: \ \mu = \mu_0$$

was assumed and tested. If the Null Hypothesis is rejected, we may then ask: What is the *true* μ of the population likely to be?

We have been concerned also with the question: Do these <u>two</u> samples come from populations with the same mean? In this case, H_0 was $\mu_1 = \mu_2$ (or $\mu_1 - \mu_2 = 0$). If the hypothesis of a zero difference is rejected, again the next question posed is: What may the true difference be between μ_1 and μ_2? Thus, after we find that a significant difference exists, we should like to know within what bounds the *true* difference might lie.

In general, therefore, after we perform a test of significance and reject the Null Hypothesis that a sample mean is really the same

as an expected mean or that the true difference is zero, we then wish to *estimate a confidence interval* for the true value. However, it is also possible to estimate confidence intervals for a population parameter without first conducting a test of significance. In this case, the interval itself is used to perform a significance test.

In considering the general problem of estimation one must remember that in an actual situation the experimenter rarely knows the parameters of a population. A sample statistic (mean, difference between means, etc.) which is an estimate of the underlying population or true parameter is observed. Because of chance, this "point" estimate probably differs from the population value. Therefore, the investigator needs to (a) estimate an "interval" which is likely to include the population parameter and (b) state the degree of confidence associated with this interval. This is comparable to estimating which of all possible population means or μ's (see Fig. 14-1) are likely to have

FIG. 14-1. Distributions of sample means from populations with different μ's.

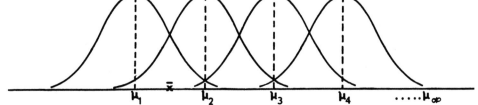

given rise to the observed $\bar{x}$. It is possible that $\bar{x}$ came from a population with μ_1, but could it not have come also from a population with μ_2?

The sample provides a point estimate that is the most likely value. The interval estimate includes all possible values for the parameter which are consistent with the data at the specified probability level.

As stated above, while interval estimation is often a sequel to a test of significance in which the Null Hypothesis is rejected, it in itself provides a significance test. For example, if a test of significance between two means at the .05 level is applied [H_0: $\mu_1 - \mu_2 = 0$] and if the observed t is greater than the $t_{.05}$ value, a zero difference is rejected as the likely true value. In such a case generally the 95% confidence interval on the true difference also will <u>not</u> include zero. Thus it is "like a significance test." Researchers may prefer confidence interval estimation to a significance test because essentially it provides significant tests relevant for many null hypotheses rather than for a single Null Hypothesis.

GENERAL THEORY AND METHOD FOR INTERVAL ESTIMATION

We know from the normal distribution of sample means around a true mean, expressed by the variate

$$z = \frac{\bar{x} - \mu}{\sigma/\sqrt{n}} \left(\text{or } \frac{\bar{x} - \mu}{SE_{\bar{x}}} \right)$$

that 95 out of 100 sample means will fall within an interval of 1.96 S.E. units on either side of the population mean. This probability can be indicated symbolically as:

$$P \left(-1.96 \le \frac{\bar{x} - \mu}{SE_{\bar{x}}} \le 1.96 \right) = .95$$

(See also Fig. 14-2.)

It can be shown that this statement is mathematically equivalent to the statement:

$$P(\bar{x} - 1.96 \ SE_{\bar{x}} \le \mu \le \bar{x} + 1.96 \ SE_{\bar{x}})$$

In other words, in repeated samples, the *probability* that the *random interval*

$$\left[\left(\begin{matrix} \bar{x} - 1.96 \ SE_{\bar{x}} \\ \uparrow \end{matrix} \right) \quad \text{and} \quad \left(\begin{matrix} \bar{x} + 1.96 \ SE_{\bar{x}} \\ \uparrow \end{matrix} \right) \right]$$

$$\begin{matrix} \textit{lower} \\ \textit{confidence} \\ \textit{limit} \end{matrix} \qquad\qquad \begin{matrix} \textit{upper} \\ \textit{confidence} \\ \textit{limit} \end{matrix}$$

will contain μ is .95. We can define these limits, therefore, as the sample mean <u>minus</u> 1.96 times the Standard Error of the Mean and the sample mean <u>plus</u> 1.96 times the Standard Error of the Mean.

With this general introduction, let us point out some important principles in confidence interval estimation:

(1) First, observe that the confidence interval is symmetrical because the interval is constructed by assuming that the observed sample mean ($\bar{x}$) is at the interval center, to which is <u>added</u> and <u>subtracted</u> the Standard Error of the Mean (multiplied by a factor).

(2) In the above example, the factor is 1.96, which represents the $z_{.05}$ value in the normal curve (for the 95% confidence interval). But if s^2 is used as an estimate of σ^2 in the Standard Error formula, and if n is 30 or less, then we must replace $z_{.05} = 1.96$, with $t_{.05}$ (for the appropriate degrees of freedom). And since $t_{.05}$ will be *larger* than $z_{.05}$ for a small n, the confidence interval may be *wider*.

(3) If we wish to be 99% instead of 95% sure of including the true mean, we construct a 99% confidence interval by using $z_{.01} = 2.58$ or $t_{.01}$ (df) (instead of $z_{.05} = 1.96$ or $t_{.05}$). Therefore the 99% confidence interval must be *wider* than the 95% (the penalty for being more certain). The comparison in width is ($2 \times \underline{2.58}$

FIGURE 14-2

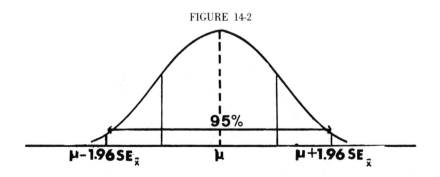

× S.E.) versus (2 × 1.96 × S.E.). Note the 2, since the term is both added and subtracted to the sample outcome.

(4) The width of the confidence interval is determined not only by the size of the factor as described in (2) and (3) above, but also by the size of the Standard Error. The S.E. can be decreased by increasing n, the size of the sample or experiment.

(5) In general, then, the confidence interval on any true (population) parameter can be constructed from the

> Sample value or statistic
> ± [(factor) × (Standard Error of the Statistic)]

where the factor is determined by (a) the level of confidence (i.e., 95% or 99%) we wish to achieve in including the true parameter within the interval and (b) the appropriate sampling statistic (i.e., z or t).

(6) Note that it is incorrect to state that "the probability that the population mean will vary between the two limits is .95." The reason is that the population parameter (i.e., μ) is fixed and not random; μ is either in the interval or not. Rather it is the interval (around the variable x̄) that is random. Other correct interpretations are: "This procedure will, in 95 out of 100 times, provide an interval which includes μ," or "The procedure which leads me to state that μ lies between the two numbers will result in my making 95 correct statements out of 100, on the average."

CONFIDENCE INTERVAL ON A TRUE PROPORTION (QUALITATIVE DATA)

Let us return to the example of the sex difference in cancer deaths of children under 1 year of age (Chapter 4) to illustrate the application of this method. The 1795 deaths were distributed as follows: 987 (55%) male and 808 (45%) female. Our question was: does the 55% of male cancer deaths differ significantly from the percent of male infants in the population (51%)? Using the z (Standard normal deviate) test, the Null Hypothesis was rejected at the P = .001 level:

$$z = \frac{\bar{x} - \mu}{\sigma/\sqrt{n}}$$

or

$$\frac{\hat{p} - p}{SE_{\hat{p}} \text{ or } \sqrt{\frac{pq}{n}}} = \frac{.55 - .51}{\sqrt{\frac{(.51)(.49)}{1795}}} = \frac{.04}{.012}$$

$$z = 3.4, P < .001$$

Difference is significant.

Therefore the true proportion of cancer deaths that are male is probably not .51 (the proportion of male infants in the population), i.e., the data suggest a sex difference in cancer risk. But just how much greater is the excess risk for males? Or, stated in another fashion, what is the true proportion of male cancer deaths under 1 year of age likely to be? It can be .55 (the sample proportion). But might it not be .54 or .56 with the observed .55 arising just by sampling variation?

To answer this question, we set up a 95% confidence interval on the true proportion, following the above general form:

$$\text{Obs. sample proportion} \pm z_{.05} (SE_{\hat{p}})$$

where *ideally*

$$SE_{\hat{p}} = \sqrt{\frac{pq}{n}}$$

Remember, however, that the true proportion p is not known (the expected p = .51 was rejected). Therefore the sample proportion $\hat{p}$ (.55) is used as its best estimate in the S.E. formula for determining confidence limits (C.L.):

$$\therefore 95\% \text{ C.L. on p} = \hat{p} \pm 1.96 \sqrt{\frac{\hat{p}\hat{q}}{n}}$$
$$\uparrow$$

[factor determined by level of confidence (e.g., 95%) for the normal distribution]

$$= .55 \pm 1.96 \sqrt{\frac{(.55)(.45)}{1795}}$$
$$= .55 \pm 1.96 (.012) = .55 \pm .0235$$

$$95\% \text{ C.L.} = \underset{\substack{lower \\ limit}}{.526} \qquad \underset{\substack{upper \\ limit}}{.574}$$

From the 95% C.L., we see that the true proportion of cancer deaths that are male is likely to be anywhere from .526 to .574. These limits do not include .51, the expected proportion under the Null Hypothesis, rejected by the z test. Thus the result agrees with the significance test.

Where samples are of small size, especially where (n × p) or (n × q) is <5, binomial confidence limits should be used (see Fig. 14-3).

FIG. 14-3. 95 percent confidence interval for the Binomial distribution. (Adapted with permission from Court, *Psychological Statistics: An Introduction*, Homewood, Ill., The Dorsey Press.) Shows graphically the 95% confidence interval for p computed from the binomial distribution for various observed proportions. To use this graph for estimating a confidence interval, locate along the base line the observed p̂ or $(1 - \hat{p})$, whichever is smaller. The limits of the 95 percent confidence interval are then obtained from the vertical scale for the points at which the ordinate above p̂ crosses the two curves corresponding to n. If $1 - \hat{p}$ is used, the confidence limits must be subtracted from 1.00.

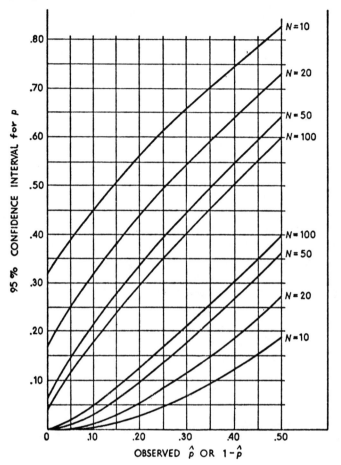

CONFIDENCE INTERVAL ON A TRUE MEAN (QUANTITATIVE DATA)

The confidence interval on the true mean (μ) for quantitative data is calculated in a manner analogous to p for qualitative data. However, quantitative data usually have two parameters, the mean (μ) and the variance (σ^2). If as the result of a significance test a hypothetical mean is rejected as the true mean of the population from which the sample was taken, this does <u>not</u> influence the estimate of the variance of the population. Therefore the Standard Error formula is the same for a significance test as for confidence interval estimation. The confidence interval on a true mean is:

Obs. sample mean ($\bar{x}$)

$\pm$ z (Standard Error of the Mean, $SE_{\bar{x}}$) or

t (Est. $SE_{\bar{x}}$)

Thus, 95% C.L. on

$$\mu = \bar{x} \pm z_{.05}\left(\frac{\sigma}{\sqrt{n}}\right) \quad \text{or} \quad t_{.05}\left(\frac{s}{\sqrt{n}}\right)$$

Note that (a) it is usually necessary to use s^2 (the sample variance) as an estimate of σ^2 (the population variance) and (b) therefore, as stated before, t must be used instead of z.

A modification of the normal approach above so as to take into account the fact that the Standard Error of the observed proportion depends on the true proportion will give limits closely similar to the binomial confidence limits, and these limits will, in general, not be symmetrical about the observed proportion.

For samples larger than 30, however, the t values are similar to z.

As an example, suppose we wish to compare the mean of mouth temperatures of a sample of 5 male patients (let us say that the sample mean $\bar{x} = 100.2°$ and the sample standard deviation $s = .47°$) with an expected mean of $98.42°$ for the population (in Table 9-3) of healthy young men and the population S.D. is unknown. The t test is

$$\frac{\bar{x} - \mu}{s/\sqrt{n}} = \frac{100.2° - 98.42°}{.47°/\sqrt{5}} = \frac{1.78°}{.21°}$$

Obs. $t_{4df} = 8.5$, $P < .001$

Difference is significant. Therefore, $98.42°$ is rejected as the mean of the population of patients from which the sample was taken. We want now to make an interval estimate for the true population mean, μ. Suppose we wish to be 99% sure that the estimated interval will include the true mean (μ). The 99% C.L. on μ are:

Obs. sample mean ($\bar{x}$)

$$\pm\ t_{.01,4df} \ (\text{Est. } SE_{\bar{x}} = s/\sqrt{n})$$

for 99% C.L.

$$= 100.2° \pm 4.6 \ (.21°)$$
$$= 100.2° \pm (0.97°)$$
$$= 99.23° \qquad 101.17°$$

lower limit   *upper limit*

These confidence limits on the true μ may be considered too wide for practical use. If a narrower confidence interval is desired, it may be possible to achieve this in either of two ways: (1) by accepting a lower confidence level (95%), thus *decreasing* the size of the factor by which the standard error is multiplied ($t_{.05,4df} = 2.78$ instead of $t_{.01,4df} = 4.6$), or (2) by *increasing* the sample size, n. This reduces the estimated $SE_{\bar{x}}$ (from the formula $s/\sqrt{n}$). It also reduces the critical t value by increasing the degrees of freedom with which the variance is estimated.

CONFIDENCE INTERVAL ON A TRUE DIFFERENCE BETWEEN TWO PROPORTIONS (QUALITATIVE DATA)

We turn now to the estimation of the true <u>difference</u> between groups. Let us use the sulfanilamide problem from earlier chapters. Recall that the z test (Normal deviate test) for a difference in percentage or proportion

of deaths under two treatment regimens was as follows, where p' represents the overall (common) estimate of p:

$$z = \frac{(\hat{p}_1 - \hat{p}_2) - 0}{SE_{\hat{p}_1-\hat{p}_2}} = \frac{(.733 - .900) - 0}{\sqrt{\dfrac{p'q'}{n_1} + \dfrac{p'q'}{n_2}}}$$

$$= \frac{-.167}{\sqrt{\dfrac{(.855)(.145)}{60} + \dfrac{(.855)(.145)}{160}}}$$

$$z = \frac{-.167}{.053} = -3.1, \ P \sim .0019$$

The difference is significant; the null hypothesis is rejected.

Suppose we now wish to obtain 95% confidence limits on the true difference between population proportions p_1 and p_2. Our formula for the 95% C.L. is then:

Obs. difference $(\hat{p}_1 - \hat{p}_2) \pm z_{.05} \ (SE_{\hat{p}_1-\hat{p}_2})$

where

$$SE_{\hat{p}_1-\hat{p}_2} = \sqrt{\frac{p_1 q_1}{n_1} + \frac{p_2 q_2}{n_2}}$$

However, as with the interval estimation for a single true proportion, these true proportions p_1 and p_2 are not known. Therefore, the Standard Error formula uses the *observed sample* $\hat{p}_1$ *and* $\hat{p}_2$ *values* as best estimates of the true proportions p_1 and p_2:

$$\therefore\ 95\% \ \text{C.L.} = (\hat{p}_1 - \hat{p}_2) \pm 1.96 \ \sqrt{\frac{\hat{p}_1 \hat{q}_1}{n_1} + \frac{\hat{p}_2 \hat{q}_2}{n_2}}$$

Note that since the Null Hypothesis has been rejected the implicit assumption is that $p_1 \neq p_2$; therefore, an overall proportion p' is <u>not</u> used in the S.E. formula for the confidence interval on the true difference[1]:

Our results are:

$(.733 - .900)$

$$\pm 1.96 \ \sqrt{\frac{(.733)(.267)}{60} + \frac{(.900)(.100)}{160}}$$

$$= -.167 \pm 1.96 \ (.030)$$
$$= -.167 \pm .059$$
$$= -.226 \qquad -.108$$

lower limit   *upper limit*

$$\frac{|\leftarrow 95\% \ \text{C.I.} \rightarrow|}{-.226 \qquad\qquad -.108 \qquad\qquad 0}$$

---

[1] Note that this is only an approximate procedure for setting limits on the true difference between proportions. Exact procedures exist relative to differences between a particular transform of such proportions, specifically log (p/q), but this subject will not be treated here.

The above 95% confidence interval on the true difference includes only negative values. In accord with the significance test, *zero* is not a likely true difference.

CONFIDENCE INTERVAL ON A TRUE DIFFERENCE BETWEEN TWO INDEPENDENT MEANS (QUANTITATIVE DATA)

To illustrate confidence interval estimation for a difference between two independent quantitative means, let us use data on the temperatures of two samples of men: healthy individuals and tuberculous cases. The data are summarized in Table 14-1. Note that both

TABLE 14-1. *Data on Temperatures of Healthy and Tuberculous Men*

	Healthy Men	Tuberculous Men
Sample size (n)	25	25
Sample mean ($\bar{x}$)	98.4°	99.3°
Standard deviation of individuals (s)	0.5°	1.2°
Est. Standard Error of Mean $\left(\text{Est. SE}_{\bar{x}} = \dfrac{s}{\sqrt{n}}\right)$	$\dfrac{0.5°}{\sqrt{25}} = .10°$	$\dfrac{1.2°}{\sqrt{25}} = .24°$

the sample mean and sample S.D. values are larger for tuberculous men than for healthy men. A graph of these data would look like Fig. 14-4.

An assumption of equal population variances is required for the *t*-test. However, the validity of the *t*-test is not seriously impaired where the population variances are only slightly dis-

similar or where the sample sizes are fairly large and equal. Therefore, we shall proceed with the *t*-test without testing for homogeneity of variances (F-test).[1] Is the difference between means significant? Since $n_1 = n_2$, our estimated $\text{SE}_{\bar{x}_1 - \bar{x}_2}$ formula is simple:

$$\begin{aligned} t &= \frac{(\bar{x}_1 - \bar{x}_2) - 0}{\text{Est. SE}_{\bar{x}_1 - \bar{x}_2}} \\ &= \frac{(\bar{x}_1 - \bar{x}_2) - 0}{\sqrt{(\text{Est. SE}_{\bar{x}_1})^2 + (\text{Est. SE}_{\bar{x}_2})^2}} \\ &= \frac{(0.9) - 0}{\sqrt{(.24)^2 + (.10)^2}} = \frac{.9°}{.26°} \\ t_{48\text{df}} &= 3.4,\ P < .001 \end{aligned}$$

Difference is significant.

The 95% confidence limits on the true difference between the means $(\mu_1 - \mu_2)$ are

Obs. difference $(\bar{x}_1 - \bar{x}_2) \pm t_{.05} (\text{Est. SE}_{\bar{x}_1 - \bar{x}_2})$
$$\begin{aligned} &= (\bar{x}_1 - \bar{x}_2) \\ &\quad \pm t_{.05,48\text{df}} \sqrt{(\text{Est. SE}_{\bar{x}_1})^2 + (\text{Est. SE}_{\bar{x}_2})^2} \\ &= 0.9° \pm 1.96\ (.26°) \\ &= 0.9° \pm (.51°) \\ &= 0.39° \qquad 1.41° \\ &\quad\ \textit{lower} \qquad \textit{upper} \\ &\quad\ \textit{limit} \qquad\ \textit{limit} \end{aligned}$$

Thus, tuberculous men are likely to have an excess mean temperature of from 0.39° to 1.41°.

Table 14-2 summarizes these data for normal and tuberculous men and also presents 95% Confidence Limits on the true mean temperatures for each group of men. Note that the confidence intervals of healthy and tuberculous men do not overlap, a finding in accord with the 95% C.I. on the true difference, which does not embrace zero.

FIGURE 14-4

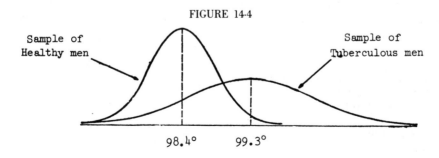

Sample of Healthy men

Sample of Tuberculous men

98.4°   99.3°

---

[1] Procedures do exist for testing normal means without the assumption of equality of variances; this has been a stimulating and controversial subject among statisticians, and there is no universal agreement as to which is the correct procedure.

TABLE 14-2. *Confidence Limits*

	Normal Men	Tuberculous Men
Sample size (n)	25	25
Sample mean ($\bar{x}$)	98.4°	99.3°
Standard Deviation of individuals (s)	0.5°	1.2°
Est. Standard Error of Mean ($SE_{\bar{x}} = s/\sqrt{n}$)	0.10°	0.24°
95% C.I. on true mean = $\bar{x} \pm t_{.05}$ (Est. $SE_{\bar{x}}$) with (n − 1) df	98.2°-98.6°	98.8°-99.8°
95% C.I. on true difference = $(\bar{x}_1 - \bar{x}_2) \pm t_{.05}$ (Est. $SE_{\bar{x}_1-\bar{x}_2}$) with ($n_1 + n_2 - 2$) df		0.39°-1.41°

CONFIDENCE INTERVAL ON A TRUE DIFFERENCE BETWEEN PAIRED MEANS (QUANTITATIVE DATA)

Similarly we can estimate a confidence interval for the true difference between paired means (μ_d) by the formula:

Obs. mean difference ($\bar{d}$) $\pm t$ (Est. $SE_{\bar{d}}$)

Recall that in Chapter 13 we answered the question, "Is there a significant difference in mean temperatures of fingers and toes?" We compared data on fingers and toes for 6 individuals by using the *t*-test, Difference Method:

$$t = \frac{\bar{d} - 0}{\text{Est. } SE_{\bar{d}}}$$

$$= \frac{\bar{d} - 0}{\left(\dfrac{s_d}{\sqrt{\text{No. of pairs}}}\right)}$$

$$= \frac{3.87° - 0}{\left(\dfrac{2.27°}{\sqrt{6}}\right)}$$

$$= \frac{3.87°}{.93°}$$

Obs. $t_{5df} = 4.2$, P < .01

Difference is significant. Null Hypothesis is rejected.

What is the interval estimate for the true mean difference? 95% C.L. on the true mean difference are:

Obs. d $\pm t_{.05,5df}$ (Est. $SE_{\bar{d}}$)
$= 3.87° \pm 2.57$ (.93°) $= 3.87° \pm (2.39°)$
$= 1.48°$ 6.26°
   lower   *upper*
   limit   *limit*

Thus the likely true mean difference lies between 1.48° and 6.26°, an interval which does not include zero. This result agrees with the *t*-test above.

Table 14-3 summarizes the various formulas for estimating confidence intervals for qualitative and quantitative data. The principles are reviewed below.

TABLE 14-3. *Confidence Limits on True Parameters*

Qualitative Data	Quantitative Data
95% Confidence Limits* on *true mean*	
$\hat{p} \pm$ exactly 1.96, or 2 $SE_{\hat{p}}$ where $SE_{\hat{p}} = \sqrt{\dfrac{\hat{p}\hat{q}}{n}}$	$\bar{x} \pm t_{.05}$ (Est. $SE_{\bar{x}}$) where Est. $SE_{\bar{x}} = s/\sqrt{n}$ with (n − 1) df
95% Confidence Limits* on *true difference between means*	
$(\hat{p}_1 - \hat{p}_2) \pm 2(SE_{\hat{p}_1-\hat{p}_2})$ where $SE_{\hat{p}_1-\hat{p}_2} = \sqrt{\dfrac{\hat{p}_1\hat{q}_1}{n_1} + \dfrac{\hat{p}_2\hat{q}_2}{n_2}}$	1. Independent samples: $(\bar{x}_1 - \bar{x}_2) \pm t_{.05}$ (Est. $SE_{\bar{x}_1-\bar{x}_2}$) where Est. $SE_{\bar{x}_1-\bar{x}_2} = \sqrt{\dfrac{s_p^2}{n_1} + \dfrac{s_p^2}{n_2}}$ with ($n_1 + n_2 - 2$) df If $n_1 = n_2$, then Est. $SE_{\bar{x}_1-\bar{x}_2} = \sqrt{(\text{Est. } SE_{\bar{x}_1})^2 + (\text{Est. } SE_{\bar{x}_2})^2}$ 2. Paired samples: $\bar{d} \pm t_{.05}$ (Est. $SE_{\bar{d}}$) where Est. $SE_{\bar{d}} = s_d/\sqrt{n}$ with (no. of pairs − 1) df

* To obtain 99% C.L., use $z_{.01} = 2.58$ (or $t_{.01}$ for appropriate df).

SUMMARY OF PRINCIPLES ON CONFIDENCE INTERVAL ESTIMATION

1. Whether or not we reject the Null Hypothesis we may still ask: With what true parameter values are the data compatible?

2. The sample outcome provides a "point" estimate. While this might be close to the true value, we know that other, perhaps more distant, population values also could have given rise to the observed outcome just by sampling variation. Therefore, we construct an interval which contains the sample outcome.

3. The width of this interval may be adjusted by the investigator since it depends on: (a) The size of the sample (n); the larger the sample, the narrower the interval. (b) The level of confidence with which the investigator wishes to assert that the interval includes the true parameter; the higher the confidence level, the wider the interval.

4. The confidence interval is usually (but not always) equivalent to a test of all possible null hypotheses including the instant Null Hypothesis. In general, if the confidence interval includes zero as a possible true difference (that is, if the lower limit is a negative value and the upper limit is positive), then the critical ratio will not be significant (the Null Hypothesis will be accepted). Conversely, if zero is not included in the interval estimate for the true difference, the critical ratio will be significant (the Null Hypothesis will be rejected).

5. The true parameter is a fixed value. The interval obtained by this estimation method, however, is a random variable which reflects sampling variation.

6. The distinction between the term ($\bar{x} \pm$ 1.96 S.D.) and ($\bar{x} \pm 1.96$ SE$_{\bar{x}}$) must be kept clearly in mind. If a population or sample is normally distributed, then about 95% of all individuals will fall between the mean value and 1.96 S.D.'s on either side. On the other hand, if we are interested in the *true mean* value of the population, then $\bar{x} \pm 1.96$ SE$_{\bar{x}}$ will give us 95% confidence limits on this parameter (see Problem 11-9).

PROBLEMS

Problem 14-1

Check all correct lettered answers (none, one, or more than one may be correct):

Results are often reported in the medical literature as the sample Mean ± one sample Standard Deviation (S.D.). It is a good procedure to report the S.D. because:

(a) It is a measure of variability of individuals.

(b) It is used to determine the Standard Error of the Mean.

(c) It influences the 95% confidence limits on the true mean.

(d) It varies with sample size.

Answer

(a), (b), and (c) *Correct.*

(d) *Not correct.* The Standard Deviation of individuals is not systematically influenced by sample size. The S.D. is an inherent property of the population and, therefore, of samples from it. If there are more elements in the sample, then there are more deviations around the mean and the numerator of the variance formula tends to increase but concomitantly the denominator increases. (Remember that variance is the <u>average</u> squared deviation around the mean:

$$s^2 = \frac{\Sigma\,(x - \bar{x})^2}{n - 1}\Bigg)$$

In contrast, the Standard Error, S.E., tends to decrease as n increases, as can be seen from its formula, $\sigma/\sqrt{n}$ or $s/\sqrt{n}$.

Problem 14-2

(a) If the 95% Confidence Limits on the true difference ($\mu_1 - \mu_2$) in weight gain are −20 mg and 10 mg, will the *t*-test on the difference between $\bar{x}_1$ and $\bar{x}_2$ be significant?

(b) In the above problem, what can be said about the true difference in weight gains under the two treatments?

Answer

(a) It will *not* be significant because the confidence interval includes a <u>zero difference</u> as one of the possible true differences.

(b) There could be no true difference, <u>or</u> either treatment could be better. While there *may* be a true difference there is insufficient evidence to assert that it exists.

Problem 14-3

Check all correct lettered answers. (None, one, or more than one may be correct):

Weight gain for Treatment Group A = 35 gms and for Treatment Group B = 30 gms. 95% Confidence Limits for the true difference in weight gain between the two groups are: −5 gms, +15 gms. One can conclude that:

(a) Treatment A is better than Treatment B.

(b) A difference in weight gain has been disproved.

(c) A larger sample will prove that Treatment A is better than Treatment B.

(d) There is insufficient evidence to conclude that there really is a difference between Treatments A and B.

Answer

Only answer (d) is correct. The 95% confidence interval on the true difference goes from a − value to a + value:

Thus, zero is one of the possible true differences. This is equivalent to finding that the null hypothesis, H_0: $(\mu_1 - \mu_2) = 0$, cannot be rejected.

(a) *Not correct.* <u>One</u> possible true difference is that Treatment A is better than Treatment B since the interval does include positive values. But it is also likely that Treatment B may be better than Treatment A or that there is no true difference. (Remember, it is necessary to look at the *entire* interval before making a decision.)

(b) *Not correct.* Although zero is a possible true difference, a difference in weight gain has not been disproved. A true difference (either positive or negative) is also likely.

(c) *Not correct.* While it is possible that a larger sample will prove that Treatment A is better than Treatment B, the reverse may be found. We are certain only that with a larger sample one is more likely to find a significant difference if in fact a true difference exists.

(d) *Correct.* We have not been able to reject the null hypothesis. Therefore, we cannot accept the alternative hypothesis that a true difference exists.

Problem 14-4

In a random sample of 100 children under 10 years of age in a county, 80% were found to have been immunized against poliomyelitis. What is the true proportion of immunized 10 year olds in the county likely to be?

Answer

95% C.L. on true proportion = $\hat{p} \pm z_{.05} (SE_{\hat{p}})$ where our best estimate of

$$SE_{\hat{p}} = \sqrt{\frac{\hat{p}\hat{q}}{n}}$$

$$= \sqrt{\frac{(.8)(.2)}{100}} = .04$$

Since $z_{.05}$ is 1.96 or approximately 2,

$$95\% \text{ C.L. on true } p = .80 \pm 2 \, (.04)$$
$$= .80 \pm .08$$
$$= .72 \qquad .88$$

lower	*upper*
limit	*limit*

Note: In this example we are considering the sample of 100 children to be a very small proportion of the total number of children in the county. A correction formula exists which takes into account the fraction of the total population being sampled, but the correction is negligible for small sampling fractions.

Problem 14-5

Results of an experiment:
Treatment A, 100 cases, survival rate is 50%
Treatment B, 100 cases, survival rate is 40%

Compute 95% and 99% confidence limits on the true <u>difference</u> in survival rates for treatments A and B. Would 99% C.L. be *wider* or *narrower* than 95%?

Answer

95% C.L. on the true difference $(p_1 - p_2) =$ Obs. $(\hat{p}_1 - \hat{p}_2) \pm z_{.05} (SE_{\hat{p}_1 - \hat{p}_2})$ where our best estimate[1] of

---

[1] Note that here, since we are setting limits on the difference between p_1 and p_2, we are not assuming that $p_1 = p_2 = p$ and therefore do not use the S.E. formula with p', the common estimate of p:

$$\sqrt{\frac{p'q'}{n_1} + \frac{p'q'}{n_2}}$$

However, in the present instance $\hat{p}_1$ and $\hat{p}_2$ are close and do not differ significantly; therefore, it would have made little difference which formula was used.

$$SE_{\hat{p}_1-\hat{p}_2} = \sqrt{\frac{\hat{p}_1\hat{q}_1}{n_1} + \frac{\hat{p}_2\hat{q}_2}{n_2}}$$

$$= \sqrt{\frac{(.5)(.5)}{100} + \frac{(.4)(.6)}{100}} = .07$$

Since $z_{.05}$ is approximately 2

$$95\% \text{ C.L.} = .10 \pm 2\,(.07)$$
$$= .10 \pm (.14)$$
$$= -.04 \qquad .24$$
$$\quad\;\; lower \qquad upper$$
$$\quad\;\; limit \qquad limit$$

Since the limits include zero, one cannot say that Treatment A is better than Treatment B.

99% C.L. would be *wider*, since we use $z_{.01} = 2.58$ (instead of $z_{.05} = 1.96$).

$$99\% \text{ C.L.} = .10 \pm 2.58\,(.07)$$
$$= .10 \pm (.18)$$
$$= -.08 \qquad .28$$
$$\quad\;\; lower \qquad upper$$
$$\quad\;\; limit \qquad limit$$

Problem 14-6

TABLE 14-4. *Weight Gain in Children*

	Group A	Group B
n	36	36
Mean	50 gms	70 gms
s	18 gms	24 gms

(a) What are the estimated Standard Errors of the Means (not assuming equality of variances)?

(b) What are the corresponding 95% Confidence Limits on the true means?

(c) Is there a significant difference in average weight gain between the two groups?

Answer

(a) The estimated Standard Error of the Mean, est. $SE_{\bar{x}}$, is $s/\sqrt{n}$. For Group A,

$$SE_{\bar{x}_1} = \frac{s_1}{\sqrt{n_1}} = \frac{18 \text{ gms}}{\sqrt{36}} = 3 \text{ gms}$$

For Group B,

$$SE_{\bar{x}_2} = \frac{s_2}{\sqrt{n_2}} = \frac{24 \text{ gms}}{\sqrt{36}} = 4 \text{ gms}$$

(b) The 95% C.L. on a true mean $= \bar{x} \pm t_{.05}$ (Est. $SE_{\bar{x}}$). $t_{.05}$ for $n - 1$ (or 35) df is approximately 2. For Group A,

$$95\% \text{ C.L.} = 50 \pm 2\,(3)$$
$$= 50 \pm 6$$
$$= 44 \text{ gms} \qquad 56 \text{ gms}$$
$$\qquad lower \qquad\qquad upper$$
$$\qquad limit \qquad\qquad limit$$

For Group B,

$$95\% \text{ C.L.} = 70 \pm 2\,(4)$$
$$= 70 \pm 8$$
$$= 62 \text{ gms} \qquad 78 \text{ gms}$$
$$\qquad lower \qquad\qquad upper$$
$$\qquad limit \qquad\qquad limit$$

(c) Since the above 95% Confidence Intervals on the two means do not overlap (see Fig. 14-5), we can conclude that the difference between the true means is significant. Had overlapping occurred, significance could still have obtained and we would proceed with a *t*-test on the observed difference. The *t*-test is shown below:

$$t = \frac{(\bar{x}_1 - \bar{x}_2) - 0}{\text{Est. } SE_{\bar{x}_1-\bar{x}_2}}$$

Since $n_1 = n_2$ we do not have to compute a pooled variance and can use as our formulas:

$$\text{Est. } SE_{\bar{x}_1-\bar{x}_2} = \sqrt{(\text{Est. } SE_{\bar{x}_1})^2 + (\text{Est. } SE_{\bar{x}_2})^2}$$
$$= \sqrt{(3)^2 + (4)^2} = 5 \text{ gms}$$
$$\therefore t = \frac{(50 - 70) - 0}{5} = \frac{-20 \text{ gms}}{5 \text{ gms}} = -4$$
$$df = (n_1 - 1) + (n_2 - 1)$$
$$= 35 + 35 = 70$$

Obs. $t = |4| \gg t_{.05,70df} = 1.96$

Difference is significant.

A third method of answering the question is to obtain 95% confidence limits on the true difference (see Fig. 14-6).

$$95\% \text{ C.L. on } \mu_1 - \mu_2 = (\bar{x}_1 - \bar{x}_2)$$
$$\pm t_{.05}\,(\text{Est. } SE_{\bar{x}_1-\bar{x}_2})$$
$$= -20 \pm 2\,(5)$$
$$= -20 \pm 10$$
$$= -30 \text{ gms} \qquad -10 \text{ gms}$$
$$\qquad lower \qquad\qquad upper$$
$$\qquad limit \qquad\qquad limit$$

FIG. 14-5. *Confidence intervals on true means.*

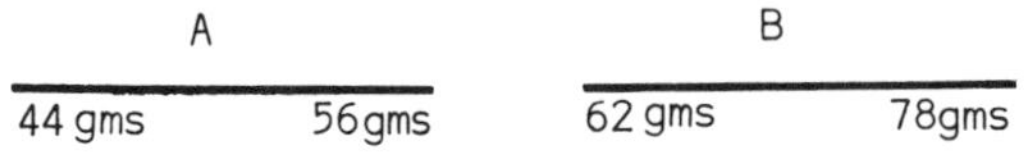

A	B
44 gms 56 gms	62 gms 78 gms

FIGURE 14-6

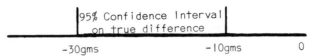

95% Confidence Interval
on true difference

-30gms   -10gms   0

This method also indicates that zero is a very unlikely true difference.

(Note that in parts (a) and (b) different S.E. and C.I. would have been obtained had we pooled variances for the two samples on the assumption of equality.)

Problem 14-7

The mean difference in diastolic blood pressure before and after treatment of 100 hypertensive patients is 10 mm Hg, and the Standard Deviation of the Difference is 5 mm Hg. What is the true difference before and after treatment likely to be?

Answer

Since these are measurements on the same individuals, they are "paired data": 95% C.L. on true difference $= \bar{d} \pm t_{.05}$ (Est. $SE_{\bar{d}}$) with df = no. of pairs $- 1$.

$$SE_{\bar{d}} = \frac{s_d}{\sqrt{\text{No. of pairs}}} = \frac{5}{\sqrt{100}} = .5 \text{ mm Hg}$$

$t_{.05}$ for no. of pairs $- 1$ (or 99) df is approximately 2.

$$\therefore 95\% \text{ C.L.} = 10 \pm 2 \ (.5)$$
$$= 10 \pm (1.0)$$
$$= 9.0 \text{ mm Hg} \qquad 11.0 \text{ mm Hg}$$
$$\qquad \quad \textit{lower} \qquad \qquad \textit{upper}$$
$$\qquad \quad \textit{limit} \qquad \qquad \textit{limit}$$

(Note that this confidence interval on the true difference does not include a difference of zero. Therefore, the difference is significant.)

Problem 14-8

(a) On what factors does the width of the 95 per cent confidence interval on a true parameter depend?

(b) If one wished to be "more certain" (e.g., 99% instead of 95% confident) about the limits of a true proportion, would this increase or decrease the width of the interval of estimation? Explain.

Answer

(a) The width of the confidence interval is

dependent upon the Standard Error. In turn, the Standard Error depends upon the population variance (σ^2 or pq) and the size of the sample (n).

The size of the sample (or degrees of freedom) influences the "precision" of our sample variance (s^2) and in turn the shape of the t-distribution so that the value of the factor ($t_{.05}$) which enters into the interval construction is also affected.

(b) It would increase the width of the interval. To be more certain that the true parameter (p) is included, the 99% confidence interval must extend 2.58 $SE_{\hat{p}}$'s instead of 1.96 $SE_{\hat{p}}$'s on either side of the sample proportion: $\hat{p} \pm 2.58 \ (SE_{\hat{p}})$ instead of $\hat{p} \pm 1.96 \ (SE_{\hat{p}})$ for the 95% confidence interval.

Problem 14-9

How do the widths of the confidence intervals using t and z compare?

Answer

Critical t values are never smaller than critical z values, although the difference can be small when the variance is estimated with many degrees of freedom. The higher critical value for t does not necessarily lead to a wider confidence interval, however, than would have resulted through the use of z coupled with the true variance. If the sample variance is by chance sufficiently small, then the estimated S.E. multiplied by t could be smaller than the true S.E. multiplied by z. On the average, however, use of t will lead to <u>wider</u> confidence intervals than will use of z.

Problem 14-10

Check all correct lettered answers (none, one, or more than one may be correct).

The 95% confidence interval for the true mean:

(a) Will include the true mean with 95% probability since the true mean is a random variable.

(b) Will include the true mean 95% of the time.

(c) Depends on sample size and population standard deviation.

(d) Is wider than the 99% confidence interval.

Answer

Only (b) and (c) are *correct*.

(a) *Not correct*. The 95% C.L. when computed correctly will include the true mean with 95% probability. However, it is not correct that the true mean is a random variable; rather it is a fixed quantity or parameter. It is the sample mean and the interval around it that are random variables.

(b) *Correct*.

(c) *Correct*. Both the sample size (n) and population Standard Deviation (σ) enter into the Standard Error formula and thus affect the width of the interval.

(d) *Not correct*. The 99% confidence interval is wider than the 95%. To be more certain (99% sure) that the true mean is included in the interval requires that the interval be wider.

Problem 14-11

In *Science*, 120:1000, 1954, evidence is given with regard to incidence of lung tumors in albino mice exposed to smoke of cigarette papers. The experiment consisted of 38 mice exposed to a fixed schedule of burning cigarette paper in a specially designed chamber and of 36 control mice in the same environment except for the smoke. There were 8 carcinomas and 5 adenomas in the experimental mice and 5 carcinomas and 6 adenomas in the controls. The conclusions in part are as follows: "There is a very slight preponderance of tumors in the experimental over the control mice, which is not significant by statistical analysis. . . . The results of this experiment indicate that cigarette paper has little or no effect on the generation of lung tumors in albino mice."

(a) Compute the confidence limits on the true difference between the tumor rates in the experimental and control mice.

(b) Would these limits support the conclusion stated, in your judgment?

Answer

(a) We first rewrite the data as a table (Table 14-5) for easier comprehension. 95%

TABLE 14-5

	With Tumors	Without Tumors	Total	Rate with Tumors	
Cigarette paper	13	25	38	.342	Difference is .036
Control	11	25	36	.306	
	24	50	74	.324	

C.L. on the true difference are $(\hat{p}_1 - \hat{p}_2) \pm z_{.05} (SE_{\hat{p}_1 - \hat{p}_2})$ where

$$SE_{\hat{p}_1 - \hat{p}_2} = \sqrt{\frac{\hat{p}_1 \hat{q}_1}{n_1} + \frac{\hat{p}_2 \hat{q}_2}{n_2}}$$

$$SE_{\hat{p}_1 - \hat{p}_2} = \sqrt{\frac{(.342)(.658)}{38} + \frac{(.306)(.694)}{36}}$$

$$= .109$$

$$95\% \text{ C.L. on } \hat{p}_1 - \hat{p}_2 = .036 \pm 2 (.109)$$
$$= .036 \pm (.218)$$
$$= -.182 \qquad +.254$$

lower upper
limit   limit

(b) The conclusion that cigarette paper has "little or no effect on the incidence of lung tumors" is not justified. The confidence limits extend from a fairly large negative difference to a fairly large positive one. Cigarette paper, therefore, could have a good effect, no effect, or a substantially detrimental effect. With larger samples which could result in narrower confidence limits on the true difference, we might be able to infer more.

It would be correct, however, to state that "there is no real evidence of any difference based on these samples."

Problem 14-12

What is your interpretation of the results of the experiment shown in Table 14-6?

TABLE 14-6. *Postoperative Effect on Plasma Ascorbic Acid for 105 Cases; Readings on the Same Individuals*

All Cases, No. = 105	(1) Preoperative Value, mg/100 ml	(2) Postoperative Value, mg/100 ml	(3) *Difference* (postoperative- preoperative), mg/100 ml
Mean	0.43	0.36	−0.07
Standard Error	0.036	0.028	0.015
95% Confidence Limits	0.36 to 0.50	0.30 to 0.41	−0.10 to −0.04
			$t = |4.93|$
			P = <.01 (significant)

* Data from Johns Hopkins Hospital.

Answer

This is a bit tricky. Note that the 95% C.L. on the preoperative and postoperative true means overlap (columns 1 and 2). Therefore one might be inclined to evaluate these results as showing "no significant difference." However, the data in column 3 show that (1) the Standard Error of the difference is *less* than the SE of either mean, (2) the 95% confidence limits on the true difference do *not* include zero, (3) the *t*-test on the difference between means is significant.

The explanation of this "paradox" is that the 95% C.L. on the true difference and the *t*-test are based on a Standard Error formula which has been adjusted for paired data (see Chapter 13). Since the preoperative and postoperative values refer to the same individuals and are positively correlated, the Standard Error of the difference is reduced by the term $2r\,(SE_{\bar{x}})\,(SE_{\bar{y}})$.

$$SE_{\bar{x}-\bar{y}} = \sqrt{(SE_{\bar{x}})^2 + (SE_{\bar{y}})^2 - 2r(SE_{\bar{x}})(SE_{\bar{y}})}$$

The 95% Confidence Interval on each mean, however, is correctly based on the Standard Error for that mean. This interval should not be adjusted just because some other measurement has been made on each individual.

Problem 14-13

A cooperative study of BCG vaccination of newborn infants was conducted in Denmark. One aspect of it was to examine the degree of tuberculin sensitivity after intradermal BCG vaccination in relation to the dose of vaccine and to the vaccination procedure. For a preliminary report of this study see the *British Medical Journal* for October 29, 1955.[1]

The subjects were babies born in the two municipal hospitals in Copenhagen between November, 1953, and January, 1955, for whom permission for BCG vaccination had been given by both the hospital staff and the mother.

The BCG vaccine was carefully prepared and tested to ensure a uniform product. All vaccinations were administered with a standardized procedure. Six different total doses of vaccine were given, varying from 0.15 mg. of BCG to 0.0047 mg. These doses were each

given in two different ways, as a single injection of 0.1 ml. or as two injections of 0.1 ml. each with a vaccine half as strong. Each baby had one tuberculin test during the follow-up period.

Table 14-7 gives a portion of the results of the tuberculin testing, showing the size of induration after vaccination for the highest and lowest total-dosage groups. These dosage groups are separated according to whether the baby received one or two injections.

TABLE 14-7. *Distribution of Size of Reaction to the 5-Tuberculin-Unit Test, 18–50 Weeks After Vaccination for Four Vaccination Groups*

Size of Induration (mm),* Stated Limits	Total BCG Injected (mg) and No. of Injections					
	0.15			0.0047		
	1 Injection	2 Injections	Total	1 Injection	2 Injections	Total
3–5				2	1	3
6–8	1		1	5	3	8
9–11	3	3	6	6	6	12
12–14	3	2	5	1	3	4
15–17	3	5	8	4	3	7
18–20	2	3	5		1	1
21–23	1	2	3			
24–26		2	2			
27–29	1		1			
Total examined	14	17	31	18	17	35

* Measurements recorded to nearest millimeter and then grouped in 3-mm classes.

(1) By inspection of Table 14-7, would you judge that the size of induration was related to the total dose of BCG given? Would you think that it was related to the number of injections used in giving the total dose?

(2) Table 14-8 (p. 170) shows for the 0.15 dosage group the means and standard deviations for the one- and two-injection groups and the Standard Errors of the Mean. A short cut formula was used for obtaining the standard deviations. Do a significance test on the difference between the two means (for one and two injections).

(3) Table 14-9 (p. 170) shows summary data and Fig. 14-7 (p. 171) graphs the cumulative percentage values for the total distributions (i.e., 31 babies in the 0.15 dosage group and 35 babies in the 0.0047 dosage group). The results of a significance test on the difference between the two means are also given. Do the results of the significance tests in (2) and (3) confirm your judgment in (1) concerning the comparison of the groups?

(4) For the 0.15-mg dosage total distribu-

---

[1] Guld, J., et al.: Suppurative lymphadenitis following intradermal BCG vaccination of the newborn, Brit. Med. J. 2:1048, 1955.

TABLE 14-8. *Size of Induration Where Total Milligrams of BCG Injected Was 0.15*

Size of Induration (mm), Stated Limits	Midpoint, x	One Injection			Two Injections		
		f	xf	x^2f	f	xf	x^2f
3–5	4	0	0	0	0	0	0
6–8	7	1	7	49	0	0	0
9–11	10	3	30	300	3	30	300
12–14	13	3	39	507	2	26	338
15–17	16	3	48	768	5	80	1280
18–20	19	2	38	722	3	57	1083
21–23	22	1	22	484	2	44	968
24–26	25	0	0	0	2	50	1250
27–29	28	1	28	784	0	0	0
Total		14	212	3614	17	287	5219

$$\text{Mean } \bar{x} = \frac{\Sigma xf}{\Sigma f = n} \qquad \bar{x}_1 = \frac{212}{14} = 15.14 \text{ mm} \qquad \bar{x}_2 = \frac{287}{17} = 16.89 \text{ mm}$$

$$\text{S.D.}^* = \sqrt{\frac{\Sigma x^2 f - \frac{(\Sigma xf)^2}{\Sigma f}}{n-1}} \qquad s_1 = \sqrt{\frac{3614 - \frac{(212)^2}{14}}{13}} \qquad s_2 = \sqrt{\frac{5219 - \frac{(287)^2}{17}}{16}}$$

$$= \sqrt{31.02} \qquad\qquad = \sqrt{23.42}$$

$$= 5.57 \text{ mm} \qquad\qquad = 4.84 \text{ mm}$$

$$\text{Est. SE}_{\bar{x}} = \frac{s}{\sqrt{n}} \qquad SE_{\bar{x}_1} = \frac{5.57}{\sqrt{14}} = 1.44 \text{ mm} \qquad SE_{\bar{x}_2} = \frac{4.84}{\sqrt{17}} = 1.17 \text{ mm}$$

* Short-cut formula for calculating S.D. for grouped data.

tion, the 95% confidence limits on the true mean size of induration are, using the sample variance for that dosage only, 14.24 mm and 17.96 mm. Compute the corresponding 95% confidence limits for the 0.0047-mg total group.

(5) Also calculate the 95% confidence limits on the true difference in the mean size of induration for the two dosage groups.

(6) Do the confidence limits computed agree with the results of your significance tests? What new information do they provide?

Answer

(1) By inspection, the distributions would indicate that size of induration is related to total dose of BCG given, but not to number of injections.

(2) Test of significance: Comparison of mean size of induration, one injection versus two injections for 0.15 mg.

TABLE 14-9

	Size of Induration (mm)	
	0.15-mg Dose (total)	0.0047-mg Dose (total)
Sample size (n)	31	35
Sample mean ($\bar{x}$)	16.10	10.60
Sample variance (s^2)	26.73	15.76
Sample S.D. (s)	5.17	3.97
Est. SE$_{\bar{x}}$ (s/$\sqrt{n}$)	0.93	0.67

$$\bar{x}_1 - \bar{x}_2 = 16.10 - 10.60 = 5.50 \text{ mm}$$

$$\text{Est. SE}_{\bar{x}_1-\bar{x}_2} = 1.13 \text{ from } \sqrt{s_p^2 \left(\frac{1}{n_1} + \frac{1}{n_2}\right)}$$

(but we could safely use $\sqrt{(\text{Est. SE}_{\bar{x}_1})^2 + (\text{Est. SE}_{\bar{x}_2})^2}$ formula since n_1 and n_2 are approximately equal)

$$\text{Obs. } t_{64df} = \frac{5.50}{1.13} = 4.87 \geqslant 1.96, P = .001 \qquad \text{(Difference is significant)}$$

FIG. 14-7. Cumulative percentage distribution of readings of tuberculin test by size of induration and by dosage on probability paper.

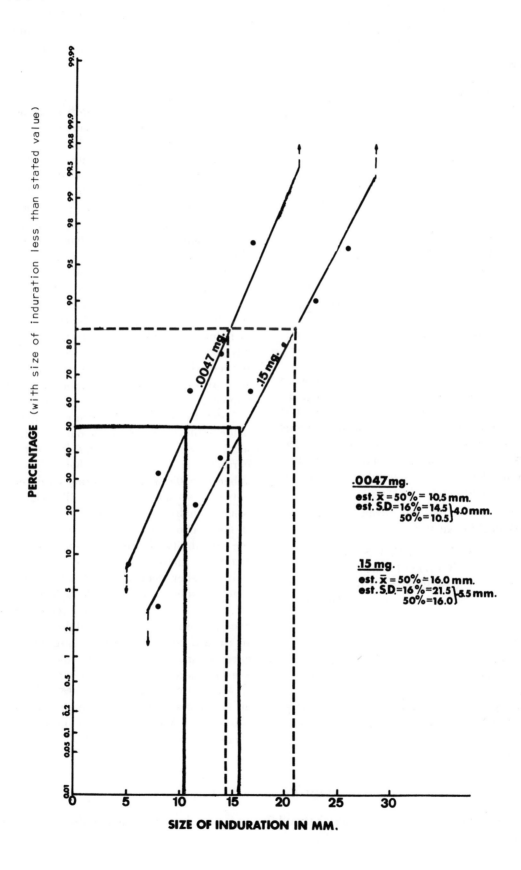

$$\bar{x}_1 = 15.14 \text{ mm}$$
$$\bar{x}_2 = 16.89 \text{ mm}$$
$$\bar{x}_1 - \bar{x}_2 = -1.75 \text{ mm}$$
$$t = \frac{(\bar{x}_1 - \bar{x}_2) - 0}{\text{Est. SE}_{\bar{x}_1 - \bar{x}_2}}$$

where

$$\text{Est. SE}_{\bar{x}_1 - \bar{x}_2} = \sqrt{s_p^2 \left(\frac{1}{n_1} + \frac{1}{n_2}\right)}$$

and

$$s_p^2 = \frac{(n_1 - 1)s_1^2 + (n_2 - 1)s_2^2}{(n_1 - 1) + (n_2 - 1)}$$
$$= \frac{(14 - 1)(31.02) + (17 - 1)(23.42)}{(14 - 1) + (17 - 1)}$$
$$= 26.83$$
$$\therefore \text{Est. SE}_{\bar{x}_1 - \bar{x}_2} = \sqrt{26.83 \left(\frac{1}{14} + \frac{1}{17}\right)}$$
$$= 1.87 \text{ mm}$$
$$\text{df} = (n_1 - 1) + (n_2 - 1)$$
$$= (14 - 1) + (17 - 1) = 29$$
$$t_{29\text{df}} = \frac{-1.75 - 0}{1.87} = -.94, \text{ P} \sim .40$$

Difference is not significant.

(3) The t-test on the difference between the means for one injection and two injections (dosage 0.15 mg) is not significant. The t-test on the difference between the means for total dosages of 0.15 and .0047 is significant. The tests confirm the judgment that size of induration may be unrelated to number of injections but is related to total dosage.

(4) 95% C.L. on true mean size for total 0.0047-mg dosage are:

$$\bar{x} \pm t_{.05, n-1\text{df}} (\text{Est. SE}_{\bar{x}})$$
$$\text{df} = 35 - 1 = 34$$
$$\therefore 95\% \text{ C.L.} = 10.60 \pm 2 \,(.67)$$
$$= 9.26 \text{ mm} \qquad 11.94 \text{ mm}$$
$$ \quad \textit{lower} \qquad\qquad \textit{upper}$$
$$ \quad \textit{limit} \qquad\qquad \textit{limit}$$

Since the 95% C.L. for true mean size for the total 0.15-mg dosage group are 14.24 mm and 17.96 mm, the confidence limits on the mean sizes for the two dosage groups do not overlap.

(5) 95% C.L. on the *true difference* in mean size are:

$$(\bar{x}_1 - \bar{x}_2) \pm t_{.05, n_1 + n_2 - 2\text{df}} (\text{Est. SE}_{\bar{x}_1 - \bar{x}_2})$$
$$\text{df} = 31 + 35 - 2 = 64$$
$$\therefore 95\% \text{ C.L.} = 5.50 \pm 2 \,(1.13)$$
$$= 3.24 \text{ mm} \qquad 7.76 \text{ mm}$$
$$ \quad \textit{lower} \qquad\qquad \textit{upper}$$
$$ \quad \textit{limit} \qquad\qquad \textit{limit}$$

Note that the confidence interval on the true difference does not include zero.

(6) The various 95% confidence intervals confirm that the size of induration is related to total dose. The confidence interval for the true mean of dosage group 0.15 mg is 14.24 mm to 17.96 mm; for dosage group 0.0047 mg it is 9.26 mm to 11.94 mm. These intervals do not overlap. Also, the confidence interval on the true difference does not include zero. Therefore, it is very likely that size of induration is in fact related to total dose.

The confidence limits enable us to state, with 95% confidence, what the true mean size of induration is likely to be. In the absence of any good reason for the results obtained to be particularly true for Copenhagen babies only, we may wish to generalize beyond them to all babies.

Note: Because of the many comparisons made (differences between one and two injections and between dosages) it is not really correct to apply the t-test without adjustment. When $\alpha = .05$, 5 out of 100 times a difference between two samples will be called significant when actually due to chance (Type I Error). If many two sample comparisons are made, the probability of calling a chance difference significant increases, i.e., the Type I Error risk is higher than .05 (see Chapter 15). One practical solution is to set the α level at, say, .01. (In this example P is .001 for the difference in induration of the total dosage groups, so we are conservative in calling this difference significant.) Other solutions involve the use of multicomparison techniques (Dunnett, C. W., J. Am. Statis. Ass. 50:1096, 1955) after an Analysis of Variance has been carried out. Analysis of Variance will be introduced in Chapter 15.

SUMMARY OF CHAPTER 14

To determine what the true mean or true difference is likely to be, estimate the 95% (or 99%) Confidence Interval:

$$(Sample\ Value) \pm [(\text{z or } t) \times (Standard\ Error\ of\ the\ Statistic)]$$

z or *t* can be .05 or .01 depending on the confidence level chosen (95% or 99%).

The formula gives *lower* and *upper limits* for the interval estimate of the parameter.

99% C.L. are always wider than the 95% C.L. on the same parameter.

A Confidence Interval corresponds to an infinity of significance tests.

	Qualitative data	Quantitative data*
95% C.L. on true mean (p or μ)	$\hat{p} \pm z_{.05}\ (SE_{\hat{p}})$	$\bar{x} \pm t_{.05}\ (Est.\ SE_{\bar{x}})$
95% C.L. on true difference between means $(p_1 - p_2)$ or $(\mu_1 - \mu_2)$	$(\hat{p}_1 - \hat{p}_2) \pm z_{.05}\ (SE_{\hat{p}_1 - \hat{p}_2})$	$(\bar{x}_1 - \bar{x}_2) \pm t_{.05}\ (Est.\ SE_{\bar{x}_1 - \bar{x}_2})$
95% C.L. on true mean difference (μ_d) (paired data)		$\bar{d} \pm t_{.05}\ (Est.\ SE_{\bar{d}})$

* Where σ^2 is known, $t_{.05}$ can be replaced by $z_{.05}$ and (Est. $SE_{\bar{x}}$) by ($SE_{\bar{x}}$).

CUMULATIVE GLOSSARY I: TERMS

Chapter 14

Confidence Interval Estimation

Determination of the interval within which a true value (population parameter) lies with a stated degree of confidence (e.g., 95 or 99 out of 100 times). (See 95% C.L. in Glossary II: Symbols.)

Confidence Limits (Interval)

The bounds (upper or lower) on a confidence interval for the estimation of a true value (population parameter).

CUMULATIVE GLOSSARY II: SYMBOLS

Chapter 14

C.L. or C.I. (95% or 99%)

Confidence limits or confidence interval on a population (true) parameter. Formula is:

sample value $\pm$ [(factor) $\times$ (Standard Error of the statistic)]

The *size of the factor* depends upon (1) the specific distribution of the sampling statistic (e.g., z or t) for the appropriate df and (2) the level of confidence (e.g., 95 or 99%). The *size of the Standard Error* depends upon (1) the size of the sample and (2) the population variance.

15
Highlights
of Miscellaneous Topics

Linear Regression (Two Variables) •
Correlation; Cause and Effect •
Analysis of Variance •
F Distribution •
Poisson Distribution •
Estimating Size of Sample Needed •
Bayes' Theorem

In this chapter, a few introductory remarks are made about a number of important topics so that the reader can become aware of these concepts. The reader is referred to more advanced texts for further exposition. The problems at the end of this chapter provide a few simple exercises on some of the methods discussed and also review methods used in earlier chapters. See if you can choose the appropriate test. Cumulative Reviews V and VI (Chapter 16) will provide a résumé of methods.

LINEAR REGRESSION (TWO VARIABLES)[1]

Regression and correlation are concerned with association in quantitative data, that is, association among measurements of *two* variables. These techniques attempt to answer the questions:

(1) Is there a relationship between the two variables?

(2) If a relationship exists, how can it be expressed? Can one variable be used to predict the other?

Suppose that on each of several individuals we can measure two quantities, x and y. Consider that so very many individuals have been measured that we can put them into subgroups, in each of which all individuals are identical in their x values but may differ in their y values. For each specified x value we

can get the average y value. The latter we can designate $E(y/x)$, the *expectation or average value of y given x*. The dependence of $E(y/x)$ on x, i.e., $E(y/x) = f(x)$, is called the *regression of y on x*.

This concept applies whether (a) the x's and y's are both subject to sampling (like heights and weights of individuals taken from some population) or (b) the x's are fixed or specified, like the dosage of some drug, with the corresponding y's then observed. Where both x's and y's might be subject to sampling, we can arrange to have only the y's subject to sampling by deliberately selecting individuals with specified x values. In statistical practice the two situations can become indistinguishable since certain analyses are made conditional on the set of x's observed as though they were fixed. (However, as will be seen later, a certain type of analysis, Correlation Analysis, is appropriate only in the bivariate case, i.e., where both x and y are subject to sampling.)

As an example, suppose that we have the set of measurements shown in Table 15-1. Let

TABLE 15-1

Height (in.)	Weight (lb)
60	135
60	120
62	140
62	130
62	135
64	145
66	150
68	150
68	160

---

[1] These methods can be expanded to more than two variables (i.e., one dependent and more than one independent variable) called *multiple regression*.

us assume that there exists a population of weights for each particular specified height. (We wish to predict weight from height.) We then call height the independent or x variable and weight the dependent or y variable. The simplest graphic representation of their relationship is in the form of a scatter diagram where the x axis is used for the independent variable and the y for the dependent (Fig. 15-1).

FIG. 15-1. Scatter diagram of weight (lb.) versus height (in.).

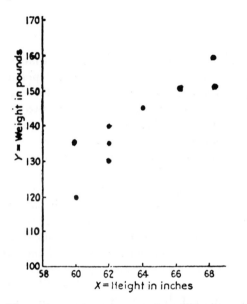

The relationship between height and weight can now be inspected visually. If as x increases y increases also, the relationship is positive. If as x increases y decreases, it is negative. Sometimes the relationship appears to be that of a straight line, i.e., *linear*.

In the simplest linear regression model, the following assumptions are made:

(1) The values for x, the independent variable, are fixed (i.e., selected by the investigator).

(2) The values for y, the dependent variable, are random.

(3) For each x there is a population of y values. These y populations have a common variance $\sigma^2_{y \cdot x}$ and their means lie on the true regression line.

Suppose that for each x value designated, such a population of y values does exist. Then we can write an equation for the *true (population) regression line* which goes through the expected or average y value for each x:

$$\mu_{y \cdot x} = A + Bx$$

where $\mu_{y \cdot x}$ is the mean of the population of y values at a given x.

A is the point at which the true regression line crosses the y axis (i.e., where x is 0). A is called the y intercept.

B is the slope of the line or the average change in y per unit change in x.

However, we rarely, if ever, have data on the entire population of y's at each x; instead we have data on a sample from each y population. Therefore we obtain, based on these y samples, estimates for A and B (called a and b) which will give us the best fitting regression line. The best fit is defined as the one which gives the smallest sum of squared vertical deviations around the sample regression line (*least squares line*)[1]:

$$y_c = a + bx$$

where y_c is the y value calculated from the regression equation.

Using another model, Fig. 15-2 shows the

FIG. 15-2. Packed blood cell volume (mm³) versus red blood cell count (millions/mm³). Reprinted by permission from *Introduction to Probability and Statistics*, fourth edition, by Henry L. Alder, and Edward B. Roessler, W. H. Freeman and Co., 1968.

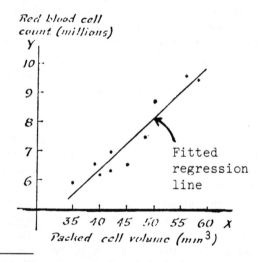

[1] In this estimate, the formula for b, the sample slope value (also called the *sample regression coefficient*), is:

$$b = \frac{\Sigma (x - \bar{x})(y - \bar{y})}{\Sigma (x - \bar{x})^2}$$

$$= \frac{\begin{pmatrix} \text{Sum of the products of the deviations of the} \\ \text{x and y pairs from their respective means} \end{pmatrix}}{\begin{matrix} \text{(Sum of the squares of the deviations of} \\ \text{x from the x mean)} \end{matrix}}$$

An alternative computational form for b is:

$$\frac{\Sigma xy - \dfrac{\Sigma x \Sigma y}{n}}{\Sigma x^2 - \dfrac{(\Sigma x)^2}{n}}$$

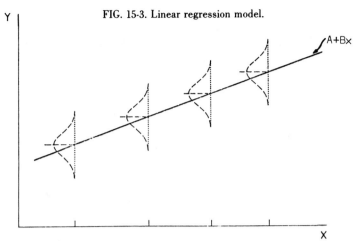

FIG. 15-3. Linear regression model.

fitting of a regression line to data dealing with packed blood cell volume (mm³) and red blood cell count (millions/mm³). In this model the x values were not fixed (selected) but vary from sample to sample. Note that in such a model one may be interested either in the regression of y on x or the regression of x on y (these are not equivalent).

An important caution for any model is that the regression line should not be extended much beyond the limits of the observational data without some basis for deciding that the simple linear relationship continues to hold.

In addition to obtaining the best fitting regression line, the Least Squares Method can be used to estimate the common variance of the y populations ($\sigma^2_{y \cdot x}$). Its sample estimate, $s^2_{y \cdot x}$, is called the *mean square deviation or variance around the estimated regression line.* The square root, $s_{y \cdot x}$, is called the *standard deviation from regression.*[2] It measures the dispersion around the regression line in the same way that the standard deviation measures the dispersion around the mean.

If one further assumption can be made, that each of the y populations is <u>distributed normally</u> (Fig. 15-3), then confidence limits can be estimated for the population values A, B, and $\sigma^2_{y \cdot x}$ and hypothesis testing carried out, e.g., that B is really not different from zero.[3]

CORRELATION; CAUSE AND EFFECT

In linear regression, there are two types of variables, a dependent and an independent variable. In correlation, neither variable is necessarily assumed to be the independent one. Correlation is used to measure the *degree* of linear relationship between the two variables. The following assumptions are made in the product moment correlation model:

(1) The regression of y on x is linear and that of x on y is linear.

(2) For each x, there exists a population of y's that is distributed normally and the variance is the same for each y population.

(3) For each y, there exists a population of x's that is distributed normally and the variance is the same for each x population.

(4) As a consequence of 1, 2, and 3 above, the marginal distributions of x alone and of y alone are also normal.

If these assumptions are satisfied, x and y are said to have a *bivariate normal distribution* (Fig. 15-4) and ρ (rho) the *population cor-*

FIG. 15-4. Model of a bivariate normal population.

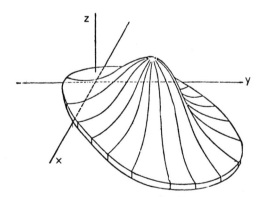

---

[2] $s_{y \cdot x}$ is usually called the standard error of estimate, but the expression is not fully appropriate here. In conformity with our previous definitions, the expression standard error of estimate should be reserved to indicate the uncertainty in the estimate of some parameter. Thus the standard error of the mean indicates how reliable or unreliable the sample mean is as an estimate of the true mean.

[3] See footnote 1 on page 178.

FIGURE 15-5

FIGURE 15-6

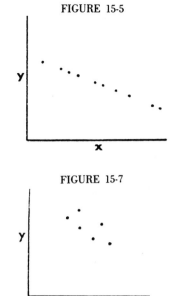

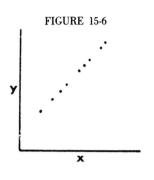

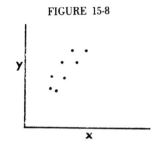

FIGURE 15-7

FIGURE 15-8

relation coefficient (Pearson's product moment) can be determined. ρ is a measure of the *degree of the linear relationship between x and y*. It is independent of any particular unit of measurement and indicates the strength of the association for any array of data in comparable terms.

Generally ρ is not known but must be estimated by the sample correlation coefficient (r), based on a sample of individuals from the population. The formula for r was given in Chapter 13 as:

$$r = \frac{\Sigma(x - \bar{x})(y - \bar{y})}{\sqrt{\Sigma(x - \bar{x})^2 \Sigma(y - \bar{y})^2}}$$

$$= \frac{\left(\begin{array}{l}\text{Sum of the products of the} \\ \text{deviations of the x and y pairs} \\ \text{from their respective means}\end{array}\right)}{\sqrt{\left(\begin{array}{l}\text{Sum of the squares of the} \\ \text{deviations of x from the x mean}\end{array}\right) \times \left(\begin{array}{l}\text{Sum of the squares of the} \\ \text{deviations of y from the y mean}\end{array}\right)}}$$

r can vary from 0 (for no linear relationship) to +1 (for a perfect positive) or to −1 (for a perfect negative linear relationship). An intermediate value indicates a less than perfect association, which is typical of most situations. For example, if all y values fall on a straight line which is non-horizontal, then the association is perfect and r is −1 or +1, depending upon the direction of the slope (i.e., negative or positive) (Figs. 15-5 and 15-6, respectively).

If there is a scatter of y values around the line, then the relationship is less than perfect (i.e., r between −1 and 0, or between 0 and +1) as in the graphs (shown in Figs. 15-7 and 15-8) because of the deviations from the line.

If x does not or cannot help at all in predicting y, then r is 0 (Fig. 15-9) or undefined (Figs. 15-10, and 15-11).

Note that, in Fig. 15-10, x does not help because all the x's are identical. In Fig. 15-11, x does not help because we know y anyway.

No generalization can be made about *curvilinear* relationships other than that when fitted

FIGURE 15-9   FIGURE 15-10   FIGURE 15-11

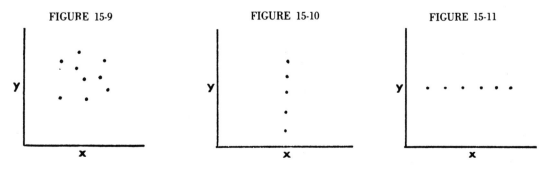

FIGURE 15-12   FIGURE 15-13   FIGURE 15-14

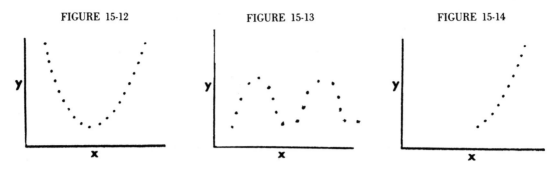

linearly they may yield 0, positive, or negative correlation, but never perfect linear correlation. For example, in Figs. 15-12 and 15-13 r is 0, whereas in Fig. 15-14, with the same curvilinear relationship as in Fig. 15-12 but only half the range, the linear component yields an r value close to +1 (i.e., x can help in predicting y). r then is a measure of how x and y vary together. r, however, is of even more use in its squared form. r^2 (*coefficient of determination*) measures the *proportion of the total variance in y*, which is associated with or can be explained by the variance in x. When r^2 is multiplied by 100, this proportion is converted to a percent.

For example, suppose that r is +0.952 for the data in Fig. 15-2 on red blood cell count and packed cell volume. Then $r^2 = (.952)^2 \times 100 = 90.6\%$. Thus 90.6% of the variability in y (the red blood cell count) can be accounted for by the variance in x (packed cell volume). The remaining variance represents the *variance* $s_{y \cdot x}^2$ due to accidental or otherwise unexplained deviations of y around the regression line.

As with the population regression coefficient (B), there are significance tests on the hypothesis that the *population correlation coefficient* rho (ρ) is zero.[1] It is important to remember that, analogous to the distinction between an important difference and a significant difference for sample means, a correlation may be significant yet so weak as to be of no practical consequence. On the other hand, correlation may appear to be strong (close to 1) yet be-

cause of the small sample size it may prove not to be significant.

There are important restrictions upon the calculation and interpretation of r. The validity of the assumptions regarding the underlying populations should be ascertained. If the populations cannot be assumed to be normal (and in certain other instances, e.g., non-linearity), then alternative non-parametric (distribution-free) correlation methods can be used, such as Kendall's Tau, Spearman's Rank Order Correlation Coefficient, etc., rather than the Pearson Product Moment Correlation Coefficient (r) just described.

Even if a correlation coefficient is large and significant, this does not prove a cause and effect relationship. Before a causal relation is asserted, various alternative interpretations of a high correlation must be ruled out (e.g., there may be a spurious correlation, or each variable may be independently related to a common third factor).

ANALYSIS OF VARIANCE

Using the *t*-test, it is possible to determine whether two sample means differ significantly. How does one determine whether more than two (say k) sample means differ significantly?

Significance testing cannot be done by repeated application of the *t*-test to pairs of sample means. Suppose we had 7 samples all drawn from the same population and were to test at the $\alpha = .05$ level all possible pairs of the sample means for significant differences.

---

[1] *t*-test for r (is rho really different from 0?):

$$t_r = \frac{r}{SE_r} = \frac{r}{\sqrt{\dfrac{1 - r^2}{n - 2}}} \quad \text{(with df n} - 2)$$

or, equivalently, for the case where only y is subject to sampling but x's are fixed, *t*-test for b (is B really different from 0?):

$$t_b = \frac{b}{SE_b} = \frac{b}{\sqrt{\dfrac{s_{y \cdot x}^2}{\Sigma (x - \bar{x})^2}}} \quad \text{(with df n} - 2)$$

This would mean that we would be making 21 (or $(7!)/(2!5!)$, the number of combinations of 7 things taken 2 at a time) possible tests, including a test comparing the highest sample mean with the lowest sample mean. As a result, the chance that the difference between these two extremes will give rise to a z value exceeding $z_{.05}$ may be much greater than 5%. One remedial measure is to require that z exceed some alternative value $z'_{.05}$ so as to take into account that it is the most extreme difference which is being tested. The more general remedial approach in which all 7 samples are simultaneously intercompared is by the F test, which generalizes the z or t test. This procedure in which all of the sample means are considered together is called the *Analysis of Variance* (ANOVA). If a significant F is obtained by this procedure, a multicomparison technique may then be employed to test which means are significantly different.

Principal assumptions for the analysis of variance model are:

(1) Each sample is randomly drawn from a normal population (necessary only for significance tests).

(2) The populations from which the different samples are drawn have the same variance.

Let us consider the simplest analysis of variance model (called "one-way"). Suppose that we take three groups of newborns, comparable with regard to birth weight, sex, race, and any other factors that might be felt to influence weight gain, and we give a different dietary formula to each group. At the end of 3 mo, the infants in each group are weighed (Table 15-2). The Null Hypothesis is that the average population weight is the same for all three groups (H_0: $\mu_1 = \mu_2 = \mu_3$). The alternative hypothesis H_a is that at least one population mean is different.

Under the Null Hypothesis (that each group was randomly drawn from the same population), σ^2 is the variance of this overall population. From the above data, it is possible to obtain two independent estimates of σ^2, or s^2:

(1) Estimate 1 is based on the variation between the sample means (*Between Groups Variation*):

Formula 1: $\quad s^2 = \dfrac{n(\Sigma(\bar{x}_i - \mathfrak{x})^2)}{k - 1}$

where k is the number of treatment groups, n is the size of each sample, $\bar{x}_i$ = the mean of each sample, and $\mathfrak{x}$ is the overall sample mean. This formula involves the square of the S.E. of the mean, called the *variance of the sample means*, which is estimated by

$$\frac{\Sigma \text{ squared deviation of each sample mean from overall mean}}{\text{No. of sample means} - 1} = \frac{\Sigma(\bar{x}_i - \mathfrak{x})^2}{k - 1}$$

$$= \frac{(\bar{x}_1 - \mathfrak{x})^2 + (\bar{x}_2 - \mathfrak{x})^2 + (\bar{x}_3 - \mathfrak{x})^2}{k - 1}$$

$$= \frac{(12.3 - 12.53)^2 + (12.7 - 12.53)^2 + (12.6 - 12.53)^2}{3 - 1}$$

$$= \frac{.0867}{2} \quad \text{or} \quad .043$$

However, it can be seen from Formula 1 above that

$$\frac{\Sigma(\bar{x}_i - \mathfrak{x})^2}{k - 1}$$

TABLE 15-2. *Weight of Infants at the End of Three Months of Feeding with Three Different Formulas (lb.)*

	Group 1	Group 2	Group 3
	12.0	12.5	12.3
	12.2	12.6	12.5
	12.4	12.8	12.7
	12.6	12.9	12.9
	$49.2 = \Sigma x_1$	$50.8 = \Sigma x_2$	$50.4 = \Sigma x_3$
Sample mean	$12.3 = \bar{x}_1$	$12.7 = \bar{x}_2$	$12.6 = \bar{x}_3$
Sample size	$4 = n_1$	$4 = n_2$	$4 = n_3$
Sample variance	$.067 = s_1^2$	$.033 = s_2^2$	$.067 = s_3^2$

$$\text{Overall mean* } \mathfrak{x} = \frac{\bar{x}_1 + \bar{x}_2 + \bar{x}_3}{3} = \frac{12.3 + 12.7 + 12.6}{3} = 12.53$$

* For unequal n_i's, we would use $\mathfrak{x} = \dfrac{n_1\bar{x}_1 + n_2\bar{x}_2 + n_3\bar{x}_3}{n_1 + n_2 + n_3}$

$$= \frac{\Sigma x_1 + \Sigma x_2 + \Sigma x_3}{n_1 + n_2 + n_3}$$

TABLE 15-3. *Analysis of Variance (One-Way Classification)*

Source of Variation	df	Sum of Squares (SS)		Mean Square = SS/df
Between Groups	$k - 1 = 2$	$n\Sigma(\bar{x}_i - \bar{x})^2$	$= .347$	Between SS/$(k - 1) = .172$
Within Groups	$N - k = 9$	$(n_1 - 1)s_1^2 + \cdots (n_k - 1)s_k^2$	$= .50$	Within SS/$(N - k) = .056$
Total	$N - 1 = 11$	$\Sigma(\bar{x}_i - \bar{x})^2$	$= .847$	
			(total sum of squared deviations)	

also is equal to s^2/n;

$$\therefore \frac{s^2}{n} = \frac{.0867}{2} = .043$$

If s^2/n is multiplied by n (or 4), the number in each treatment group, we get s^2, which is an estimate of σ^2:

$$s^2 = \frac{4(.0867)}{2} = \frac{.347}{2} = .174$$

(2) Estimate 2 is based on the variation *within* the samples (*Within Groups Variation*).

In Chapter 12, a pooled estimate of σ^2 was obtained for two samples and this estimate, s_p^2, was computed as:

$$s_p^2 = \frac{(n_1 - 1)s_1^2 + (n_2 - 1)s_2^2}{(n_1 - 1) + (n_2 - 2)}$$

In the case of three samples, s_p^2 is:

$$s_p^2 = \frac{(n_1 - 1)s_1^2 + (n_2 - 1)s_2^2 + (n_3 - 1)s_3^2}{(n_1 - 1) + (n_2 - 1) + (n_3 - 1)}$$

The general formula is:

$$s_p^2 = \frac{(n_1 - 1)s_1^2 + \cdots (n_k - 1)s_k^2}{(n_1 - 1) + \cdots (n_k - 1) = N - k}$$

In this example

$$s_p^2 = \frac{3(.067) + 3(.033) + 3(.067)}{3 + 3 + 3}$$

$$= \frac{.50}{9} = .056$$

The two s^2 values or estimates of σ^2 are presented in the traditional analysis of variance (one-way classification) table (Table 15-3), where k = number of treatment groups and N = total number of measurements. If the null hypothesis, $\mu_1 = \mu_2 = \mu_3$, is true, then both estimates of σ^2 are unbiased and differ from each other only by chance. If, however, not all the population means are equal, greater variation *between* the groups would be expected than *within* them. An F ratio is formed to test H_0:

$$F = \frac{\text{Est. of } \sigma^2 \text{ from Between Groups}}{\text{Est. of } \sigma^2 \text{ from Within Groups}}$$

$$= \frac{\text{Between SS}/(k - 1)}{\text{Within SS}/(N - k) \text{ (or } s_p^2)}$$

$$= \frac{.174}{.056} = 3.1$$

If H_0 is not true, the estimate of σ^2 from Between Groups is expected to be larger than that obtained from Within Groups. Therefore the F test performed is a one-tailed test. If the observed F exceeds the critical F at a designated level of significance, the Null Hypothesis is rejected. In order to expand our knowledge of the analysis of variance and to investigate some other applications the F distribution will now be examined further.

F DISTRIBUTION

F describes the simultaneous distribution of two independent estimates of a population variance. These estimates are expressed as a ratio:

$$F = s_1^2/s_2^2$$

Like the Chi Square distribution, the shape of the F distribution is dependent upon the df, here *two* different df values, the df value for the numerator and that for the denominator (Table 15-4 and Fig. 15-15).

Note that where there are only two samples, then the df in the numerator which pertains to the between sample variance is $k - 1 =$

FIG. 15-15. F distributions.

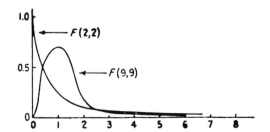

TABLE 15-4. *Short Table of Critical Values of*
the Variance Ratio, F*

P = 0.05

df'\df	1	2	3	4	5	10	20	30	∞
1	161.4	199.5	215.7	224.6	230.2	241.9	248.0	250.1	254.3
2	18.51	19.00	19.16	19.25	19.30	19.40	19.45	19.46	19.50
3	10.13	9.55	9.28	9.12	9.01	8.79	8.66	8.62	8.53
4	7.71	6.94	6.59	6.39	6.26	5.96	5.80	5.75	5.63
5	6.61	5.79	5.41	5.19	5.05	4.74	4.56	4.50	4.36
10	4.96	4.10	3.71	3.48	3.33	2.98	2.77	2.70	2.54
15	4.54	3.68	3.29	3.06	2.90	2.54	2.33	2.25	2.07
20	4.35	3.49	3.10	2.87	2.71	2.35	2.12	2.04	1.84
25	4.24	3.39	2.99	2.76	2.60	2.24	2.01	1.92	1.71
30	4.17	3.32	2.92	2.69	2.53	2.16	1.93	1.84	1.62
40	4.08	3.23	2.84	2.61	2.45	2.08	1.84	1.74	1.51
60	4.00	3.15	2.76	2.53	2.37	1.99	1.75	1.65	1.39
120	3.92	3.07	2.68	2.45	2.29	1.91	1.66	1.55	1.25
∞	3.84	3.00	2.60	2.37	2.21	1.83	1.57	1.46	1.00

Values of F equal to or greater than those tabulated occur by chance less frequently than the indicated level of P. df are degrees of freedom associated with the greater of the two variance estimates; df' are degrees of freedom associated with the smaller of the two variance estimates.

* Abridged from Table V of Fisher, R. A., and Yates, F., *Statistical Tables for Biological, Agricultural and Medical Research*, 6th ed., published by Oliver and Boyd, Edinburgh, by permission of the authors and publisher.

$2 - 1 = 1$. The denominator has the df of $(n_1 - 1) + (n_2 - 1)$. In this case, $F = t^2$.[1]

To evaluate an observed F in Analysis of Variance, the variance estimate between groups is always placed in the numerator and that within groups in the denominator. There

---

[1] The relationship between t and F when there are only two samples can be obtained as follows. From before we know that F equals a ratio of two estimates of the population variance, if in fact the two samples come from the same population:

$$F = \frac{\text{The between samples estimate of the variance}}{\text{The within samples estimate of the variance}} = \frac{\text{Between SS}/(k-1)}{s_p^2}$$

With k = 2,

$$F = \frac{[n_1(\bar{x}_1 - \bar{x})^2 + n_2(\bar{x}_2 - \bar{x})^2]/(k-1)}{s_p^2}$$

where $\bar{x}$ = the overall mean. The t which is obtained from the ordinary comparison of two independent samples is

$$t = \frac{(\bar{x}_1 - \bar{x}_2) - 0}{\text{Est. SE}_{\bar{x}_1 - \bar{x}_2}}$$

$$\therefore t^2 = \frac{(\bar{x}_1 - \bar{x}_2)^2}{s_p^2 \left(\frac{1}{n_1} + \frac{1}{n_2}\right)}$$

$$= \frac{[(\bar{x}_1 - \bar{x}) - (\bar{x}_2 - \bar{x})]^2}{s_p^2 \left(\frac{1}{n_1} + \frac{1}{n_2}\right)}$$

(Note: Since $\bar{x}$ is added and subtracted, the value in the bracket does not change.)
This expression simplifies to

$$t^2 = \frac{[(\bar{x}_1 - \bar{x}) - (\bar{x}_2 - \bar{x})]^2 \left(\frac{n_1 n_2}{n_1 + n_2}\right)}{s_p^2}$$

$$t^2 = \frac{[n_1(\bar{x}_1 - \bar{x})^2 + n_2(\bar{x}_2 - \bar{x})^2]/1}{s_p^2}$$

$$\therefore t^2 = F$$

(See above formula for F, with k = 2.)

is a different F table for each level of significance; i.e., if we wish that value such that 5% of the area of the $F_{(5,10)}$ curve is to the right of it, we would find that the critical F is 3.33 (Table 15-4). If, however, we wish the value above which 1% of the area of the $F_{(5,10)}$ curve falls we have to consult another table. That is, each F table involves two sets of df and the desired level of significance. As an example, for our data on weights F is 3.1. The df in the numerator is 2, and in the denominator 9. $F_{(2,10)}$* in a P = .05 table is 4.10 > 3.1. Therefore, the variance between treatment means is not significantly higher than expected. If our example had yielded a significant F, we could then employ a multicomparison technique to determine which means are significantly different.

Note that in the illustration above we have deliberately set the sample sizes n_i (n_1, n_2, n_3) equal so as to take advantage of the fact that then the true variances of the $\bar{x}_i$ also would be equal. But the F-test approach when properly used also extends to unequal n_i.

There are two main uses of the F distribution:

(1) It is the basis of the Analysis of Variance where more than two sample means are tested. For this purpose two independent sample estimates of σ^2 are compared.[1] Thus, even though the Null Hypothesis in the Analysis of Variance concerns the equality of means, the significance test itself involves a ratio of variance estimates based upon the reasoning that, if the means are not all equal, the variance estimate in the numerator will be much larger than in the denominator. Therefore a one-tailed test is used.[2]

(2) It is also important for testing the assumption which underlies many statistical tests (such as the t-test) that two population variances are equal. The two sample variance estimates, s_1^2 and s_2^2, form the F ratio, s_1^2/s_2^2.

---

* Closest value to $F_{(2,9)}$.

[1] It should be pointed out that we are referring here to the simplest model of Analysis of Variance. The reader is referred to more advanced texts on the design of experiments.

[2] An F-test can also be used in place of the t-test by using t^2 as an F with the numerator 1 df and with the denominator having the df of t. Where a one-sided t-test is achieved, the tail probability for such an F should then be halved, provided the observed departure from the Null Hypothesis is in the anticipated direction.

Here we may have no theoretical basis for assuming which of the two population variances should be the larger; we should then use a two-tailed F-test. A two-tailed F-test is achieved by taking the ratio of the larger to the smaller sample variance and doubling the corresponding F table tail probability. Thus, significance at the .05 level obtains when such a variance ratio is greater than the critical F shown in a P = .025 table.

POISSON DISTRIBUTION

Poisson distribution, like the binomial, is a discrete distribution. A random variable, x, has a Poisson distribution with parameter λ (lambda) if

$$P(X = x) = \frac{e^{-\lambda}\lambda^x}{x!}$$

where x = a count, 0, 1, 2, . . . ; e = 2.7183 (base of natural logarithms); and λ is both the mean and the variance (square of the standard deviation) of the distribution, i.e., $\lambda = \mu = \sigma^2$.

Applications of the Poisson Process

(1) The Poisson process describes the sampling distribution from a population of isolated counts in a continuum of time or space. If the mean occurrence of an isolated event is λ, then the probability of its occurrence 0, 1, 2, 3, . . . times in a random sample is given by the above formula. The Poisson process can then be used to describe the distribution of:

(a) Sample counts of radioactive disintegration per minute.

(b) Agar plates by number of colonies per plate.

(c) Samples of red blood cells per chamber.

Suppose we were to examine microscope slides of a culture of microorganisms where the expected number (λ) is 1 per square centimeter. What is the probability that we would observe 5 or more in a square centimeter? This question can be answered with the aid of Table 15-5. That is, we set $\lambda = 1.0$ and x as 0, 1, . . . , ∞. Then the Probability of 5 or more microorganisms is 1 − the Cumulative Probability where x = 4, or 1 − .9963 = 0037.

(2) Poisson distribution is also used as a limiting form of the binomial when p is very small (i.e., when the event is very rare) but n is so large that n × p (the mean number) is

TABLE 15-5. *Poisson Probability Function for* λ = 1.0

x	Probability	Cumulative Probability $\left(\sum_0^x \text{Prob.}\right)$
0	.367879	.367879
1	.367879	.735758
2	.183940	.919698
3	.061313	.981011
4	.015328	.996339
5	.003066	.999405
6	.000511	.999916
7	.000073	.999989
⋮	⋮	⋮
∞		1.000000
	1.000000	

a finite constant equal to λ. Suppose that the usual fatality rate for a disease is very small (p = .001) and in a series of 1000 cases 6 deaths are observed. What is the probability of 6 or more deaths, given a fatality rate of .001? Here n × p equals (1000) × (.001) = 1.0, which is so small that the normal distribution cannot be used as a satisfactory approximation to the binomial. Instead the Poisson is used, where λ = n × p = 1.0. From Table 15-5, it is seen that the Probability of x ⩾ 6 is 1 − the Cumulative Probability where x = 5, or 1 − .9994 = .0006. Therefore, the occurrence of 6 or more deaths is indeed rare.

Tables are available for using observed x values to set confidence limits on λ (similar to binomial confidence limits on p) and for testing for significance the difference between the observed x values.

ESTIMATING SIZE OF SAMPLE NEEDED

In earlier chapters, sample size was discussed from the standpoint of its effect on the magnitude of the Standard Error for data already collected. However, before we begin a survey or conduct an experiment, we may wish to have some estimate of the minimum size of the sample needed to obtain the desired information with specified precision.

As an example, suppose that we wish to know the minimum sample size needed to determine p, the proportion of children in the population vaccinated against poliomyelitis? We make use of the familiar formula from Chapter 4:

$$z = \frac{\hat{p} - p}{SE_{\hat{p}}} = \frac{\hat{p} - p}{\sqrt{pq/n}}$$

where $\hat{p}$ = observed sample proportion and we wish to solve for n.

Before the investigator proceeds he must make three specifications:

(1) First, how <u>closely</u> does he want to estimate p? Suppose he wants to estimate p within a distance delta, where δ = .04. That is, he wants his sample to yield a $\hat{p}$ value within δ = .04 units of the true p, i.e.,

$$\hat{p} - p = \delta = .04$$

(2) Second, how <u>sure</u> does he wish to be of estimating p so closely? Suppose he wishes to be 95% certain that $\hat{p}$ will be within the distance δ of the true p, i.e.,

$$z_{\text{alpha } (\alpha)} = z_{.05}$$

(3) Third, approximately what does he anticipate the <u>value of p</u> to be? If no estimate can be made, the most conservative approach is to set p at .5 since S.E. will then be a maximum.

In the above example, then

$$z_{.05} = \frac{\hat{p} - p}{SE_{\hat{p}}} = \frac{\delta}{\sqrt{pq/n}}$$

Squaring both sides,

$$(z_{.05})^2 = \frac{\delta^2 n}{pq}$$

Solving for n,

$$n = (z_{.05})^2 (pq)/\delta^2$$

In the case of p = .5, q = .5,

$$n = (z_{.05})^2 (.25)/\delta^2$$

And since $z_{.05} \sim 2$ and δ = .04

$$n \sim (2)^2 (.25)/(.04)^2$$

or

$$n \sim 1/(.04)^2$$

so

$$n \sim 625$$

Note that in the case of p = .5 and $z_{.05}$ we can use the simple formula $n \sim 1/\delta^2$.

The same procedure is followed for quantitative data. Here we use (from Chapter 11)

$$z = \frac{\bar{x} - \mu}{\sigma/\sqrt{n}} \quad \text{or} \quad \frac{\delta}{\sigma/\sqrt{n}}$$

Proceeding as above, we obtain

$$n = \frac{z^2\sigma^2}{\delta^2}$$

It is necessary here to know σ, the standard deviation of the population, based on past experience. Where σ is not known, a pilot study could be useful, or we may purposely use a conservatively high value for σ, similar to the use of $p = .5$ in the binomial case.

As an example, suppose the standard deviation of a population is estimated at 30 mm. Our permissible error δ is 10 mm, and we wish to be 99% confident that we will be within this distance of the true μ (i.e., $z_\alpha = z_{.01}$). Then

$$n = \frac{(2.58)^2(30)^2}{(10)^2} \quad \text{and} \quad n \sim 60$$

Note that the necessary sample size can also be determined by a specification of the desired S.E. of the estimate and the anticipated standard deviation (σ) of the population. The sample size is then given by

$$n = \frac{\sigma^2}{(SE)^2}$$

The above examples illustrate how to determine the sample size necessary for estimating a parameter. Methods also exist for the determination of sample size when the purpose of the experiment is to demonstrate treatment effects, e.g., that a difference exists between survival rates under two treatment regimens. Here the experimenter must specify not only the desired level of assurance against a false claim of a non-zero difference (at significance level α, the so-called Type I or α error) but also the protection desired against failure to detect a specified true difference in effects. (This kind of failure is called a Type II or β error.) For this purpose tables are available which take into account the *power of the test* $(1 - \beta)$ for various assumed true differences and α levels.[1]

. To demonstrate an extreme outcome, we have a slightly different problem. Suppose we have a disease which has invariably been fatal in the past. We have a new treatment which we think can be curative, even if in only a small percentage of patients. If we can produce even a single cure we will have proved our case. Then how many persons shall we test to be (95%) sure of producing at least one cure if the cure rate is as low as a p, say, of .02?

From the first term of the binomial formula with $p = .02$, the probability of no cures among 148 individuals ($n = 148$, $r = 0$) is 5.03%, and among 149 individuals 4.93%. So if we use 149 individuals we would be 95.07% sure of producing at least 1 cure.

We might also use the Poisson approach, since p is small. When λ, the expected or mean number of successes, is 2.997, we find from appropriate tables that the probability of 0 successes is 0.05, and of 1 or more successes 0.95. Since $\lambda = np$ and p is .02, solving for n we obtain

$$n = \frac{\lambda}{p} = \frac{2.997}{.02}$$
$$n = 149.9$$

This is about the same sample size as that obtained using the binomial approach.

BAYES' THEOREM

This theorem, which will be defined below, provides another application of probability to medical practice. Usually the physician knows the *conditional*[2] probability of a particular symptom complex or positive test <u>given a particular disease</u> P(S/D) or P(+/D). However, he wants to know for the individual patient the *conditional* probability of the disease <u>given the symptom complex or positive test</u> P(D/S) or P(D/+). How can Bayes' Theorem help?

To illustrate, suppose it is known that the prevalence of a particular disease in the general population is .002. If a person is selected at random and we ask, "What is the probability that he has the disease?" our answer would be .002. If, however, he is given a laboratory test specific for the disease and the results are positive, our estimate of the probability that he has the disease has to be modified. Let us assume that if a person has the disease this laboratory test is positive 80% of the time (*true positive*). If a person does <u>not</u> have the disease, it is positive 10% of the time (*false*

---

[1] See Snedecor, G. W., and Cochran, W. G., *Statistical Methods*, 6th ed., Iowa State Press, 1967, pp. 111–114 and 221–223.

---

[2] See Chapter 2 for definition of Conditional Probability.

FIGURE 15-16

P(Disease given a + test)

$$= \frac{\text{P(Disease)} \cdot \text{P(+ test given the disease is present)}}{[\text{P(Disease)} \cdot \text{P(+ test given the disease is present)}] + [\text{P(No Disease)} \cdot \text{P(+ test given the disease is not present)}]}$$

or

$$\text{P(D/+)} = \frac{\text{P(D)} \cdot \text{P(+/D)}}{[\text{P(D)} \cdot \text{P(+/D)}] + [\text{P}(\overline{\text{D}}) \cdot \text{P(+/}\overline{\text{D}})]} = \frac{(.002)(.80)}{(.002)(.80) + (.998)(.10)}$$

$$= .0158 \text{ or } 1.6\%$$

positive). We can list all of these probabilities as follows. Let

P(D) = The probability that the disease is present for any random person (the prevalence ratio of the disease) = .002

P($\overline{\text{D}}$) = The probability that the disease is not present for any random person = .998

P(+/D) = The probability of a positive test <u>given</u> that the disease exists, i.e., *sensitivity* of the test = .80 (true positive)

P(+/$\overline{\text{D}}$) = The probability of a positive test <u>given</u> that the disease does not exist[1] = .10 (false positive)

P(D/+) = The probability of the disease <u>given</u> that the test is positive (i.e., the probability of interest)

Then according to Bayes' Theorem the probability of the disease given the symptom complex or positive test is shown in Fig. 15-16.

The Bayes' theorem probability for the person's having the disease is only 1.6%, but it may be sufficiently high to warrant the physician following this diagnostic avenue further. He will do so as an intuitive act usually, rather than as a deliberate following of Bayes' rules.

PROBLEMS

Problem 15-1

Table 15-6 presents results from a series of extensive experiments designed to ascertain the size and sources of error in bacteriological grading of milk. The results given here are concerned only with the process of counting colonies on plates. Twelve plates were counted twice by each of 12 observers, two of whose

---

[1] The probability of a <u>negative</u> test given that the disease does not exist is called the *specificity* of the test = 1 − .10 = .90 (true negative).

TABLE 15-6. *Plate Counts of Milk*

Plate Number	1st Count of Observer		2nd Count of Observer	
	C	J	C	J
R1	346	333	344	336
R4	205	188	209	176
R6	52	35	54	39
R7	137	126	142	116
R10	158	145	146	143
R12	240	220	250	231
P2	63	51	55	53
P3	167	159	158	152
P5	81	65	93	92
P8	174	160	182	158
P9	146	101	142	112
P11	138	103	138	116

Source of data: Johns Hopkins University School of Hygiene and Public Health.

results are recorded below. Six of the plates had been put up with raw and six with pasteurized milk. The first time they were counted the plates were labeled 1 through 12. They were taken away and renumbered 13 to 24 in an order different from that previously used. Thus, although the same plate was counted twice by each observer, the impression was given that 24 different plates were being provided. Each observer entered the count on a slip of paper which was removed after the first 12 plates were counted, so that if suspicion were aroused that the same 12 plates were being recounted no reference could be made to the previous figures obtained.

Make graphs which will show (1) how well the two technicians agree with each other and (2) the consistency of each technician.

Discuss the interpretation of these graphs.

Answer

This exercise illustrates the value of a scatter diagram for visualizing the relationship between two variables. A series of two observations on the same plate are plotted as coordinates of a single point. If the two observations are in perfect agreement the point will

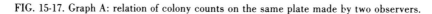

FIG. 15-17. Graph A: relation of colony counts on the same plate made by two observers.

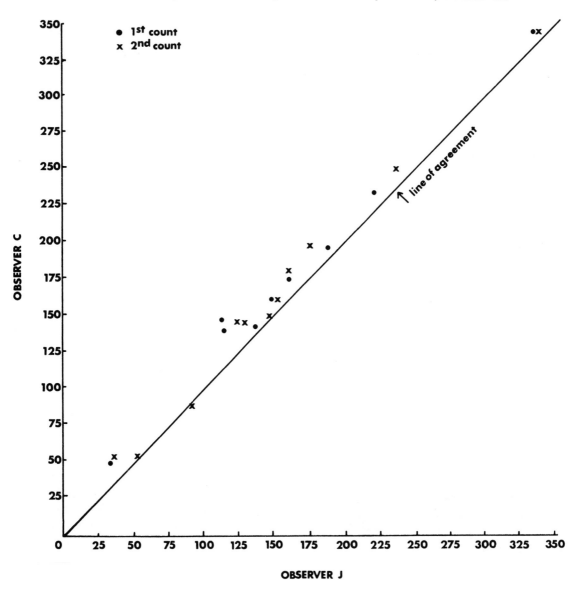

fall on a line (*line of agreement*) which makes a 45° angle with either axis.

(1) In Fig. 15-17 (Graph A) *interobserver variation* is shown. The observations of C and J for the same plate are the coordinates of each point. (Although the first and second counts could have been averaged for each observer, they were plotted separately to point up the extent of the deviation between C and J on a single reading.) It is noted that all but one of the points fall above the line of agreement, indicating that the counts of C are systematically higher than those of J. If the points had fallen below the line it would have indicated that the counts of J were higher than those of C. It should be noted that it is

not possible to tell from the data which observer is more *accurate* (i.e., closer to the true value).

(2) In Fig. 15-18 (Graph B) it is possible to examine *intraobserver* variation. The first and second counts for each observer constitute the coordinates of each point. For each observer, there appear to be about as many points above the line of agreement as below, reflecting a random error in measurement. Since C's points are closer to the line of agreement than J's it would appear that C is more consistent in his counting; note that in plate number P5 (Table 15-6) J's two measurements are in somewhat serious disagreement.

An F test can be used to determine whether

FIG. 15-18. Graph B: relation of first and second colony count for each observer.

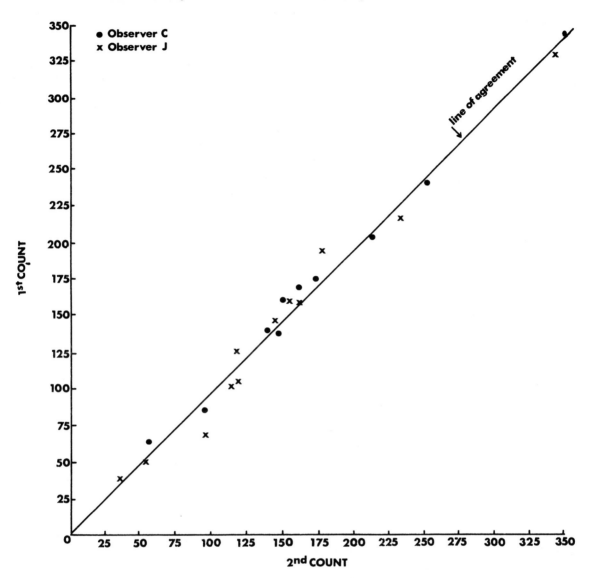

there is a significant difference in the consistency of the two observers.

Problem 15-2

Regression of y with respect to x refers to the mean change in y with a unit change in the independent variable x. *True or False?* If *false*, state the reason.

Answer

True. This relation can be expressed by the regression coefficient (b), which is the slope of the regression line. The slope is defined as the average change in y, the dependent variable, for each unit change in x, the independent variable. (See Fig. 15-19.)

FIGURE 15-19

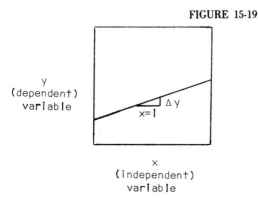

$$b = \frac{change\ in\ y}{unit\ change\ in\ x}$$

$$= \frac{\Delta y}{1}$$

FIGURE 15-20

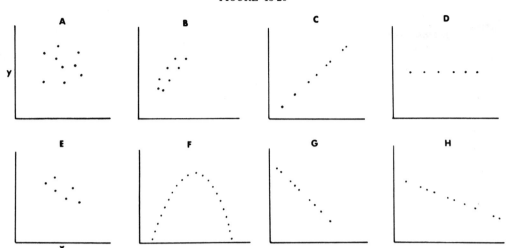

Problem 15-3

If two variables are highly correlated, a cause and effect relationship has been established. *True or False?* If *false*, state the reason.

Answer

False. The relation may be spurious or each variable may be independently related to a common third factor. Or it may be that we have confused which factor is the cause, and which the effect.

Problem 15-4

Indicate for each of the scatter diagrams A through H in Fig. 15-20 whether the correlation coefficient (r) is approximately 0, between 0 and −1, between 0 and +1, approximately −1, or approximately +1, or undefined.

Answer

(A) Approximately 0; x does not seem to help much in predicting y.

(B) Between 0 and +1.

(C) Approximately +1. (y values fall closely about a line with a positive slope.)

(D) Undefined   (y values fall closely about a horizontal line. Therefore the slope is zero; x is of no value in predicting y, and the prediction of y would be the same whether or not we knew x.)

(E) Between 0 and −1.

(F) 0. (The relationship is a curvilinear one which in this particular case will yield a zero least squares slope.)

(G) Approximately −1. (y values fall closely about a line with a negative slope.)

(H) Same as G.

Problem 15-5

A correlation coefficient (r) can be calculated validly for any set of data on two variables. *True or False?* If *false*, state the reason.

Answer

False. A correlation coefficient (r) (also called Pearson's Product Moment Coefficient) can be properly calculated only when both x and y are subject to random sampling from some bivariate population, with the x, y pairs chosen independently of each other. If the x's (or the y's) are fixed and then the y's (or x's) chosen, the correlation coefficient will be invalid. Where the sampling-from-a-bivariate-population condition is met, difficulties can still attend interpretation of a sample correlation coefficient, as for example when the population is not normal or the regressions are not linear. In some of these situations, non-parametric (distribution-free) measures of correlation can still be useful (e.g., Kendall's Tau or Spearman's Rank Order Correlation Coefficient).

Problem 15-6

Analysis of variance (ANOVA) is the technique of partition of the variance into component parts in order to evaluate the sources of variation. This technique is useful for the simultaneous comparison of means of several treatment groups. The F distribution plays a key role in ANOVA. *True or False?* If *false,* state the reason.

Answer

True. All statements in the paragraph are correct.

Problem 15-7

The basis of the reading of Standard Deviation as well as Mean in some scintillation (Geiger) counters is that radioactive counts/minute follow the Poisson distribution. *True or False?* If *false,* state the reason.

Answer

True. Since the distribution is Poisson, the variance equals the mean (i.e., $\sigma^2 = \mu = \lambda$). Since the Standard Deviation (σ) is the square root of the mean, the Geiger counter can be graduated to show both the count and its square root.

Problem 15-8

Ten samples of equal volume were taken from a bacterial culture and spread on agar plates. The numbers of colonies developing on the ten plates were

14, 15, 13, 21, 15, 14, 26, 16, 20, 13

Theoretical considerations lead us to expect that the number of colonies on a plate should follow a particular distribution where the mean and variance are equal and where these parameters depend on the density of bacteria in the original suspension.

(a) What is the theoretical distribution called?

(b) Calculate the mean number of colonies in the sample of 10.

(c) Would you be at all likely to get such a sample mean if the true mean were equal to 15?

Answer

(a) The theoretical distribution is Poisson, in which the variance (σ^2) is equal to the mean λ.

(b) The mean number of colonies in the sample:

$$\bar{x} = \frac{\Sigma x}{n} = \frac{167}{10} = 16.7$$

(c) We use the Normal deviate test to compare the sample mean, 16.7, with the expected population mean, 15.

$$z = \frac{\bar{x} - \lambda}{SE_{\bar{x}}} \qquad \text{where } SE_{\bar{x}} = \frac{\sigma}{\sqrt{n}}$$

Since the population mean, λ, is the same as the variance (σ^2), we know that $\sigma = \sqrt{15}$, and (since σ is known) the Normal deviate or z-test is then appropriate:

$$SE_{\bar{x}} = \frac{\sqrt{15}}{\sqrt{10}} = 1.225$$

$$\therefore z = \frac{16.7 - 15}{1.225} = \frac{1.7}{1.225} = 1.39$$

$$P = .16$$

Difference is not significant; therefore one could readily by chance alone get a sample mean $\bar{x}$ (of 16.7) so far or further from the population mean λ of 15.

Problem 15-9

Suppose from past experience it is known that the standard deviation of the weight of an organ in a certain disease following the usual treatment procedure is 4 gms. We wish to be 95% confident that we will not deviate by more than 1 gm in estimating the true mean weight of the organ using a new treatment procedure. What is the minimum size of sample needed?

Answer

We use the general formula:

$$n = \frac{z^2 \sigma^2}{\delta^2}$$

where $z_{.05} \sim 2$

$\sigma = 4$ gms

$\delta = 1$ gm

$$\therefore n \sim \frac{(2^2)(4^2)}{(1)^2} = 64$$

TABLE 15-7. *54 FEMALE STUDENTS, 1969 Hemoglobin Values, SMA4 Olivetti Printout*

V				
11·8	S			
12·0	S	14·0	S	
12·1	S	14·0	S	
12·1	S	14·0	S	
12·2	S	14·0	S	
12·6	S	14·1	S	
12·7	S	14·1	S	
12·8	S	14·2	S	
12·8	S	14·2	S	
12·9	S	14·2	S	
13·0	S	14·2	S	
13·0	S	14·2	S	
13·0	S	14·3	S	
13·0	S	14·4	S	
13·1	S	14·4	S	
13·2	S	14·4	S	
13·2	S	14·4	S	
13·3	S	15·0	S	
13·4	S	15·0	S	
13·4	S	15·4	S	
13·4	S	15·4	S	
13·4	S	15·5	S	
13·4	S		Z	
13·4	S	Σx	735·3000	C◊
13·4	S			
13·5	S	n	54·0000	E◊
13·6	S			
13·6	S	Σx^2	10050·6500	B◊
13·6	S			
13·7	S	$\bar{x}$	13·6166	A◊
13·7	S			
13·8	S	$\frac{(\Sigma x)^2}{n}$	10012·3350	D◊
13·8	S			

$$\Sigma x^2 - \frac{(\Sigma x)^2}{n} \qquad 38\cdot 3150 \quad A\Diamond$$

$$s^2 \qquad 0\cdot 7229 \quad A\Diamond$$

$$s \qquad 0\cdot 8502 \quad A\Diamond$$

$$\frac{s}{\sqrt{n}} = SE_{\bar{x}} \qquad 0\cdot 1156 \quad A\Diamond$$

Problem 15-10: Hemoglobin Values of Female Medical Students[1]

Table 15-7 shows a computer printout of 54 hemoglobin values[2] as determined by the SMA4 autoanalyzer. These data refer to presumably healthy female medical students. The computed sample mean ($\bar{x}$), sample variance (s^2), sample standard deviation (s), and

---

[1] This exercise was suggested by Dr. Mary Porter, Chairman, Department of Clinical Pathology, Medical College of Pennsylvania (formerly Woman's Medical College), to illustrate to sophomore MCP students the application of biostatistics to their own laboratory values.

[2] A frequency distribution of these values shows a preference for certain numbers, and especially for even terminal digits (14 odd and 40 even); thus there is some bias in the data.

FIG. 15-21. Hemoglobin values of 54 MCP female students, 1969 (intervals of 0.5 gm %).

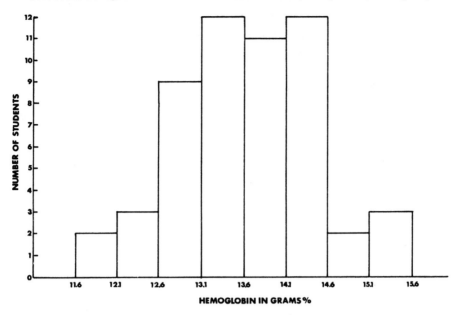

Standard Error of the Mean ($SE_{\bar{x}}$) are also shown. Note the alternative formula

$$\left[\Sigma x^2 - \frac{(\Sigma x)^2}{n} \right]$$

used for the numerator of the variance formula $\Sigma(x - \bar{x})^2$.

A histogram of the data grouped in 0.5 gm% is shown in Fig. 15-21 and the cumulative percentage frequency in Fig. 15-22. The 84%–50% and 50%–16% values are not exactly equal, but $Q_3 - Q_2$ equals $Q_2 - Q_1$. Also the median and mean coincide, as do the graphically (average) estimated and calculated stan-

FIG. 15-22. Cumulative percentage distribution of hemoglobin values (intervals of 0.5 gm %).

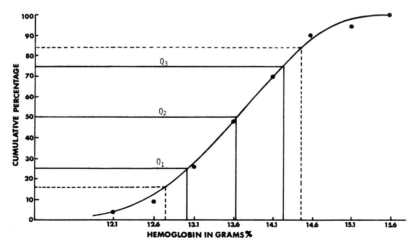

FIG. 15-23. Distribution calculated from mean and standard deviation.

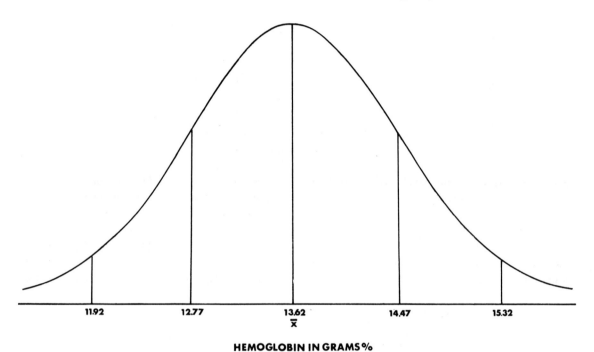

Locate Your Hemoglobin Value on the sample distribution.

Are you within the arbitrary "Normal" range ($\bar{x} \pm 2$ S.D.) ?

How many Standard Deviations are you from the mean? S.D. = .85 gms. %
(x)

$$z = \frac{x-\mu}{\sigma} = \frac{x-13.62}{.85}$$

$$z = ?$$

| 11.92 | 12.77 | 13.62 | 14.47 | 15.32 |
| | | $\bar{x}$ | | |

HEMOGLOBIN IN GRAMS%

dard deviations, characteristics of a normal distribution. Based on the calculated mean and standard deviation, a hypothetical normal curve was drawn (Fig. 15-23). Students were asked to locate their own hemoglobin value on this graph.

To determine whether the sample mean (13.62) differs significantly from Wintrobe's mean (14.0) for U. S. females,[3] a z-test was carried out (Table 15-8) using Wintrobe's value of 1.0 for σ. For purposes of this study we have treated Wintrobe's results as if they were

based on a very large sample. Our sample mean differed significantly from 14.0 but may not represent a significant departure from Wintrobe's data if they are actually based on a small study.

95% Confidence Limits were obtained on the true mean for all female medical students (assuming that MCP students are typical).

Table 15-9 shows that the mean for this female sample was significantly different (higher) than the mean for 38 college male students.

To determine whether the autoanalyzer gives the same results as the Klett method, a t-test (for paired data) was carried out on male hemoglobin values obtained by both

---

[3] Wintrobe, M., *Clinical Hematology*, 6th ed., Lea & Febiger, 1967.

TABLE 15-8. *Comparison of Hemoglobin Values for a Sample of Female Medical Students Versus U.S. Population of Females*

Population of adult females (Wintrobe): $\mu = 14.0$ gms % $\sigma = 1.0$ gm %

Is our sample mean value of 13.62 gms % significantly different from 14.0 gms %?

Distribution of Sample Means Around a True Mean

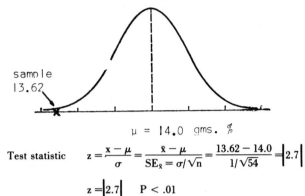

Test statistic $z = \dfrac{x - \mu}{\sigma} = \dfrac{\bar{x} - \mu}{SE_{\bar{x}} = \sigma/\sqrt{n}} = \dfrac{13.62 - 14.0}{1/\sqrt{54}} = \left|2.7\right|$

$z = \left|2.7\right|$ $P < .01$

Our sample mean value is significantly different from the expected mean of 14.0 gms %

95% Confidence Limits on true mean (μ) (assuming that the standard deviation of female medical students is different than that of the population of adult females)

$$= \bar{x} \pm t_{.05.53df} \; (\text{Est. } SE_{\bar{x}}) \quad \text{where} \left(\text{Est. } SE_{\bar{x}} = \frac{s}{\sqrt{n}} = \frac{.85}{\sqrt{54}} = .1156\right)$$

$$\therefore 95\% \text{ C.L. on } \mu = 13.62 \pm \; 1.96 \; (.1156)$$
$$= 13.62 \pm \quad .23$$
$$= 13.39, \quad 13.85 \text{ gms } \%$$
$$\quad\; lower \quad upper$$
$$\quad\; limit \quad\; limit$$

TABLE 15-9. *Comparison of Hemoglobin Values for Sample of Females Versus Males*

	Females	Males
n	54	38
$\bar{x}$	13.62 , gm %	16.13 , gm %
s^2	.72	.98
s	.85	.99

t-Distribution of Sample Differences Around a True Difference of 0 (for 90 df)

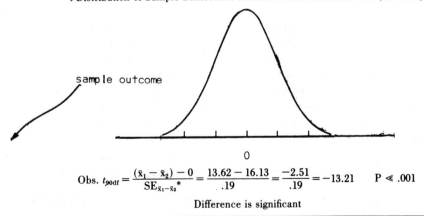

Obs. $t_{90df} = \dfrac{(\bar{x}_1 - \bar{x}_2) - 0}{SE_{\bar{x}_1 - \bar{x}_2}}* = \dfrac{13.62 - 16.13}{.19} = \dfrac{-2.51}{.19} = -13.21$ $P \ll .001$

Difference is significant

---

* Formula for $SE_{\bar{x}_1 - \bar{x}_2}$:

$$s_p^2 = \frac{(n-1)(s_1^2) + (n-2)(s_2^2)}{(n_1 - 1) + (n_2 - 1)} = \frac{(53)(.72) + (37)(.98)}{90} = .8269$$

$$SE_{\bar{x}_1 - \bar{x}_2} = \sqrt{s_p^2 \left(\frac{1}{n_1} + \frac{1}{n_2}\right)} = \sqrt{.8269 \left(\frac{1}{54} + \frac{1}{38}\right)} = .19 \text{ gm\%}$$

TABLE 15-10. *Comparison of Two Methods of Hemoglobin Determination for 38 Men (Data in gm %)*

Individual	Klett	SMA4	d (Difference)	d² (Difference)²
1	16.5	16.7	−.2	.04
2	15.2	15.8	−.6	.36
.	.	.	.	.
.	.	.	.	.
37	18.0	17.6	+.4	.16
38	12.2	12.8	−.6	.36
Total			−4.00	10.60

$$\bar{d} = \Sigma d / \text{No. of pairs} = -4.00/38 = -.1053$$

$$s_d^2 = \frac{\Sigma(d - \bar{d})^2}{\text{No. of pairs} - 1} = \left[\frac{\Sigma d^2 - \dfrac{(\Sigma d)^2}{\text{No. of pairs}}}{\text{No. of pairs} - 1}\right]^* = \frac{10.60 - \dfrac{(4.00)^2}{38}}{37} = 0.2751$$

$$s_d = \sqrt{0.2751} = 0.5245$$

$$SE_{\bar{d}} \text{ or } s_{\bar{d}} = \frac{s_d}{\sqrt{\text{No. of pairs}}} = \frac{0.5245}{\sqrt{38}} = 0.0851$$

$$\text{Obs. } t = \frac{\bar{d} - 0}{s_{\bar{d}}} = \frac{-.1053}{.0851} = -1.24$$

|1.24| is less than 1.96 (critical value at .05 level) for 37 df

Difference is not significant

* This is a short-cut computational form for s_d^2.

methods (Table 15-10). The mean difference was not significant.

Problem 15-11

Test yourself on this problem, which reviews the application of different statistical methods.

Exercise Based on a Study of the Effect of Iron Supplementation of an Infant Formula.[1]

A study is being conducted by the Department of Pediatrics at Medical College of Pennsylvania (MCP) to determine whether iron supplementation of a standard infant formula has any effect on the incidence of iron deficiency anemia, pica, lead poisoning, and infection in a lower socioeconomic group. It is a double blind study, i.e., neither the parent who receives the formula nor the professional staff involved in the care of the baby knows which formula the infant is receiving.

The mothers of all babies born on the ward service of MCP (and, for part of the time, on the affiliated services at Germantown and Episcopal Hospitals) between June, 1964, and May, 1967, were invited to participate in the study by a public health nurse. Excluded from the study were babies who weighed less than $5\frac{1}{2}$ pounds at birth, twins, babies whose mothers chose to breast-feed, and babies who were ill or had hematological problems. Following delivery at the hospital, the mother was invited to join the study. If she agreed, a history was taken which included age and education of both parents, number of adults in household, number of siblings, weekly family income, per capita expenditure for food, type of housing (owned or rented), and number of occupants per room. The baby was examined, weighed, and measured, and blood studies were performed at birth and again at 72 hours. Half of the babies were assigned to standard formula and the other half to iron-enriched formula by a previously designated randomized method. The babies were fed standard formula while in the nursery and were discharged home on study formula. The cans of formula for individual babies were labeled with the baby's study number.

Return clinic visits were scheduled at fixed intervals at each of which progress was re-

[1] Permission to use these unpublished data was granted by Dr. Doris A. Howell, Professor and Chairman, Department of Pediatrics, Medical College of Pennsylvania. This exercise was prepared principally by Dr. Judith Mausner, Medical College of Pennsylvania.

TABLE 15-11

	2–5 Weeks		20–26 Weeks	
	Standard Formula	Enriched Formula	Standard Formula	Enriched Formula
n	301	316	170	191
x̄ (gm %)	12.5	12.5	11.4	11.9
S.D. (gm %)	1.6	1.7	1.1	.9

TABLE 15-12

	2–5 Weeks		20–26 Weeks	
	Standard Formula	Enriched Formula	Standard Formula	Enriched Formula
Total no.	301	316	170	191
No. with Hgb < 10 gms %.	14	21	23	4

corded. Sufficient formula was dispensed to last from one visit to the next for the first year of life. After that, formula was supplied if the mother desired, but most babies were given pasteurized milk. Strained foods were added to the diet according to the usual dietary routine. No special dietary instructions were given. Mothers were instructed not to give vitamin or iron supplements.

Infant formula was provided free as an inducement toward participation. Inducement was later extended to include free taxi vouchers for clinic visits to further reduce attrition.

1. Assume that you are on the staff of this project. Comment on the advantages and drawbacks of each of the following methods of assigning formula to the babies. Which would you recommend?

(a) One formula comes in cans with yellow labels, and the other in cans with blue labels. Instruct the nurses to distribute an equal number of blue and yellow cans each week.

(b) Assign babies to cans with blue or yellow labels by use of a table of random numbers.

(c) Relabel cans so that all appear similar and can be identified only by code. Assign the coded numbers to babies by use of a table of random numbers.

The mean hemoglobin values (in g %) and standard deviation for both groups of babies at 2–5 weeks and 20–26 weeks of age are listed in Table 15-11.

2. Would you expect to find significant differences between the two groups in the early weeks of life? If such differences existed, what conclusions would you draw?

3. Is the difference in the mean hemoglobin values at 20–26 weeks for the two groups statistically significant? Is this difference likely to be clinically important?

4. The proportion of a group with "abnormal" values is also of interest in addition to the mean. We will somewhat arbitrarily take 10 gms % of hemoglobin as the lower limit of acceptability or "normality." Table 15-12 shows the proportion with hemoglobin under 10 gms % for both age groups.

Using the data of Table 15-12, test for the significance of the difference between the proportions with hemoglobin under 10 gms % in each of the two age groups. Does this affect your answer in part 3 about the clinical importance of the difference in formulas?

5. Table 15-13 recapitulates the number of babies in the study at 20–26 weeks versus

TABLE 15-13

Formula	No. at 2–5 Weeks	No. at 20–26 Weeks
Standard	301	170
Enriched	316	191

those at 2–5 weeks for both groups. Test whether there is a significant difference in the dropout rates for the two groups. If there were significant differences in dropout rates, what would the implications be? If the dropout rates are similar, does this necessarily mean that attrition did not introduce bias into the study?

6. Hemoglobin values for 5 babies at both 2–5 weeks and at 20–26 weeks are given in

TABLE 15-14

Baby Number	Hgb at 2–5 Weeks	Hgb at 20–26 Weeks
1	16.3 gms %	11.9 gms %
2	14.1	12.1
3	10.8	10.9
4	13.0	11.0
5	15.1	10.8

Table 15-14. Did the average hemoglobin value for these babies change significantly over this time period?

Answer

1. (a) This is an easy method for distributing formula, but poor because: (1) A nurse may develop notions about which formula is in blue and which in yellow cans. She may assign small babies to what she thinks is the enriched formula. (2) If differences between the groups on the two formulas become apparent, the clinic staff and/or mothers in the study may be influenced and interpret signs of possible illness according to formula given.

(b) This method eliminates problem (1) above, but problem (2) still exists. The major advantage over (a) is that the two groups of infants will be more comparable at the start of study.

(c) This method is cumbersome to accomplish but is the only valid method for insuring unbiased observations by staff and parents. If differences between study and control groups develop during the course of the study, it will not affect the observations on children admitted to the later part of the study.

2. No, significant differences probably should not exist because there is insufficient time for any difference in formula to have had much of an effect. However, it is necessary to check whether the groups are initially comparable on relevant parameters (hemoglobin values).[1] If significant differences existed, this could be due to chance. (Since $\alpha = .05$, in every 100 trials, 5 will result in a "significant difference" even if no true difference exists — Type I error.) A significant difference also

---

[1] Actually it would be desirable to use any difference in initial values to obtain a more precise evaluation of the results by the technique of analysis of covariance, a subject which will not be gone into here.

could arise if there were some break in random assignment of cases.

3. *Significance Test on the Mean Hemoglobin Values at 20–26 Weeks (in gm %).*

$$n_1 = 170 \qquad n_2 = 191$$
$$\bar{x}_1 = 11.4 \qquad \bar{x}_2 = 11.9$$
$$s_1 = 1.1 \qquad s_2 = .9$$
$$s_1^2 = 1.21 \qquad s_2^2 = .81$$
$$s_p^2 = \frac{(n_1 - 1)s_1^2 + (n_2 - 1)s_2^2}{n_1 + n_2 - 2}$$
$$= \frac{169(1.21) + 190(.81)}{170 + 191 - 2}$$
$$= \frac{358.4}{359} = .998$$

$$SE_{\bar{x}_1 - \bar{x}_2} = \sqrt{s_p^2\left(\frac{1}{n_1} + \frac{1}{n_2}\right)} = \sqrt{.998\left(\frac{1}{170} + \frac{1}{191}\right)}$$
$$t = \frac{(\bar{x}_1 - \bar{x}_2) - 0}{SE_{\bar{x}_1 - \bar{x}_2}} = \frac{11.4 - 11.9}{.105}$$
$$= \frac{-.5}{.105} = -4.76$$

$$t_{critical} = t_{.05, n_1 + n_2 - 2df} = t_{.05, 359df} = 1.96$$

Conclusion: $\mu_1 \neq \mu_2$, at the 5% level of significance.

The difference in mean hemoglobin values at 20–26 weeks is statistically significant. A difference of 0.5 gm % is unlikely to be clinically important for an individual child, but a reduction of 0.5 on the average could indicate the existence of some children with highly depressed values in one group (or highly increased values in the other group).

4. *Comparison of the Proportion of Babies Having a Hemoglobin < 10 gms %.*

(a) 2–5 Weeks.

$$\hat{p}_1 = \frac{14}{301} = .047$$
$$\hat{p}_2 = \frac{21}{316} = .066$$
$$p' = \frac{35}{617} = .057$$
$$q' = 1 - p' = .943$$
$$p'q' = (.057)(.943) = .0538$$
$$z = \frac{(\hat{p}_1 - \hat{p}_2) - 0}{\sqrt{\frac{p'q'}{n_1} + \frac{p'q'}{n_2}}}$$
$$= \frac{-.019}{\sqrt{\frac{.0538}{301} + \frac{.0538}{316}}} = -1.00$$

$$P \sim .32$$

Difference is not significant.

(b) 20–26 Weeks

$$\hat{p}_1 = \frac{23}{170} = .135$$

$$\hat{p}_2 = \frac{4}{191} = .021$$

$$p' = \frac{27}{361} = .075$$

$$q' = 1 - p' = .925$$

$$p'q' = (.075)(.925) = .0694$$

$$z = \frac{(\hat{p}_1 - \hat{p}_2) - 0}{\sqrt{\dfrac{p'q'}{n_1} + \dfrac{p'q'}{n_2}}}$$

$$= \frac{.114}{\sqrt{\dfrac{.0694}{170} + \dfrac{.0694}{191}}} = 4.07$$

$$P \sim .001$$

Difference is significant.

Table 15-12 provides some evidence that iron enrichment may be of clinical value. The proportion with "abnormally" low hemoglobin is much lower in the group receiving enriched as compared to standard formula. However, attempts to provide further evidence of the value of iron enrichment were not successful. No difference between the groups was found in rates of illness or in severity of illness as measured by days of hospitalization or number of separate admissions to hospital.

5. Test of the Difference in the Dropout Rates (see Table 15-15).

$$\hat{p}_1 = \frac{131}{301} = .435$$

$$\hat{p}_2 = \frac{125}{316} = .396$$

$$p' = \frac{256}{617} = .415$$

$$q' = .585$$

$$p'q' = (.415)(.585) = .2428$$

$$z = \frac{(\hat{p}_1 - \hat{p}_2) - 0}{\sqrt{\dfrac{p'q'}{n_1} + \dfrac{p'q'}{n_2}}}$$

$$= \frac{.039}{\sqrt{\dfrac{.2428}{301} + \dfrac{.2428}{316}}} = .98$$

$$P \sim .35$$

Difference is not significant.

TABLE 15-15

Formula	No. at 2–5 Weeks	No. at 20–26 Weeks	No. of Dropouts
Standard	301	170	131
Enriched	316	191	125

A significant difference in dropout rates would raise several points for consideration. First, there might have been some break in double-blind technique. If mothers knew, or thought they knew, whether their infant was receiving the "better" formula, they might be more inclined to stay with the study than if they were not in the enriched-formula group. If nurses knew the composition of the infants' formula, they might encourage mothers of the babies in the enriched formula group to stay with the project, etc.

Alternatively, a high dropout rate among the "control" babies might occur because of a real difference in effects of the formula. If these babies did not thrive well, the mothers might get discouraged with their progress and remove them from the study. If the babies doing poorly in the control group were removed, real differences between the two formulas might be obscured.

Finally, one should note that similarity of dropout rates for the two groups is not proof of lack of bias due to attrition. It is still possible that different segments of the two groups leave the study for different reasons but that the net effect would be similar rates of loss of cases. Where dropout rates are high, we must always consider the possibility of biased values for remaining children, even where the difference in dropout rates is not significant. High dropout rates could conceal a true effect or might in some way create a false appearance of an effect. Even moderate dropout rates can make for difficulties.

6. Comparison of Hemoglobin Values at 2–5 Weeks and at 20–26 Weeks (in gms %) (See Table 15-16).

$$\bar{d} = \frac{12.6}{5} = 2.52$$

$$s^2 = \frac{14.10}{4} = 3.525$$

$$s = 1.88$$

$$SE_{\bar{d}} = \frac{1.88}{5} = .84$$

$$\text{Obs. } t = \frac{\bar{d} - 0}{SE_{\bar{d}}} = \frac{2.52}{.84} = 3.00$$

$$3.00 > 2.78 \ (t_{.05 \text{ critical for 4 df}})$$

There is a significant difference in the hemoglobin values at 2–5 weeks compared to 20–26 weeks.

TABLE 15-16

Hgb, 2–5 Wks.	Hgb, 20–26 Wks.	d	$(d - \bar{d})$	$(d - \bar{d})^2$
16.3	11.9	4.4	1.88	3.53
14.1	12.1	2.0	−.52	.27
10.8	10.9	−.1	−2.62	6.86
13.0	11.0	2.0	−.52	.27
15.1	10.8	4.3	1.78	3.17
69.3	56.7	12.6	0	14.10

SUMMARY OF CHAPTER 15

In this chapter we have acquainted the reader with a few additional techniques. These techniques and some of their principal uses follow.

Linear regression
—for obtaining the best estimate of a dependent variable when the independent variable is known and the relationship is linear.

Correlation
—for studying the degree of linear relationship between two variables.

Analysis of Variance
—for comparing *two or more* sample means.

F distribution
—for analysis of variance problems; for comparing two independent sample estimates of a population variance.

Poisson distribution
—for studying events in time or space; as an approximation to the binomial when p is very small but n is very large.

Estimating sample size
—to help the investigator determine before he embarks upon an investigation the minimum size of the sample he will need to achieve a specified precision.

Bayes' Theorem
—to estimate a conditional probability of interest given certain other probability estimates.

Note: In this chapter we have attempted to expose the reader to some additional important concepts and methods and the assumptions underlying these methods. It is not possible to develop these methods adequately and to provide appropriate problem-solving exercises without going much more deeply into these areas. However, it is important that the reader be aware that these techniques exist and that they can be useful to him in his medical practice and in his research. We hope that this material will stimulate the reader to pursue these topics further in the many excellent, more advanced texts that are available.

CUMULATIVE GLOSSARY I: TERMS

Chapter 15

Regression Line	An equation which relates the average y (the dependent variable) to the associated value for x (the independent variable). For linear regression the equation is: $$y_c = a + bx$$
Regression Coefficient	The slope (b) of the regression line. Represents the average change in y per unit change in x. (See Glossary II.)

Mean Square Deviation from Regression	Average squared vertical deviation of the y values around the regression line: $$(s_{y \cdot x}^2)$$
Standard Deviation from Regression[1]	The square root of the average squared vertical deviation of the y values around the regression line: $$(s_{y \cdot x})$$
Least Squares Method	A method of fitting a regression line to a set of data so as to minimize the sum of squared vertical deviations of the y values around that line.
Coefficient of Determination	r^2, the square of the sample correlation coefficient. Like r, a measure of the degree of association between two variables. It indicates the proportion of variance in y associated with or ex-explained by the variance in x.
Analysis of Variance (ANOVA)	A method of partitioning variance into its parts, such as *between two or more* treatment groups and *within* treatment groups so as to yield independent estimates of the population variance. The ratio of these independent estimates then can be tested using the F distribution. This provides a method of significance testing on the sample means.
F *Distribution*	The distribution followed by the ratio of two independent sample estimates of a population variance, i.e., $F = s_1^2/s_2^2$. The shape of the distribution depends on two degree of freedom values associated respectively with s_1^2 and s_2^2.
Poisson Distribution	A discrete distribution (only 0 or positive integers possible) which may be derived as the limiting form of the binomial when p is very small but n is so large that $n \times p$ approaches a small finite constant. Has one parameter λ (lambda) which represents both the mean and the variance.
Bayes' Theorem	A theorem which is useful in obtaining conditional probabilities. One application is determining the probability of a disease given a symptom complex (or positive test) P(D/S), which takes into account knowledge of the probability of the symptom complex (or positive test) given the disease P(S/D). A simplified expression is: $$P(D/S) = \frac{P(D) \cdot P(S/D)}{[P(D) \cdot P(S/D)] + [P(\bar{D}) \cdot P(S/\bar{D})]}$$

---

[1] Often inappropriately called the Standard Error of the Estimate.

CUMULATIVE GLOSSARY II: SYMBOLS

Chapter 15

b

Regression coefficient, also called the slope of the regression line

$$= \frac{\Sigma(x - \bar{x})(y - \bar{y})/(n - 1)}{\Sigma(x - \bar{x})^2/(n - 1)} = \frac{\text{Covariance of x and y}}{\text{Variance of x}}$$

Note that b is the *sample* regression coefficient which estimates B, the *population* regression coefficient.

y_c

y value predicted from the regression equation $y_c = a + bx$; therefore always falls on the regression line.

λ

(Small Greek letter lambda). The single parameter (both mean and variance) of Poisson distribution.

$\bar{\bar{x}}$

Overall mean or weighted average of two or more sample means ($\bar{x}_i$).

k

Number of treatment groups (or sample means) in an experiment.

δ

(Small Greek letter delta). The difference between two values, as for example the permissible difference between the sample estimate and the true value

16
Reviews

Cumulative Review V:Qualitative Data •
Cumulative Review VI: Quantitative Data

Note: In this final review chapter, in order to highlight the differences and similarities between significance tests we will state them in more formal terms, i.e., the explicit Null Hypothesis H_0 and some alternative hypothesis H_a. To carry out a significance test at the α level, we must test under the conditions that the Null Hypothesis is true, e.g., that μ takes some particular Null Hypothesis value in which we are interested, μ_0. Therefore our hypothesis is H_0: $\mu = \mu_0$. An alternative hypothesis might be that the true mean does not equal the hypothesized mean μ_0 but equals some alternative mean which we can designate as μ_a. Thus

$$H_a: \mu = \mu_a \neq \mu_0$$

Similarly, when testing a sample proportion

FIGURE 16-1

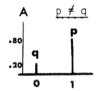 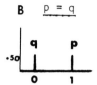

0   Attribute absent

1   Attribute present

we shall let the symbol p_0 represent the hypothesized null true proportion (comparable to μ_0) and p_a represent the true proportion under the alternative hypothesis (comparable to μ_a). Thus

$$H_0: p = p_0 \qquad H_a: p = p_a \neq p_0$$

In comparing two sample means our Null Hypothesis is that the true difference between population means μ_1 and μ_2 is 0, whereas an alternative hypothesis might be that the true difference between μ_1 and μ_2 is equal to some value, delta (δ), which is not equal to 0. Thus

$$H_0: (\mu_1 - \mu_2) = 0 \qquad H_a: (\mu_1 - \mu_2) = \delta \neq 0$$

A comparable statement for testing two sample proportions is

$$H_0: (p_1 - p_2) = 0 \qquad H_a: (p_1 - p_2) = \delta \neq 0$$

Although a few of these symbols are new, the reader should remember that the significance tests actually are carried out exactly as before when stated in a less formal manner.

CUMULATIVE REVIEW V
(Qualitative Data)
---

(1) BINOMIAL POPULATIONS

Binomial populations have two categories, p and q, where $q = 1 - p$, and therefore there is only *one* independent parameter. For example, in population A, 80% or .80 (p) have the attribute and 20% or .20 (q) do not (see Fig. 16-1).

FIGURE 16-2

 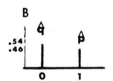

FIGURE 16-3

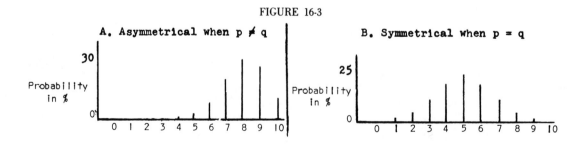

Number of successes out of 10 trials

Note: The sum of discrete probabilities equals 1 (or 100%)

FIGURE 16-4

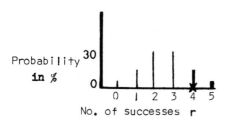

Probability **in %**

No. of successes **r**

x = the number of observed successes
P = the probability of 4 successes plus the probability of 5 successes

(2) BINOMIAL SAMPLES

In samples from binomial populations, $\hat{p}$ differs from p only by chance. For example, in sample A, 78% or .78 ($\hat{p}$) have the attribute and 22% or .22 ($\hat{q}$) do not (see Fig. 16-2).

(3) BINOMIAL SAMPLING DISTRIBUTIONS OF PROPORTIONS ($\hat{p}$)

We draw many samples of small size, for example, n = 10, from a binomial population and graph the frequency distribution of the number or proportion of successes. Against such a chance distribution the outcome in a sample of 10 is evaluated (see Fig. 16-3).

Example (for Small Samples Where n × p is < 5, or n × q is < 5)

When a new treatment is used, 4 out of 5 patients survive, i.e., $\hat{p}$ = .8. With the previous standard treatment, p = .5. Determine whether $\hat{p}$ is unusually high compared to p. A directional question such as this indicates a one-tailed test.

Significance Test

$$H_0: p = p_0 = .5 \qquad H_a: p = p_a > .5$$

Question: Is $\hat{p}$ larger than a p of .5 only by chance? Locate $\hat{p}$ on the chance distribution of sample proportions under the Null Hypothesis, and determine P, the probability of an outcome as extreme as or more extreme than that observed. Reject H_0 if P is less than the chosen level of significance. (See Fig. 16-4.)

Procedure: Use the Binomial Formula

$$\frac{n!}{r!(n-r)!} \, p^r q^{n-r}$$

P = the probability (r = 4) + the probability (r ≐ 5) where n = 5, p = .5, and q = .5 (one-tailed test).

$$P = \frac{5!}{4!1!} (.5)^4(.5)^1 + \frac{5!}{5!0!} (.5)^5(.5)^0$$
$$= 5(.5)^5 + (.5)^5 = .19$$

P ≐ .19, which is greater than the chosen level of significance (.05); therefore the Null Hypothesis is accepted. (Note that failure to obtain significance here primarily reflects inadequate study size.)

Confidence Limits

To obtain confidence limits on a true p, see Fig. 14-3, page 160.

(1) The C.L. can be used to test H_0: p = p_0. If p_0 is not within the confidence band, H_0 is rejected.

(2) The C.L. can also be used to set limits on what value p may actually take.

(4) NORMAL SAMPLING DISTRIBUTIONS OF PROPORTIONS ($\hat{p}$)

We draw many samples of large size, e.g., n = 100, from the binomial population and graph the frequency distribution of sample proportions. With large samples, the exact sampling distribution, the Binomial, is approximated by the Normal, provided p is not too close to 0 or 1. (See Fig. 16-5.)

FIGURE 16-5

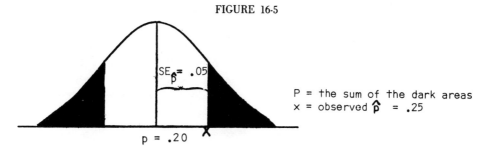

$SE_{\hat{p}}$ = .05

p = .20

P = the sum of the dark areas
x = observed $\hat{p}$ = .25

Some properties of the normal approximation to the binomial are:

(1) The average of the distribution of sample proportions is the true p, i.e., $\mu = p$.

(2) The Standard Deviation (σ) = Standard Error of Proportion $(SE_{\hat{p}}) = \sqrt{pq/n}$.

(3) Both p and n determine the size of the $SE_{\hat{p}}$ and therefore the reliability of the sample proportion as an estimate of p.

Example (for Large Samples, i.e., Where $n \times p$ and $n \times q \geqslant 5$)

A new treatment tried on 64 cases has a success rate of .25, i.e., $\hat{p} = .25$.

The previous recovery rate, based on long experience, for the standard treatment was $.20 = p$. Is the sample proportion .25 significantly different from a p of .20? Use a two-tailed test.

Significance Test

$$H_0: \ p = p_0 = .20 \qquad H_a: \ p = p_a \neq .20$$

Question: Is the true p of the population from which the sample was drawn really equal to an hypothesized p_0 of .20? Locate the observed $\hat{p}$ on the chance distribution of sample $\hat{p}$'s which is centered at p_0 under the Null Hypothesis. Determine P, the probability of an outcome as extreme or more extreme than that observed. Reject H_0 if the probability is less than the chosen level of significance (i.e., if $z_{obs.}$ is > $z_{critical}$, e.g., $z_{.05} = 1.96 = 2$). (see Fig. 16-5.)

Procedure: Use the Normal Deviate test.

$$n = 64, \ \hat{p} = .25, \ p_0 = .20$$

$$z^* = \frac{x - \mu}{\sigma} = \frac{\hat{p} - p_0}{SE_{\hat{p}}} = \frac{\hat{p} - p_0}{\sqrt{\dfrac{p_0 q_0}{n}}}$$

$$= \frac{.25 - .20}{\sqrt{\dfrac{(.20)(.80)}{64}}} = \frac{.05}{.05} = 1.00$$

Since

$$z_{obs.} = 1.00 < z_{.05} = 1.96$$

the Null Hypothesis that the true p of the popu-

---

* When numbers are small, a correction for continuity should be made:

$$z_c = \frac{\left(|\hat{p} - p_0| - \dfrac{1}{2n} \right)}{SE_{\hat{p}}}$$

lation from which the sample was drawn is .20 is accepted.

Confidence Limits

Let us assume that our sample value $\hat{p}$ is .375 instead of .25. Then our z test on H_0: $p = p_0 = .20$ is significant:

$$z = \frac{x - \mu}{\sigma} = \frac{\hat{p} - p_0}{SE_{\hat{p}}}$$

$$= \frac{\hat{p} - p_0}{\sqrt{\dfrac{p_0 q_0}{n}}} = \frac{.375 - .20}{\sqrt{\dfrac{(.20)(.80)}{64}}} = \frac{.175}{.05}$$

$$= 3.50 > 1.96 \text{ for } z_{.05}$$

It is unlikely that this sample comes from a binomial population where the true $p = .20$. What, then, is the true p likely to be?

$$95\% \text{ C.L. on } p = \hat{p} \pm z_{.05} \ (SE_{\hat{p}})$$

where $SE_{\hat{p}} \cong \sqrt{\hat{p}\hat{q}/n}$,

$$= .375 \pm 2 \sqrt{\frac{(.375)(.625)}{64}}$$

$$= .375 \pm 2(.0605) = .375 \pm .121$$

$$= .25, .50$$

95% C.I.
on true p

.20 .25   .50

Note that the 95% C.L. exclude the rejected value of .20.

(5) NORMAL SAMPLING DISTRIBUTIONS OF DIFFERENCES IN PROPORTIONS $(\hat{p}_1 - \hat{p}_2)$

In A of Fig. 16-6, we draw many independent random samples of large size, e.g., $n_1 = 100$, $n_2 = 100$, from the same binomial population and graph the frequency distribution of sample proportions. We also graph the curve of differences between the sample proportions, centered at the true difference of 0. This is the Null Hypothesis curve, which is used to evaluate a difference between two sample proportions. In B of Fig. 16-6, we draw similar curves for samples drawn from different populations. In this case, the center of the curve of sample differences, or true difference, is not 0.

Note: The Standard Deviation of the sampling distribution of differences is called the Standard Error of the Difference

$$SE_{\hat{p}_1 - \hat{p}_2} = \sqrt{\frac{p'q'}{n_1} + \frac{p'q'}{n_2}}$$

FIGURE 16-6

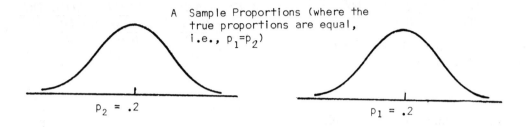

Normal Approximation to
<u>Distributions of Sample Proportions and of Sample Differences</u>

A Sample Proportions (where the
true proportions are equal,
i.e., $p_1 = p_2$)

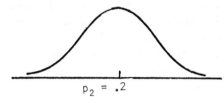

$p_2 = .2$ $p_1 = .2$

B Sample Proportions (where $p_1 \neq p_2$)

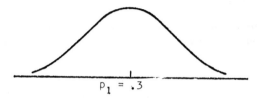

$p_2 = .2$ $p_1 = .3$

A   Sample Differences (where $p_1 = p_2 = .2$)
This is the Null Hypothesis Curve

B. Sample Differences (where
$p_1 \neq p_2$, $p_1 = .3$, $p_2 = .2$)

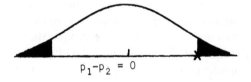

$p_1 - p_2 = 0$

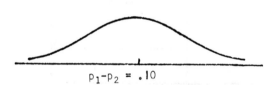

$p_1 - p_2 = .10$

(x = observed sample difference)

where p' is the estimated true proportion of the population. It is based on the overall observed proportion (under the Null Hypothesis of no true difference).

Example

100 patients with a particular disease who received treatment A have a recovery rate of 0.4. Another 100 with the same disease, who received treatment B have a recovery rate of 0.2. Is this consistent with equality of the true recovery rate for A and B?

Significance Test

$H_0: (p_1 - p_2) = 0$ $H_a: (p_1 - p_2) = \delta \neq 0$

Question: Does $(\hat{p}_1 - \hat{p}_2)$ differ from 0 only by chance? Locate the observed difference on the chance distribution of differences between sample proportions centered around a true difference of 0. Determine the probability (P)

of an outcome as extreme as or more extreme than that observed. Reject H_0 if P is less than the chosen level of significance.

Note: We <u>always</u> test against the Null Hypothesis curve of sample differences (Fig. 16-6A).

Procedure: Use the Normal Difference Test.

$$n_1 = 100, \ n_2 = 100, \ \hat{p}_1 = .4, \ \hat{p}_2 = .2$$

$$z^* = \frac{(\hat{p}_1 - \hat{p}_2) - 0}{SE_{\hat{p}_1 - \hat{p}_2}} = \frac{(\hat{p}_1 - \hat{p}_2) - 0}{\sqrt{\frac{p'q'}{n_1} + \frac{p'q'}{n_2}}}$$

* When numbers are small, a correction for continuity should be made: subtract $\frac{1}{2}$ from the numerator of the larger fraction and add $\frac{1}{2}$ to the numerator of the smaller fraction. For example, instead of

$$\hat{p}_1 - \hat{p}_2 = \left(\frac{40}{100} - \frac{20}{100}\right)$$

we would use, in the formula for z_c:

$$z_c = \left(\frac{39.5}{100} - \frac{20.5}{100}\right) \Big/ .065$$

$$p' = \frac{40 + 20}{100 + 100} = \frac{60}{200} = .3$$

$$q' = 1 - p' = .7$$

$$z = \frac{(.40 - .20) - 0}{\sqrt{\frac{(.3)(.7)}{100} + \frac{(.3)(.7)}{100}}} = \frac{.20}{.065} = 3.1$$

Since $z_{obs.}$ is $> z_{.05} = 1.96$, the difference is significant and H_0 is rejected.

Confidence Limits

The confidence limits may be used either to test H_0 or to obtain C.L. on the true difference.

95% C.L. on $p_1 - p_2 = (\hat{p}_1 - \hat{p}_2) \pm z_{.05} (SE_{\hat{p}_1 - \hat{p}_2})$

Here we do <u>not</u> assume that $p_1 = p_2$, so $SE_{\hat{p}_1 - \hat{p}_2}$ is estimated by

$$\sqrt{\frac{\hat{p}_1 \hat{q}_1}{n_1} + \frac{\hat{p}_2 \hat{q}_2}{n_2}}$$

$$95\% \text{ C.L.} = .20 \pm 2 \sqrt{\frac{(.4)(.6)}{100} + \frac{(.2)(.8)}{100}}$$

$$= .20 \pm 2(.063)$$

$$= .07, .33$$

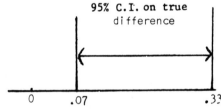

95% C.I. on true difference

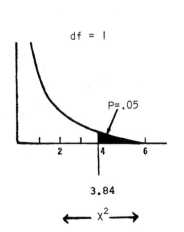

Note: The confidence interval ordinarily will not include 0 if the difference is significant using the Normal Difference Test.

(6) CHI SQUARE DISTRIBUTION

The shape of the Chi Square Distribution in Fig. 16-7 varies according to the number of independent values (degrees of freedom) contributing to the distribution. The total area under each curve = 1.

A. CONTINGENCY TABLES – COMPARISON OF SAMPLE DISTRIBUTIONS WITH EACH OTHER
χ^2 Test of Two Sample Proportions[1]
(2 × 2 Tables)

Example

Among patients with a severe disease, 20 out of 100 who receive Treatment A survive while 40 out of 100 receiving Treatment B survive. Is the survival rate different for Treatment A than Treatment B?

Note: This is the same example as that used for the Normal Difference Test of Two Sample Proportions; see (5).

Significance Test

$$H_0: (p_1 - p_2) = 0 \qquad H_a: (p_1 - p_2) = \delta \neq 0$$

Question: Are p_1 and p_2 really equal? Do $\hat{p}_1$ and $\hat{p}_2$ differ only by chance? Locate the observed χ^2 on the χ^2 distribution with 1 df and determine P, the probability of an outcome as extreme or more extreme, under the Null Hypothesis. If P is less than the chosen level of significance (e.g., $\alpha = .01$), reject the Null Hypothesis.

Procedure: The example above can be set up as a 2 × 2 contingency table (two rows and two columns)

$$\chi^2_{obs.} = \sum \frac{(O - E)^2}{E}$$

---

[1] Also called a test of association. Expected numbers must be ≥ 5.

FIGURE 16-7

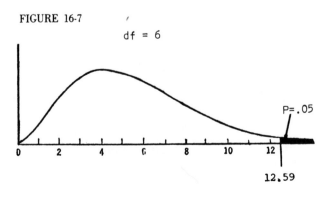

df = 1

df = 6

P=.05

P=.05

3.84

12.59

$\longleftarrow \chi^2 \longrightarrow$

$\longleftarrow \chi^2 \longrightarrow$

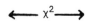

TABLE 16-1

	Number			
	Alive	Dead	Total	Proportion alive
Treatment A	20	80	100	$.20 = \hat{p}_1$
Treatment B	40	60	100	$.40 = \hat{p}_2$
	60	140	200	$.30 = p'$

$p' = $ Estimated common p under the assumption $p_1 = p_2 = p$

with $(r - 1)(c - 1)$ df, or 1 df since $r = 2$ and $c = 2$. ($O = $ observed number and $E = $ expected number for each cell.) (See Table 16-1.)

Note: Where numbers are small, use Yates' correction for continuity:

$$\chi_c^2 = \sum \frac{\left(|O - E| - \frac{1}{2}\right)^2}{E}$$

Expected no. alive for each group

$$= \left(\frac{\text{Total alive}}{\text{Total number}}\right)$$
$\times$ total number in each group
$$= \frac{60}{200} \text{ (or } p') \times \text{ total number in each group}$$

The expected number of dead are computed similarly.

	Alive		Dead	
	O	E	O	E
Treatment A	20	30	80	70
Treatment B	40	30	60	70
	60	60	140	140

Obs. $\chi_{1df}^2 = \sum \dfrac{(O - E)^2}{E} = \dfrac{(20 - 30)^2}{30}$

$\quad + \dfrac{(40 - 30)^2}{30} + \dfrac{(80 - 70)^2}{70}$

$\quad + \dfrac{(60 - 70)^2}{70}$

$\quad = \dfrac{100}{30} + \dfrac{100}{30} + \dfrac{100}{70} + \dfrac{100}{70}$

$\quad = 9.52 > \chi_{.01, 1df}^2 = 6.64$

Thus $P < .01$, and the difference is significant. (See Fig. 16-8.)

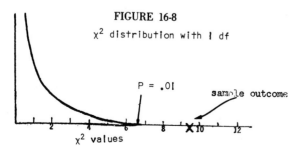

FIGURE 16-8

χ^2 distribution with 1 df

P = .01

sample outcome

χ^2 values

χ^2 Test of More than Two Sample Proportions (Multiple Samples or Multiple Categories), (r $\times$ c Tables)

Example

Among patients with a particular disease, 35 of 100 with Treatment A survive, 75 of 100 with Treatment B survive, and 40 of 100 with Treatment C survive. Is the survival rate different under the three treatments?

Significance Test

$\quad H_0: p_1 = p_2 = p_3 = p$
$H_a:$ Not all p_i's are equal, i.e.,
$\quad p_1$ and p_2 may be the same but
$\quad$ they differ from p_3.

Question: Do the sample proportions $\hat{p}_i$ differ only by chance? Locate the observed χ^2 on the Chi Square Distribution for the appropriate degrees of freedom and determine P, the probability of an outcome as extreme or more extreme, under the Null Hypothesis. If P is less than the chosen level of significance, reject H_0.

Procedure[1]:

$$\chi_{obs.}^2 = \sum \frac{(O - E)^2}{E}$$

with $(r - 1)(c - 1)$ df, or $(3 - 1)(2 - 1) = 2$ df. (See Table 16-2.)

TABLE 16-2

	Number			Proportion Alive
	Alive	Dead	Total	
Treatment A	35	65	100	.35
Treatment B	75	25	100	.75
Treatment C	40	60	100	.40
	150	150	300	$.50 = p'$

[1] For multicomparisons (r $\times$ 2 contingency tables), see Ryan, T. A., Significance Tests for Multiple Comparisons of Proportions, Variances, and Other Statistics, Psychol. Bull. 47:318, 1960.

Expected no. alive for each group

$$= \left(\frac{\text{Total alive}}{\text{Total number}}\right)$$

$\times$ total number in each group

$$= \frac{150}{300} \text{ (or p') } \times \text{ total number in each group}$$

The expected number of dead are computed similarly.

	Alive		Dead	
	O	E	O	E
Treatment A	35	50	65	50
Treatment B	75	50	25	50
Treatment C	40	50	60	50
	150	150	150	150

$$\text{Obs. } \chi^2_{\text{2df}} = \frac{(35-50)^2}{50} + \frac{(75-50)^2}{50}$$

$$+ \frac{(40-50)^2}{50} + \frac{(65-50)^2}{50}$$

$$+ \frac{(25-50)^2}{50} + \frac{(60-50)^2}{50}$$

$$= \left(\frac{1900}{50}\right) = 38$$

$$38 > \chi^2_{.01,2df} = 9.21, \ P \ll .001$$

Difference is significant. (See Fig. 16-9.)

FIGURE 16-9

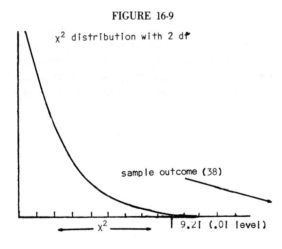

B. χ^2 TEST OF GOODNESS OF FIT OF A SAMPLE DISTRIBUTION TO A POPULATION DISTRIBUTION

Example 1

Could the observed (sample) distribution have arisen from a particular hypothetical population?

Blood groups are distributed as shown in Table 16-3 in the general population and in

TABLE 16-3

Blood Group	General Population Proportion	Cancer Patients No.	Cancer Patients Proportion
O	.45	40	.40
A	.40	45	.45
B	.10	9	.09
AB	.05	6	.06
	1.00	100	1.00

100 gastric carcinoma patients. Do gastric carcinoma patients have the same blood group distribution as the general population?

Significance Test

H_0: Gastric carcinoma patients have blood groups distributed the same as the general population

H_a: The blood groups are distributed differently in gastric carcinoma patients and the general population

Question: Are blood groups distributed the same in gastric carcinoma patients as in the general population? Locate the observed χ^2 on the Chi Square Distribution with the appropriate df, and determine P, the probability of an outcome as extreme or more extreme, under the Null Hypothesis. If P is less than the chosen level of significance, reject H_0 and accept H_a.

Procedure:

$$\chi^2 = \sum \frac{(O-E)^2}{E} \quad \text{with } (r-1) \text{ df*}$$

(See Table 16-4.)

TABLE 16-4

Blood Group	Observed No.	Expected No.	O − E	(O − E)²	(O − E)²/E
O	40	45	−5	25	25/45
A	45	40	+5	25	25/40
B	9	10	−1	1	1/10
AB	6	5	+1	1	1/5
	100	100	0		1.48

* In Goodness of Fit tests, an additional df is subtracted for each population parameter estimated from the data (e.g., if a normal distribution is fitted to an observed distribution and the parameters μ and σ are estimated from the data, 2 additional df are subtracted).

$$\text{Obs. } \chi^2_{3df} = \sum \frac{(O-E)^2}{E} = \frac{25}{45} + \frac{25}{40} + \frac{1}{10} + \frac{1}{5}$$
$$= 1.48$$
$$1.48 < \chi^2_{.05,3df} = 7.82, \text{ P} > .05$$

Difference between distributions is not significant (i.e., the fit is sufficiently good).

Example 2

The Goodness of Fit test can be used to compare an <u>observed proportion</u> with an <u>expected proportion</u>. In this case, the observed and expected distributions consist of only two categories. We use the example from the z-test on page 204 where a success rate of .25 for a new treatment tried on 64 cases is compared with an expected recovery rate of .20 based on the standard treatment. (See Table 16-5.)

TABLE 16-5

	Standard Treatment, Expected Proportion	New Treatment			
		Obs. Prop.	Obs. No. (O)	Exp. No. (E)	$(O-E)^2/E$
Success	.20	.25	16	12.8	$(3.2)^2/12.8$
Failure	.80	.75	48	51.2	$(-3.2)^2/51.2$
	1.00	1.00	64	64.0	

Significance Test

H_0: The distribution of outcomes for the new treatment is the same as that for the standard treatment

H_a: The new treatment is associated with a different outcome distribution than the standard

Question: Are outcomes distributed the same under the new treatment as under the standard treatment? Locate the observed χ^2 on the Chi Square distribution with 1 df and determine P, the probability of an outcome as extreme or more extreme, under the Null Hypothesis. If P is less than the chosen level of significance, reject H_0 and accept H_a.

Procedure:

$$\chi^2_{1df} = \sum \frac{(O-E)^2}{E}$$
$$= \frac{(3.2)^2}{12.8} + \frac{(-3.2)^2}{51.2} \sim 1.0 < 1.96 \therefore \text{P} < .05$$

Therefore, we observe the same result as with the z-test. (Remember, for 1 df, $\chi^2 = z^2$.) Since the result is not significant, we need not repeat the test with Yates' correction for continuity. If Yates' correction were used:

$$\chi^2_c = \sum \frac{[|O-E| - 0.5]^2}{E}$$
$$= \frac{(2.7)^2}{12.8} + \frac{(-2.7)^2}{51.2} = .71$$

Result not significant.

C. PAIRED CHI SQUARE TEST FOR NON-INDEPENDENT SAMPLE PROPORTIONS

This is McNemar's test for sample proportions which are <u>not</u> independent.

Example

A group of 80 patients are screened on two procedures for a disease. Is there a significant difference in the proportions of positive reactors for each of the two procedures?

Significance test

H_0: $(p_1 - p_2) = 0$ $\qquad$ H_a: $(p_1 - p_2) = \delta \neq 0$

Question: Are p_1 and p_2 really equal? Do $\hat{p}_1$ and $\hat{p}_2$ differ only by chance? Locate the observed χ^2 on the χ^2 distribution with 1 df and determine P, the probability of an outcome as extreme or more extreme, under the Null Hypothesis. If P is less than the chosen level of significance (e.g., $\alpha = .05$), reject the Null Hypothesis.

Procedure: McNemar's test (χ^2_{1df}): Ties are eliminated, and only those pairs with discrepant results on the two procedures are considered, e.g., categories B and C in Table 16-6.

TABLE 16-6

		Second Procedure		
		Positive	Negative	Total
First procedure	Positive	A = 40	B = 10	50
	Negative	C = 20	D = 10	30
	Total	60	20	80

$$\hat{p}_1 = \frac{50}{80} = .625 \qquad \hat{p}_2 = \frac{60}{80} = .75$$

Hypothetical Populations

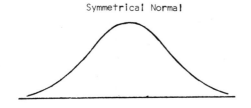

Symmetrical Normal   Symmetrical Non-normal

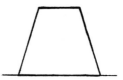

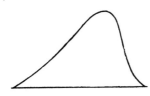

Non-symmetrical with left tail skew   Log Normal

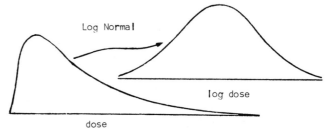

log dose

dose

$$\hat{p}_1 - \hat{p}_2 = \frac{B-C}{N} = \frac{10-20}{80} = -.125$$

$$\chi^2 = \frac{(B-C)^2}{B+C} = \frac{(10-20)^2}{10+20} = \frac{100}{30} = 3.33$$

$$\chi^2_c = \frac{(|B-C|-1)^2}{B+C} = \frac{(|10-20|-1)^2}{10+20}$$

$$= \frac{81}{30} = 2.70$$

$$3.33 \text{ or } 2.70 < 3.84 \text{ for } \chi^2_{.05,1df}$$

∴ There is no significant difference in the proportions positive for the two procedures.

CUMULATIVE REVIEW VI
(Quantitative Data)

(1) QUANTITATIVE POPULATIONS

These are populations of measurement of data such as temperatures or heights. These distributions of continuous populations can be of any shape, as is shown in Fig. 16-10.

See also Table 16-7 for summary measures of quantitative populations.

TABLE 16-7. *Summary Measures of Populations*

Measure	Interpretation
Mean (μ)	Arithmetic mean, $\Sigma x/N$
Variance (σ^2)	Measure of variability: average squared deviation around mean: $$\frac{\Sigma(x-\mu)^2}{N}$$
Standard deviation (σ)	Square root of variance: $$\sqrt{\frac{\Sigma(x-\mu)^2}{N}}$$
Coefficient of variation (C.V.)	$\sigma/\mu \times 100$ (dimensionless). Expresses S.D. as a percent of the mean
Median	Middle value of ordered data
Mode	Most frequent value
Range	Difference between the highest and lowest values
Quartiles, percentiles	Values that divide ordered data into 4 equal parts, 100 equal parts

FIGURE 16-11

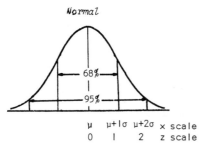

Normal

68%

95%

μ $\mu+1\sigma$ $\mu+2\sigma$ x scale
0   1   2   z scale

where $z = \frac{x-\mu}{\sigma}$

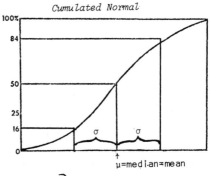

Cumulated Normal

100%
84
50
25
16
0

σ σ

μ=median=mean

84%-50%
50%-16% } Values on the abscissa = σ

FIGURE 16-12

Sample from Normal Population   Sample from Log Normal Population

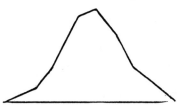
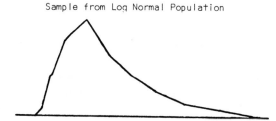

If the population is normally distributed, then μ and σ describe it completely. Any observation (x) from a normal distribution can be located on the Standard Normal Curve by the number of Standard Deviations (σ) it is from μ (i.e., $x - \mu$). Use the Standard Normal Deviate

$$z = \frac{x - \mu}{\sigma}$$

(See Fig. 16-11.)

(2) QUANTITATIVE SAMPLES

Like the binomial sample, the quantitative sample tends to be a replica of the parent population (Fig. 16-12). The sample mean ($\bar{x}$) estimates the population mean (μ); the sample standard deviation or (s) estimates the population standard deviation (σ):

$$\bar{x} = \frac{\Sigma x}{n} \quad \text{and} \quad s = \sqrt{\frac{\Sigma (x - \bar{x})^2}{n - 1}}$$

If the sample is from a Normal Population (see Fig. 16-12), the S.D. can be estimated as Sample Range/K. K is a constant whose value depends on the number in the sample (see Table 11-3).

(3) NORMAL SAMPLING DISTRIBUTIONS OF MEANS ($\bar{x}$)

We draw many random samples of large size, e.g., n = 30, from a quantitative population and graph the frequency distribution of the sample means. This curve is used for testing the significance of a sample mean (see Fig. 16-13). Note that the distribution of random sample means generally follows the Normal distribution, no matter what the shape of the original population, as $n \to$ becomes sufficiently large (Central Limit Theorem).[1]

The center of the distribution of sample means is the true μ. The S.D. of the distribution or $SE_{\bar{x}}$ is $\sigma / \sqrt{n}$. Both σ and $\sqrt{n}$ determine the size of the $SE_{\bar{x}}$ and therefore the reliability of the sample mean as an estimate of μ.

The probability under the Null Hypothesis of an outcome as extreme as or more extreme than that observed is determined from

$$z = \text{Standard Normal deviate}$$
$$= \frac{x - \mu}{\sigma} \quad \text{(general form)}$$

where x is the sample mean ($\bar{x}$), μ is the population mean, and S.D. $= \sigma_{\bar{x}}$ or $SE_{\bar{x}} = \sigma / \sqrt{n}$. Thus

$$z = \frac{\bar{x} - \mu}{\sigma / \sqrt{n}}$$

Example

Is a sample mean ($\bar{x}$) of 10 mm significantly different from $\mu = 13$ mm where n, the sample size, is 25 and σ^2 is <u>known</u> to be 25 mm?

---

[1] There is a technical requirement that the average value of Σx^2 be finite.

FIGURE 16-13

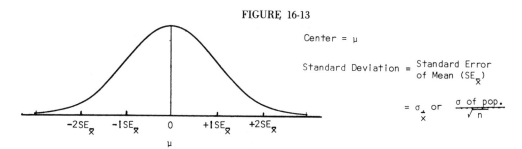

Center = μ

Standard Deviation = Standard Error of Mean ($SE_{\bar{x}}$)

$= \sigma_{\bar{x}}$ or $\frac{\sigma \text{ of pop.}}{\sqrt{n}}$

Significance Test

$$H_0: \mu = \mu_0 = 13 \qquad H_a: \mu = \mu_a \neq 13$$

Question: Is $\bar{x}$ really equal to μ (i.e., does an $\bar{x}$ of 10 mm differ from a true mean of 13 mm only by chance)? Locate $\bar{x}$ on the chance distribution of sample $\bar{x}$'s around the hypothesized μ_0. Determine P, the probability of an outcome as extreme or more extreme, under the Null Hypothesis. Reject H_0 if the probability is less than the chosen level of significance, i.e., if $z_{obs.}$ is $> z_{critical}$.

Procedure: Use the Normal Deviate test.

$$\mu_0 = 13, \ \bar{x} = 10, \ \sigma^2 = 25 \ (\sigma = 5), \ n = 25$$
$$z = \frac{\bar{x} - \mu_0}{\sigma/\sqrt{n}} = \frac{10 - 13}{5/\sqrt{25}} = \frac{-3}{1} = -3$$

Since the absolute value of $z_{obs.}$ is $3 > z_{.05} = 1.96$, the Null Hypothesis that the observed mean of 10 has come from a population whose mean (μ) is 13 is rejected.

Confidence Limits

The confidence limits may be used to test H_0 or to obtain C.L. on the μ for which $\bar{x}$ is an estimate.

$$\begin{aligned} \text{95\% C.L. on } \mu &= \bar{x} \pm z_{.05} \ (SE_{\bar{x}}) \\ &= \bar{x} \pm z_{.05} \ (\sigma/\sqrt{n}) \\ &= 10 \pm 2(1) = 8.0 \text{ mm}, 12.0 \text{ mm} \end{aligned}$$

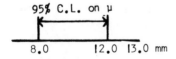

Note: The 95% C.L. do not include a μ of 13.

(4) *t*-DISTRIBUTION FOR TESTING SAMPLE MEANS ($\bar{x}$)

The *t*-distribution is a distribution of sample means where the <u>population variance σ^2 is not known</u> and instead the sample variance estimate, s^2, is used in the $SE_{\bar{x}}$ formula. Thus, instead of using

$$z = \frac{\bar{x} - \mu}{\sigma/\sqrt{n}} \quad \text{(normal distribution)}$$

we use

$$t = \frac{\bar{x} - \mu}{\text{Est. } SE_{\bar{x}}} = \frac{\bar{x} - \mu}{s/\sqrt{n}}$$

The *t*-distribution for small samples (e.g., for $n = 30$ or less) has more area in the tails than the Normal. Therefore a sample mean must be more standard errors of the mean away from μ to be significant, i.e., t must be larger than z for $P < .05$. The shape of the *t*-distribution depends on the $n - 1$ df which enter into s^2. It approaches the Normal as the df increase. Over 30 df, $t \sim z$. (See Fig. 16-14.)

Example

Is a sample mean ($\bar{x}$) of 10 mm significantly different from $\mu = 13$ mm where n, the sample size, is 25 and $s^2 = 36$? (σ^2 is not known.)

Significance Test

$$H_0: \mu = \mu_0 = 13 \qquad H_a: \mu = \mu_a \neq 13$$

Question: Is $\bar{x}$ really equal to μ (does an $\bar{x}$ of 10 mm differ from a true mean of 13 mm only by chance)? Locate $\bar{x}$ on the chance distribution of sample $\bar{x}$'s around μ_0. Determine P, the probability of an outcome as extreme or more extreme, under the Null Hypothesis. Reject H_0 if the probability is less than the chosen level of significance, i.e., if $t_{obs.} > t_{critical}$, e.g.,

$$t_{.05[(n-1)df=24]} = 2.1$$

Procedure: Use the *t*-test.

$$\mu_0 = 13, \bar{x} = 10, \ s^2 = 36, \ (s = 6), \ n = 25$$
$$t = \frac{\bar{x} - \mu_0}{\text{Est. } SE_{\bar{x}}} = \frac{\bar{x} - \mu_0}{s/\sqrt{n}} = \frac{10 - 13}{6/\sqrt{25}} = \frac{-3}{1.2} = -2.5$$

Since the absolute value of $t_{obs.} = 2.5 > 2.1$, $P > .05$, and H_0 is rejected.

FIGURE 16-14

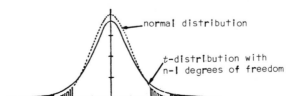

Confidence Limits

The confidence limits may be used either to test H_0 or to obtain C.L. on the true μ.

$$95\% \text{ C.L. on } \mu = \bar{x} \pm t_{.05(n-1df)} \text{ (Est. SE}_{\bar{x}})$$
$$= 10 \pm t_{.05,24df} \text{ (Est. SE}_{\bar{x}})$$
$$= 10 \pm (2.1)\,(1.2) = 10 \pm 2.5$$
$$= 7.5, 12.5$$

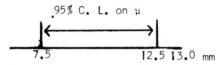

95% C. L. on μ

7.5   12.5 13.0 mm

The 95% C.L. do not include 13, so H_0 is rejected.

(5) NORMAL SAMPLING DISTRIBUTION OF DIFFERENCES BETWEEN INDEPENDENT MEANS $(\bar{x}_1 - \bar{x}_2)$

We draw two independent random samples, e.g., $n_1 = 25$, $n_2 = 25$, and determine the difference between the sample means. We repeat this operation many times, and graph the frequency distribution of differences. In A of Fig. 16-15, the two samples are drawn from the same population, and in B of the same figure from two different populations.

Note: We always test against the Null Hypothesis curve (the curve on the left of Fig. 16-15).

Example

Does a sample mean of 8 mm differ significantly from an independent sample mean of 5 mm where n_1 is 10, n_2 is 10, and you <u>know</u> that $\sigma_1^2 = \sigma_2^2 = 5$?

Significance Test

$H_0: (\mu_1 - \mu_2) = 0$ $H_a: (\mu_1 - \mu_2) = \delta \neq 0$

Question: Are μ_1 and μ_2 really equal? Do $\bar{x}_1$ and $\bar{x}_2$ differ only by chance? Locate the observed difference on the chance distribution of sample differences centered around a true difference of 0 (curve A). Determine P, the probability of a difference as extreme or more extreme, under the Null Hypothesis. Reject H_0 if the probability is less than (α) the chosen level of significance, i.e., reject H_0 if $z_{obs.}$ is $> z_{.05} = 1.96$ or 2.

Procedure: Use the Normal Difference test.

$$\bar{x}_1 = 8, \ \bar{x}_2 = 5, \ n_1 = 10, \ n_2 = 10, \ \sigma_1^2 = \sigma_2^2 = 5$$
$$z_{obs.} = \frac{(\bar{x}_1 - \bar{x}_2) - 0}{SE_{\bar{x}_1 - \bar{x}_2}} = \frac{(\bar{x}_1 - \bar{x}_2) - 0}{\sqrt{\dfrac{\sigma^2}{n_1} + \dfrac{\sigma^2}{n_2}}}$$
$$= \frac{8 - 5}{\sqrt{\dfrac{5}{10} + \dfrac{5}{10}}} = \frac{3}{1} = 3$$

Since $z_{obs.}$ is $> z_{.05}$, we reject the hypothesis that the true difference is 0.

Confidence Limits

The confidence limits may be used either to test H_0 or to obtain confidence limits on the true $\mu_1 - \mu_2$.

$$95\% \text{ C.L. on } \mu_1 - \mu_2 = (\bar{x}_1 - \bar{x}_2) \pm z_{.05} \, (SE_{\bar{x}_1 - \bar{x}_2})$$
$$= (8 - 5) \pm 2\,(1)$$
$$= 3 \pm 2 = 1, 5 \text{ mm}$$

95% C.L. on $\mu_1 - \mu_2$

0 1   5 mm

The 95% C.L. do not include 0 so H_0: $\mu_1 - \mu_2 = 0$ is rejected.

(6) t-DISTRIBUTION FOR TESTING DIFFERENCES BETWEEN INDEPENDENT SAMPLE MEANS $(\bar{x}_1 - \bar{x}_2)$

For a distribution of $(\bar{x}_1 - \bar{x}_2)$ differences where the <u>population variance</u> σ^2 is not known

FIG. 16-15. Distribution of differences between means of two samples: (A) From the same population $(\mu_1 = \mu_2 = \mu)$; (B) from different populations $(\mu_1 \neq \mu_2)$.

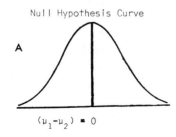

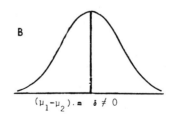

Null Hypothesis Curve

A $(\mu_1 - \mu_2) = 0$

B $(\mu_1 - \mu_2) = \delta \neq 0$

and must be estimated from the sample variances s_1^2 and s_2^2, use the t rather than the normal distribution, i.e., instead of

$$z = \frac{(\bar{x}_1 - \bar{x}_2) - 0}{\sqrt{\dfrac{\sigma^2}{n_1} + \dfrac{\sigma^2}{n_2}}}$$

use

$$t = \frac{(\bar{x}_1 - \bar{x}_2) - 0}{\sqrt{\dfrac{s_p^2}{n_1} + \dfrac{s_p^2}{n_2}}}$$

In the special case where $n_1 = n_2$,

$$t = \frac{(\bar{x}_1 - \bar{x}_2) - 0}{\sqrt{\dfrac{s_1^2}{n_1} + \dfrac{s_2^2}{n_2}}}$$

Note: $s_p^2 =$ pooled variance estimate based on s_1^2 and s_2^2.

Assumptions: (1) Each sample is randomly drawn from a normal population, and (2) the populations represented by the different samples have the same variance.

A. EXAMPLE ($n_1 = n_2$)

Does a sample mean of 8 mm differ significantly from one of 5 mm where n_1 is 10, n_2 is 10, $s_1^2 = 7$, and $s_2^2 = 3$?

Significance Test

H_0: $(\mu_1 - \mu_2) = 0$ H_a: $(\mu_1 - \mu_2) = \delta \neq 0$

Question: Are μ_1 and μ_2 really equal? Do $\bar{x}_1$ and $\bar{x}_2$ differ only by chance? Locate the observed difference on the chance distribution of sample differences centered around a true difference of 0. Determine P, the probability of an outcome as extreme or more extreme, under the Null Hypothesis. Reject H_0 if the probability is less than the chosen level of significance, i.e., if $t_{obs.}$ is $> t_{critical}$, e.g.,

$$t_{.05[(n_1-1)+(n_2-1)=18df]} = 2.1$$

Note: If $(n_1 - 1) + (n_2 - 1)$ is 30 or more, the z distribution approximates the t distribution and may be used instead.

Procedure: Use the t distribution of differences between independent sample means.

$\bar{x}_1 = 8$, $\bar{x}_2 = 5$, $n_1 = 10$, $n_2 = 10$, $s_1^2 = 7$, $s_2^2 = 3$

$$t_{obs.} = \frac{(\bar{x}_1 - \bar{x}_2) - 0}{\text{Est. SE}_{\bar{x}_1 - \bar{x}_2}}$$

$$= \frac{(\bar{x}_1 - \bar{x}_2) - 0}{\sqrt{(\text{Est. SE}_{\bar{x}_1})^2 + (\text{Est. SE}_{\bar{x}_2})^2}}$$

$$= \frac{(\bar{x}_1 - \bar{x}_2) - 0}{\sqrt{\dfrac{s_1^2}{n_1} + \dfrac{s_2^2}{n_2}}}$$

$$t_{obs.} = \frac{(8 - 5) - 0}{\sqrt{\dfrac{7}{10} + \dfrac{3}{10}}} = \frac{3}{1} = 3$$

Since $t_{obs.}$ is $3 > t_{.05,18df} = 2.1$, we reject the hypothesis that the true difference is 0.

Confidence Limits

The confidence limits may be used either to test H_0 or to obtain limits on the true $\mu_1 - \mu_2$.

95% C.L. on $\mu_1 - \mu_2 = (\bar{x}_1 - \bar{x}_2)$
$$\pm t_{.05[(n_1-1)+(n_2-1)df]} \times$$
$$(\text{Est. SE}_{\bar{x}_1 - \bar{x}_2})$$
$$= (8 - 5) \pm (2.1)(1)$$
$$= 3 \pm 2.1$$
$$= 0.9, 5.1 \text{ mm}$$

95% C.L. on $\mu_1 - \mu_2$

```
           |←----------------→|
   0      0.9              5.1 mm.
```

The 95% C.L. do not include 0, so H_0 is rejected.

B. EXAMPLE ($n_1 \neq n_2$)

Does a sample mean of 8 mm differ significantly from an independent sample mean of 5 mm where $n_1 = 10$, $n_2 = 20$, $s_1^2 = 7$, and $s_2^2 = 3$?

Significance Test

H_0: $(\mu_1 - \mu_2) = 0$ H_a: $(\mu_1 - \mu_2) = \delta \neq 0$

Question: Are μ_1 and μ_2 really equal? Do $\bar{x}_1$ and $\bar{x}_2$ differ only by chance? Locate the observed difference on the chance distribution of sample differences centered around a true difference of 0. Determine P, and reject H_0 if $t_{obs.} > t_{critical}$.

Procedure: Use the t test of $(\bar{x}_1 - \bar{x}_2)$ differences, particularly if $(n_1 - 1) + (n_2 - 1)$ is 30 or less. Estimate σ^2 from s_{pooled}^2 (i.e., weighted average of s_1^2 and s_2^2).

$$s_p^2 = \frac{(n_1 - 1)s_1^2 + (n_2 - 1)s_2^2}{(n_1 - 1) + (n_2 - 1)}$$

$$= \frac{9(7) + 19(3)}{9 + 19} = \frac{63 + 57}{28} = 4.3$$

$$t_{obs.} = \frac{(\bar{x}_1 - \bar{x}_2) - 0}{\text{Est. SE}_{\bar{x}_1 - \bar{x}_2}} = \frac{(\bar{x}_1 - \bar{x}_2) - 0}{\sqrt{s_p^2 \left(\frac{1}{n_1} + \frac{1}{n_2} \right)}}$$

$$= \frac{(8 - 5) - 0}{\sqrt{\frac{4.3}{10} + \frac{4.3}{20}}} = \frac{3}{.8} = 3.75$$

$$t_{critical} = t_{.05[(n_1-1)+(n_2-1)=28df]} = 2.0$$

Since $t_{obs.} > t_{.05,28df}$, we reject the hypothesis that the true difference is 0.

Confidence Limits

The confidence limits may be used to test H_0 or to obtain limits on the true $\mu_1 - \mu_2$.

$$95\% \text{ C.L. on } \mu_1 - \mu_2 = (\bar{x}_1 - \bar{x}_2)$$
$$\pm t_{.05(n_1+n_2-2df)} \times$$
$$(\text{Est. SE}_{\bar{x}_1-\bar{x}_2})$$
$$= (8 - 5) \pm (2.0)\ (.8)$$
$$= 3 \pm 1.6 = 1.4, \ 4.6 \text{ mm}$$

The 95% confidence limits do not include 0, so H_0 is rejected.

(7) DIFFERENCES BETWEEN MEANS OF PAIRED SAMPLES (NON-INDEPENDENT DATA)

With paired samples, we have a situation where two samples are not independent and may be correlated, i.e., matched pairs, "before" and "after" readings on the same patient, etc.

Example

The table below shows measurements (in mm) for 6 individuals before and after treatment. Is there a significant difference between the "before" and "after" mean values?

Individual	Before (y)	After (x)
1	14	15
2	12	13
3	13	14
4	14	16
5	18	17
6	13	15
Mean	14	15

A. t-TEST, ADJUSTING $SE_{\bar{x}-\bar{y}}$

Significance Test

$$H_0: \ (\mu_x - \mu_y) = 0 \qquad H_a: \ (\mu_x - \mu_y) = \delta \neq 0$$

Question: Are μ_x and μ_y really equal? Do $\bar{x}$ and $\bar{y}$ differ only by chance? Adjust $SE_{\bar{x}-\bar{y}}$ to take the non-independence of the samples into account, and then perform the usual t-test with df = number of pairs − 1.

Procedure: Use the t-test, adjusting $SE_{\bar{x}-\bar{y}}$.

$$t_{obs.} = \frac{(\bar{x} - \bar{y}) - 0}{SE_{\bar{x}-\bar{y}}}$$

and the

$$SE_{\bar{x}-\bar{y}} = \sqrt{(SE_{\bar{x}})^2 + (SE_{\bar{y}})^2 - 2r(SE_{\bar{x}})(SE_{\bar{y}})}$$

where r is the product moment correlation coefficient.

An alternative procedure gives the same mathematical result without requiring the calculation of r. (See "*t*-Test, Difference Method," next.)

B. t-TEST, DIFFERENCE METHOD ($\bar{d}$)

Obtain the difference (d) for each x, y pair, and consider it a new variate (see Fig. 16-16, p. 216).

Significance Test

$$H_0: \ (\mu_x - \mu_y) = 0, \text{ or } \mu_d = 0$$
$$H_a: \ (\mu_x - \mu_y) = \delta \neq 0, \text{ or } \mu_d = \delta \neq 0$$

Question: Are μ_x and μ_y really equal? Does $\bar{d}$ differ from 0 only by chance? Locate the sample difference $\bar{d}$ on the distribution of sample mean differences (3) centered at 0. Reject H_0 if $t_{obs.} > t_{critical}$ with (no. of pairs − 1) df.

Procedure: Use the t-test, Difference Method. (See Table 16-8, p. 216.)

$$s_d^2 = \frac{\Sigma(d - \bar{d})^2}{\text{No. of pairs} - 1} = \frac{6}{6 - 1} = 1.2$$
$$s_d = \sqrt{1.2}$$

$$\text{Est. SE}_{\bar{d}} = \frac{s_d}{\sqrt{\text{No. of pairs}}} = \frac{\sqrt{1.2}}{\sqrt{6}} = .45$$

$$t_{obs.} = \frac{\bar{d} - 0}{\text{Est. SE}_{\bar{d}}} = \frac{1}{.45} = 2.2$$

which is less than

$$t_{critical} = t_{.05(no.\ pairs-1df)} = t_{.05,5df} = 2.57$$

∴ Difference is not Significant.

FIGURE 16-16

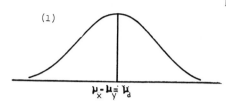

(1)

In the Population

The distribution of the *population of differences* (d) for x, y pairs centered at a true difference of μ_d:

S.D. of population $= \sigma_d$

$$= \sqrt{\frac{\Sigma(d - \mu_d)^2}{\text{No. of pairs (in the population)}}}$$

(2)

$$\bar{x} - \bar{y} = \bar{d}$$

In the Sample

The distribution of *one sample of differences* (d) for x, y pairs with a mean difference of $\bar{d}$.

S.D. of sample $= s_d = \sqrt{\frac{\Sigma(d - \bar{d})^2}{\text{No. of pairs (in the sample)} - 1}}$

(3)

$$\mu_d = 0$$

The Null Hypothesis Distribution

The sampling distribution of *many mean differences* ($\bar{d}$), centered around a hypothetical true difference μ_d of 0.

S.D. of sampling distribution $= SE_{\bar{d}}$

$$= \frac{s_d}{\sqrt{\frac{\text{No. of pairs}}{\text{(in each sample)}}}}$$

Confidence Limits

The confidence limits may be used to test H_0 or to obtain limits on the true mean difference.

95% C.L. on $\mu_d = \bar{d} \pm t_{.05, \text{ no. pairs}-1df} \times$
(Est. $SE_{\bar{d}}$)
$= 1 \pm 2.57(.45) = 1 \pm 1.16$
$= -0.16, +2.16$

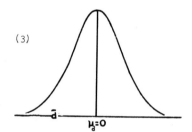

95% C.L. on μ_d

-0.16 0 $+2.16$ mm

The interval includes zero and therefore agrees with *t*-test (not significant).

C. SIGN TEST

Significance Test

If on the average the true paired difference were 0, under a symmetrical model[1] we would expect as many positive differences as negative differences, i.e., the probability of a + difference is equal to the probability of a − difference = 50%. Use the binomial formula with p = .5 to calculate the probability of ob-

[1] Our Null Hypothesis in making the sign test is actually that x and y are identically distributed, so that the true average difference is zero and, further, the x − y values are symmetrically distributed around zero.

TABLE 16-8. *Values in Millimeters*

Individual	Before (y)	After (x)	(x − y) = (d)	(d − $\bar{d}$)	(d − $\bar{d}$)²
1	14	15	+1	0	0
2	12	13	+1	0	0
3	13	14	+1	0	0
4	14	16	+2	+1	1
5	18	17	−1	−2	4
6	13	15	+2	+1	1
Total	84	90	+6 = Σd	0	6 = Σ(d − $\bar{d}$)²
Mean	14	15	+1 = $\bar{d}$	(check)	

taining a sample proportion of $+$ (or $-$) signs as extreme as that observed or more extreme. If a difference is 0, ignore it, i.e., reduce the sample size by the number of 0 differences (or ties). The Binomial formula is

$$\frac{n!}{r!(n-r)!}\, p^r q^{n-r}$$

Procedure: Sign Test: In the above example, $n = 6$, $p = .5$, and we observed $5 +$ differences and no ties. Therefore, P, the probability of an outcome as extreme or more extreme (two-tailed), under the Null Hypothesis, is:

$$\text{The sum of}\begin{cases}P(6) + P(5) = \dfrac{6!}{6!0!}\,(.5)^6(.5)^0 \\[2pt] \qquad + \dfrac{6!}{5!1!}\,(.5)^5(.5)^1 \\[2pt] \qquad = .016 + .094 = .11 \\[2pt] P(0) + P(1) = \dfrac{6!}{0!6!}\,(.5)^0(.5)^6 \\[2pt] \qquad + \dfrac{6!}{1!5!}\,(.5)^1(.5)^5 \\[2pt] \qquad = .016 + .094 = .11\end{cases} = .22$$

Since $P = .22 > P = .05$, the difference is not significant.

Notes on the Sign Test

(1) The Sign Test is a non-parametric test, i.e., it does not require the assumption of the t-test that the differences are normally distributed.

(2) If the assumption of normality is valid, then, for detecting a true difference between means, the sign test is less likely than the t-test to lead to rejection of the Null Hypothesis when untrue.

(3) A two-tailed sign test cannot yield significant results at the .05 level unless there are at least 6 non-zero (non-tied) pairs.

(4) If the number of non-zero pairs is large, then [(no. pairs) $\times$ (.5)] will be ≥ 5 and the normal approximation to the binomial (i.e., normal sampling distribution of proportions) or z test may be used for the sign test.

(8) TEST OF MORE THAN TWO SAMPLE MEANS (ANALYSIS OF VARIANCE)

Where more than two sample means are to be evaluated, e.g., three treatment groups and a placebo group, we cannot validly perform a t test comparing all possible pairs of means at the $t_{.05}$ level, as this would include a test comparing the highest sample mean and the lowest sample mean. This extreme comparison would yield a t value greater than $t_{.05}$ with probability much in excess of .05. Therefore we use the analysis of variance technique.

Significance Test

$$H_0: \mu_1 = \mu_2 = \mu_3 \ldots \mu_k$$
$$H_a: \text{Not all } \mu_i\text{'s are equal}$$

Assumptions: (1) Each sample is randomly drawn from a normal population, and (2) the populations represented by the different samples have the same variance.

Procedures:

(a) Partition the variance into its components, i.e., partition the sum of squared deviations or the "sum of squares" (SS) into "between" and "within" sample components.

(b) Use these subdivisions of the SS to derive two independent estimates of the population variance.

(c) Use the F ratio[1] to compare these estimates:

$$F = \frac{\text{Estimate of } \sigma^2 \text{ from variance } \textit{between} \text{ sample means}}{\text{Estimate of } \sigma^2 \text{ from variance } \textit{within} \text{ sample means}}$$

$$= \frac{(\text{Between means SS})/(k-1)}{(\text{Within means SS or residual SS})/(N-k)}$$

$$= s^2_{\text{pooled}}$$

(d) Do a one-tailed F test since if the samples are not from the same population, we would expect more variability *between* the samples than *within* them and consequently a larger numerator in the observed F compared to the denominator.

(e) Reject H_0 if F_{observed} exceeds F_{critical}. Then use a multicomparison technique to determine which sample means are significantly different.

(9) BIVARIATE DATA

Here we are concerned with the simultaneous distribution of measurements of *two*

---

[1] F distribution with df in numerator and denominator.

FIGURE 16-17

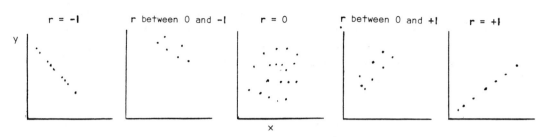

variables. We wish to evaluate the relationship between these variables.

A. CORRELATION OR DEGREE OF ASSOCIATION

How are x and y related? Through use of the sample correlation coefficient or (r) we can obtain a quantitative measure of the degree of *linear* relationship. r is independent of any particular unit of measurement. It indicates the *strength* of association for any array of data.

r can be used <u>only</u> when x and y are assumed to arise from a bivariate population and has special applicability when the bivariate population is normal. Under other circumstances, non-parametric correlation methods can be used.

r can vary from 0 (no linear relationship) to +1 for a perfect positive or −1 for a perfect negative linear relationship. If as x increases y does also, the relationship is positive. If as x increases y decreases, it is negative. The relationship is "perfect" if all y values fall on a straight line which is non-horizontal. (See Fig. 16-17.)

Assuming that the bivariate population is normal, we can test the null assumption that the population correlation coefficient (ρ) (rho) is zero.

Note: A sample correlation coefficient may be statistically significant but be too weak to be of use. It may also be strong (close to +1 or −1) but because of sample size may not be significant when tested. Even if it is significant this does not imply cause and effect, as there may be spurious correlation, or each variable may be related independently to a common third factor.

B. REGRESSION

If after visual inspection x and y in Fig. 16-18 appear to have a linear relationship, we can fit a regression line to the data (assuming that the y populations for each x value have equal variances).

The line which best fits the data is the one which gives the <u>least</u> <u>sum of squared vertical deviations</u> around the line.

The fitted sample regression line is described by the equation $y_c = a + bx$, where a is the y intercept and b is the slope or average change in y per unit change in x.

Note: The regression line should never be extended much beyond the limits of the observational data unless there is good reason to suppose that the linear relationship continues to hold.

FIGURE 16-18

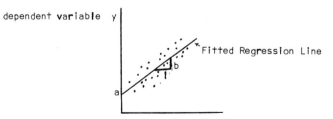

17
Miscellaneous Exercises

The purpose of this last chapter of the text is to challenge the reader to test his understanding of basic statistics by solving a "mixed bag" of short exercises.[1] It is relatively simple to solve a problem where the analytic method is suggested by the chapter heading. It is more difficult, and at the same time more realistic, to be required to select the appropriate method (or methods) without such hints.

Here are some guidelines as to how to approach a statistical problem:

(1) First, be very clear in your mind that you understand specifically what question is being asked.

(2) Be certain that the question is answerable by the data given. For this set of exercises you can assume that this preliminary screening has been done for you. But when presented with a practical problem it will be necessary for you to decide not only what the question of interest is, but also whether it can be answered validly by the data, i.e., that the design of the experiment is sound, that the appropriate type of measurement has been made or the appropriate unit has been enumerated, and that no bias has been introduced in the collection of this information.

(3) Be certain that the question being asked is, in your judgment, clinically important, for example, that only those differences which you consider large enough to matter in the outcome of patient care are being tested for statistical significance.

(4) You now proceed to the method of statistical analysis. The first major question here is: Are the data (a) *qualitative* (i.e., categorical, such as "allergic" or "non-allergic") or (b) *quantitative* (i.e., measurement data of height, time, weight, or another continuous variable)? This distinction is of basic importance because, although there are many similarities

in the approach to the two types of data, there are specific differences in method with a larger number of parameters involved in most quantitative distributions.

(5) The second major methodologic question is: Do these data represent the distribution of individuals in a population (or sample), or do they represent the distribution of a statistic derived from samples, such as a distribution of sample means around a true mean or a distribution of sample differences around a true difference between population means? With qualitative data the problem is almost always concerned with a sampling distribution because the population itself is readily described (by p). With quantitative data, many problems are concerned with the *description* of the distribution of the population (or sample) of individuals because of the larger number of parameters involved in such a description. Other problems are concerned with the sampling distribution of estimates of these parameters (sample means, standard deviations, etc.) for the purpose of *inference* regarding the population (true) value.

(6) The size of the sample or experiment is another important consideration in the method. If the population proportions multiplied by the size of the sample, i.e., $(n \times p)$ and $(n \times q)$ are 5 or more, then large sample methods, such as the normal distribution of sample. proportions, can be used instead of the binomial expansion in solving qualitative problems. Similarly, if the standard deviation of the quantitative population is unknown and must be estimated from the sample, then the t-distribution must be used in estimating the standard error of the sample mean, unless the sample size is greater than 30, in which case the normal distribution is adequate.

In the solutions to the exercises that follow, these basic statistical criteria are listed to help you approach the problem in a systematic

---

[1] This chapter was suggested by Colin White, Yale University School of Medicine, who also provided the data for many of the exercises.

fashion. More complete tables than those used in the previous chapters are available in the Appendix.

As a gentle warning, the last two problems present two common errors in statistical evaluation and interpretation of data.

PROBLEM 17-1

Match the type of sampling with the sampling procedure in the following.

Type of Sampling

A. Biased sampling.
B. Simple random sampling.
C. Systematic sampling.
D. Matched (case control) sampling.

Sampling Procedure

(1) 100 cases drawn from a clinic file on the basis of a randomly selected last digit of the case number (e.g., every case ending with the digit 2).

(2) 100 cases drawn from a clinic file on the basis of a table of random numbers.

(3) 100 cases drawn from a clinic file with same age, sex, color, and socioeconomic status as found in 100 patients in a study of malignant hypertension.

(4) 100 cases drawn from a clinic file on the basis of two randomly selected first letters of the surname (e.g., every patient whose surname begins with the letters B or M).

Answers

(1) C   Such sampling is usually not biased unless the last digit is assigned on the basis of position in family or other selective factor.
(2) B
(3) D
(4) A   Because of the association of surname with ethnic group, "alphabetic" sampling is almost always biased.

PROBLEM 17-2

A. Comparison of Group Means by the *t*-test.
B. Analysis of Variance.
C. Chi Square Analysis.
D. Evaluation of a Mean Difference.

E. Rank Order Correlation.
F. Product Moment Correlation.

In each of the following studies, which of the above statistical tests would be appropriate for analyzing the data recorded?

(1) A comparison of the systolic blood pressure recorded in normal subjects who had been recumbent for 5 min with their hands at their sides and after the arm had been raised to drain the venous blood.

(2) A comparison of the gain in weight over a period of 1 month for one group of infants given a supplemented diet and another group given a standard diet.

(3) A comparison of data on reaction time after administration of three tranquilizers and a placebo. Patients in a large ward were randomly allocated into four groups for the different treatment.

(4) The relation between serum uric acid levels and serum creatinine levels in presumably healthy pregnant women in their second trimester.

(5) The relation between psychiatric clinic man-hours per 1000 population and the median per capita income in each state.

(6) A comparison of the presence of Australian antigen in the serum of children with Down's syndrome and of other children in an institution for the mentally retarded.

Answer

(1) D   The evaluation of a mean (paired) difference would be involved here since the two samples are not independent.

(2) A   The *t*-test of group means would be appropriate since the measurements are on two independent samples.

(3) B   Analysis of Variance is needed since data have been collected on four groups of patients and all four samples means must be considered together. If F is significant, we could then compare treatments by a multi-comparison technique (see Chapter 15).

(4) F   These data probably meet the assumptions of the product moment correlation coefficient model: that the two variables have a bivariate normal distribution (see Chapter 15).

(5) E   Here we can be almost certain that the two variables are not normally distributed, and therefore a non-parametric (distribution-free) method, such as rank order correlation is preferred.

(6) <u>C</u> These data are qualitative, and therefore the Chi Square analysis is appropriate.

PROBLEM 17-3

It is desired to survey the health needs of a multiethnic population residing in a large census tract to be served by a new Health Maintenance Organization. The census tract consists of 100 blocks. Approximately 200 households are to be sampled. Match the sampling procedure with the type of sampling listed below, and discuss its merits.

Type of Sampling

A. Simple Random Sampling.
B. Two-Stage Stratified Sampling.
C. Area Cluster Sampling.
D. Systematic Sampling.

Sampling Procedure

(1) The 100 blocks are classified on the basis of ethnicity and median rent into five fairly homogenous subgroups of 20 blocks each. Four blocks are selected randomly from each subgroup, and 10 households are selected from each of these 20 blocks.

(2) Five blocks are selected randomly from the 100 blocks and 40 households then selected randomly from each of these five blocks.

(3) 200 households are selected randomly from all households in the area.

(4) Every n^{th} household in the tract is selected, yielding 200 households.

Answer

(1) <u>B</u> This is probably the best method of sampling the households. Stratification will tend to assure that households from each ethnic subgroup are included in the sample and will tend to reduce the sampling variance. Selecting households from only 20 blocks will reduce the survey costs [see (3) below].

(2) <u>C</u> This is not a desirable method because not all ethnic subgroups may be included in the five randomly chosen blocks.

(3) <u>A</u> Simple random sampling should result in a fairly "representative" sample. However, the principal difficulty with this method is the expense involved in: (a) establishing an adequate sampling frame of households for the entire census tract and (b) traveling to

households scattered throughout the tract. The sampling variance will tend to be larger than with stratification.

(4) <u>D</u> In addition to the problem of travel cost as in (3), there is possible bias (e.g., if every n^{th} house is a corner house with higher rentals).

PROBLEM 17-4

A. Biological Variation.
B. Validity.
C. Precision.
D. Observer Variation.
E. Bias.

Which of the above terms can be correctly used to describe a characteristic of each of the following five studies?

(1) Blood samples were supplied as coded duplicates to a laboratory technician who analyzed them for serum cholesterol level, being unaware either of the presence of check samples or identity of pairs.

(2) Bacterial counts on 12 plates were read by each of three technicians.

(3) A study was carried out at Harvard University where physiologic data were obtained on "normal" young men with regard to pulse rate, blood pressure, weight, height, etc. The data on any one factor were recorded by the same observer.

(4) Records of children from 10 private elementary schools in a particular city were used as the sampling frame to estimate the status of immunization against poliomyelitis of all children aged 6 through 10 in a large city.

(5) A study is carried out of the effects of ethanol ingestion, in which an observer's description of the degree of intoxication is compared to the plasma osmolality for each patient.

Answer

(1) <u>C</u> Since the technician has recorded results for duplicates from the same sample, it is possible to determine the closeness (precision) of repeated measurements.

(2) <u>D</u> The differences here between the counts for the 12 plates, each read by three observers, reflect observer variation.

(3) <u>A</u> Since all data on any one factor have been recorded by the same observer, differences observed from student to student could be attributed to biological variation.

(4) <u>E</u> Private school children are not necessarily representative of the general school population in a city. They may have had special advantages in health care, resulting in a higher percentage immunized than would appear in a sample drawn from all types of schools in the city.

(5) <u>B</u> On the assumption that plasma osmolality is highly correlated with plasma ethanol concentration and the degree of intoxication in a patient,[1] an observer's findings could be validated by the plasma osmolality.

PROBLEM 17-5

An investigator is interested in the relationship between two variables (such as blood urea nitrogen and serum creatinine) A and B in uremic patients in general. Which of the two studies below is more appropriate?

Study

(1) 16 simultaneous measurements of A and B on the same individual.

(2) 16 simultaneous measurements of A and B on 16 different individuals.

Answer

Study 2 is more appropriate for inference for all uremic patients. In study 1 the 16 measurements all pertain to the same individual and therefore can be used to draw conclusions with respect to that individual only; inference for uremic patients in general is not possible.

PROBLEM 17-6

A. P. Shapiro, et al. report (Development of Bacteriuria in a Hypertensive Population, Ann. Intern. Med. 74:861–868, 1971) that 20% of hypertensive outpatients will have urine with a positive reaction to a catalase test on initial screening. Among such patients with positive catalase 30% turn out to have bacteriuria.

(a) What proportion of hypertensive patients can be predicted to have bacteriuria when first seen?

[1] Robinson, A., et al.: Ethanol Ingestion—Commonest Cause of Elevated Plasma Osmolality? New Eng. J. Med. 248:1253, June, 1971.

(b) What assumption is made in the above answer?

Answer

Type of data: Qualitative, given a probability for a positive catalase test among hypertensive outpatients and a conditional probability for the presence of bacteriuria.

Method: Use definition of conditional probability, and apply the multiplication rule to obtain the compound probability.

Solution

(a) The probability of a hypertensive outpatient having a positive catalase test = .20. The probability that a patient already having a positive catalase test will have bacteriuria = .30. Therefore, the probability of a patient having bacteriuria is: $.20 \times .30 = .06$.

Conclusion: 6% of the hypertensive patients can be predicted to have bacteriuria when first seen.

(b) It assumes that it is not possible for a patient with a <u>negative</u> catalase test to have bacteriuria. The authors state that, because of the association of non-catalase producing enterococci with other urinary tract infections and inflammations resulting in production of catalase, "in only a rare instance was a negative catalase test associated with an infected urine." If such false negatives are not very rare, a more complicated analysis would be necessary.

PROBLEM 17-7

In a random sample of 150 men from a certain population there are 120 who smoke. Find the 99% confidence limits for the true percent of smokers in the population from which the sample was drawn.

Answer

Type of data: Qualitative; presents a sample outcome and a desired confidence level.

Method: Use the formula for the interval estimate for the true proportion.

Solution

99% C.L. on true $p = \hat{p} \pm z_{.01} \, (\mathrm{SE}_{\hat{p}})$

$$= \hat{p} \pm z_{.01} \, \sqrt{\frac{\hat{p}\hat{q}}{n}}$$

$$\hat{p} = \frac{120}{150} = .8$$

$$\hat{q} = \frac{30}{150} = .2$$

$$\therefore 99\% \text{ C.L.} = .8 \pm 2.58 \sqrt{\frac{(.8)(.2)}{150}}$$

$$= .8 \pm .08$$

$$= .72 \text{ and } .88$$

The true proportion of smokers is likely to lie between .72 and .88 (with 99% confidence).

PROBLEM 17-8

Assume that the gestation period for women follows a normal distribution, with a mean of 280 days and standard deviation of 10 days. In what proportion of cases would you expect gestation periods of:
(a) 300 days or more?
(b) 313 days or more?

Answer

Type of data: Quantitative; gives the parameters (mean and standard deviation) of the normal distribution of a population of individuals.

Method: Obtain areas of the standard normal curve where

$$z = \frac{x \text{ (observed value)} - \mu \text{ (mean value)}}{\sigma \text{ (Standard Deviation of population)}}$$

Solution

(a) $z = \dfrac{x - \mu}{\sigma} = \dfrac{300 - 280}{10} = 2$

That is, 300 days is 2 standard deviations beyond the mean. The area between μ and $\pm 2\sigma = .9545$, while the area beyond in both tails is .0455. The area in one tail (beyond 300) is one-half of .0455 or .0228 or 2.28%. A gestation period of 300 days or more is likely in 2.28% of the cases.

(b) $z = \dfrac{313 - 280}{10} = 3.3$

When $z = 3.3$, the area in both tails is approximately .0010. The area beyond 313 is one-half of this, i.e., .0005 or .05%. A gestation period of 313 days or more is likely in .05% of the cases.

PROBLEM 17-9

The effect of fresh orange juice was compared with that of an equivalent amount of synthetic ascorbic acid in treating guinea pigs suffering from scurvy. The response measured was the length in mm of the odontoblasts at the end of a six-week period.

(a) Test the hypothesis that the means of the populations from which the samples were drawn are the same. State the significance level you propose to use; accept or reject the Null Hypothesis; and interpret your findings.

(b) Find the 99% confidence limits on the true difference between the population means.

Length of odontoblasts in mm

Orange juice	Ascorbic acid
8.2	4.2
9.4	5.2
9.7	5.8
9.7	6.4
10.0	7.0
14.5	7.3
15.2	10.0
16.1	11.2
17.6	11.2
21.5	11.5

Answer

Type of data: Quantitative; shows the distributions of two independent samples.

Method: Use the *t*-test between two independent means where the population variance is not known and $n_1 = n_2$ (based on the distribution of chance differences between two independent sample means around a true difference of 0).

Solution

(a) Assume the Null Hypothesis, which states that the two samples were drawn from populations with the same mean. Use a 5% significance level. (See Table 17-1).

TABLE 17-1

	Data in mm	
	Group A	Group B
n	10	10
$\bar{x}$	13.19	7.98
$s^2 = \dfrac{\Sigma(x - \bar{x})^2}{n - 1}$	19.63	7.54
$\dfrac{s^2}{n} = (\text{Est. SE}_{\bar{x}})^2$ (since $s/\sqrt{n} = \text{Est. SE}_{\bar{x}}$)	1.96	.75

$$t = \frac{(\bar{x}_1 - \bar{x}_2) - 0}{\text{Est. SE}_{\bar{x}_1 - \bar{x}_2}}$$

and since $n_1 = n_2$,

$$\text{Est. SE}_{\bar{x}_1 - \bar{x}_2} = \sqrt{(\text{Est. SE}_{\bar{x}_1})^2 + (\text{Est. SE}_{\bar{x}_2})^2}$$
$$t = \frac{(13.19 - 7.98) - 0}{\sqrt{1.96 + .75}} = \frac{5.21}{1.65} = 3.16$$

Degrees of freedom $= n_1 + n_2 - 2 = 18$
Critical $t_{.05, 18df} = 2.10$
Obs. $t = 3.16 > 2.10$ $\therefore P < .05$
Reject H_0

Conclusion: From the above test statistic, one would conclude that the means of the populations from which these samples were drawn are significantly different. It would seem likely that the difference observed is due to the difference in treatment between the two groups, orange juice giving the greater length of odontoblasts.

(b) 99% Confidence Limits on the true difference between the means of the two populations:

$$99\% \text{ C.L.} = (\bar{x}_1 - \bar{x}_2) \pm t_{.01, 18df} (\text{Est. SE}_{\bar{x}_1 - \bar{x}2})$$
$$= 5.21 \pm 2.88 \ (1.65)$$
$$= 5.21 \pm 4.75$$
$$= 0.46 \text{ mm} \qquad 9.96 \text{ mm}$$
$$\quad \ \ \textit{lower} \qquad\qquad \textit{upper}$$
$$\quad \ \ \textit{limit} \qquad\qquad \ \ \textit{limit}$$

PROBLEM 17-10

The disease cystic fibrosis is caused by an autosomal recessive gene and is manifested in the homozygous condition.

(a) Given that a family is identified because of the occurrence of the disease in one child, what is the probability that the next child will manifest the disease?

(b) What is the likelihood that, of 4 children, 2 or more will be affected if both parents are carriers?

Answer

Type of data: Qualitative; gives information about the genetics of cystic fibrosis which can be used to determine an expected proportion.

Method: We make use of the multiplication and addition rules for calculating probability and of the binomial distribution of sample proportions around an expected proportion (small sample method) since $n \times p$ (or $n \times q$) is <5.

Solution

(a) Although the occurrence of the disease in one child identifies each parent as having a recessive gene for cystic fibrosis, it in no way affects the probability of the next child manifesting the disease. According to Mendelian law, we must calculate a joint probability, i.e., the probability of a recessive gene from the father and a recessive gene from the mother, by use of the multiplication rule:

$$\text{Prob. (homozygous recessive)} = P_F \times P_M$$
$$= \tfrac{1}{2} \times \tfrac{1}{2} = \tfrac{1}{4}$$

Therefore, there is a 25% chance that the second child will manifest the disease.

(b) Use the binomial formula

$$\frac{n!}{r!(n-r)!} \, p^r q^{n-r}$$

where $n = 4$, $p = \tfrac{1}{4}$, and $q = \tfrac{3}{4}$.

The problem is to find the probability of 2, 3, or 4 affected children.

$$P \ (r = 2) = \frac{4!}{2!2!} \left(\frac{1}{4}\right)^2 \left(\frac{3}{4}\right)^2 = \frac{54}{256}$$
$$P \ (r = 3) = \frac{4!}{3!1!} \left(\frac{1}{4}\right)^3 \left(\frac{3}{4}\right)^1 = \frac{12}{256}$$
$$P \ (r = 4) = \frac{4!}{4!0!} \left(\frac{1}{4}\right)^4 \left(\frac{3}{4}\right)^0 = \frac{1}{256}$$

$$P \ (r = 2, 3, \text{ or } 4) = \frac{67}{256}$$
$$\text{(by the addition rule)}$$

The probability that 2 or more of 4 children will manifest the disease is $67/256 = .26$.

PROBLEM 17-11

Is there an association between the use of pooled plasma and the development of jaundice? In the data below, patients who received pooled plasma are compared with those who received whole blood (whole blood was taken from a single donor for each patient in whom it was used).

Answer

Type of data: Qualitative; shows outcomes of two independent samples.

Method: Since all expected numbers ≥ 5, use large sample methods, either (a) the Chi Square test for a 2×2 contingency table, or (b) the test based on the normal distribution of chance differences between two sample proportions centered at a true difference of 0.

Solution

(a) Chi Square contingency test: see Table 17-2.

TABLE 17-2

Transfusion	Number of Patients Who		
	Developed Jaundice	Did Not Develop Jaundice	Total
Whole blood	2 (8.1)*	246 (239.9)	248
Pooled plasma	13 (6.9)	201 (207.1)	214
Total	15	447	462

* ( ) = expected numbers obtained from overall p' and q' times the total number in each group where $p' = \frac{15}{462} = .0325$, $q' = \frac{447}{462} = .9675$.

$$\chi^2 = \sum \frac{(O - E)^2}{E}$$
$$= \frac{(2 - 8.1)^2}{8.1} + \frac{(13 - 6.9)^2}{6.9}$$
$$+ \frac{(246 - 239.9)^2}{239.9} + \frac{(201 - 207.1)^2}{207.1}$$
$$= 10.32$$

Degrees of freedom $= (r - 1)(c - 1) = 1$
Critical χ^2 for P $= .01$, 1 df $= 6.63$
Obs. $\chi^{2*} = 10.32 > 6.63$ ∴ P $< .01$

Conclusion: Reject H_0 and conclude that there is an association between the use of pooled plasma and the development of jaundice.

(b) Normal Difference test:

$n_1 = 248$ $n_2 = 214$

$\hat{p}_1 = \frac{2}{248} = .00806$ $\hat{p}_2 = \frac{13}{214} = .06074$

$p' = \frac{15}{462} = .0325$ $q' = \frac{447}{462} = .9675$

$$z = \frac{(\hat{p}_1 - \hat{p}_2) - 0}{\sqrt{\frac{p'q'}{n_1} + \frac{p'q'}{n_2}}}$$
$$= \frac{(.00806 - .06074) - 0}{\sqrt{(.0325)(.9675)\left(\frac{1}{248} + \frac{1}{214}\right)}} = -3.19$$

---

* If Yates' correction is used,

$$\chi_c^2 = \sum \frac{\left(|O - E| - \frac{1}{2}\right)^2}{E} = 8.54$$

However, the conclusion is the same.

Critical $z_{.01} = 2.58$
Obs. z $= |3.19| > 2.58$ ∴ P $< .01$

Conclusion: Reject H_0. Same result as with method (a) since $\chi_{1df}^2 = z^2$. If the continuity correction for z is used, the results would be the same as χ^2 with Yates' correction.

PROBLEM 17-12

A survey is being planned to determine the number of grams of protein eaten each day, on the average, by the adults in a defined population. The standard deviation of the daily intake is estimated as 15 gms. If we wish to have a 95% chance of obtaining a mean which is within 5 gms of the correct value, how many subjects should we study?

Answer

Type of data: Quantitative; presents an estimated standard deviation σ of a population of individuals, an allowable error δ and a confidence level.

Method: Use the formula for calculating n, given the above specifications.

Solution

$$n = \frac{z^2\sigma^2}{\delta^2}$$

where $z_{.05} \sim 2$, $\sigma = 15$ gms, and $\delta = 5$ gms. Then

$$n = \frac{(2)^2(15)^2}{(5)^2} = 36$$

Conclusion: A sample size of 36 would give us a 95% chance of obtaining an estimate of the population mean that is within 5 gms of the correct value.

PROBLEM 17-13

If samples of size 25 are drawn from a normally distributed population with mean of 20 mg and standard deviation of 4 mg, within what range will the middle 90% of the sample means fall?

Answer

Type of data: Quantitative; presents the parameters (mean and standard deviation) of a normally distributed population and the theoretical distribution of samples from this population.

Method: Use the normal distribution of sample means around a true mean and obtain areas of the standardized normal curve where

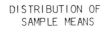

$$z = \frac{\text{(Obs. sample mean)} - \text{(Population mean)}}{\text{Standard Error of the mean}}$$

$$= \frac{\bar{x} - \mu}{SE_{\bar{x}}}$$

Solution

μ (population mean) $= 20$ mg
σ (population standard deviation) $= 4$ mg
n (size of samples) $= 25$
$SE_{\bar{x}} = \sigma/\sqrt{n} = 4/\sqrt{25} = .8$

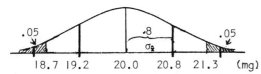

DISTRIBUTION OF
SAMPLE MEANS

From the tables of areas of the normal curve: to provide an area in both tails $= 1 - .90 = .10$ (i.e., $P = .10$), z must be 1.64.

Substituting in

$$z = \frac{\bar{x} - \mu}{SE_{\bar{x}}}$$

and solving for $\bar{x}$:

$$\bar{x} = \mu + z(SE_{\bar{x}})$$
$$= 20 + 1.64(.8)$$
$$= 21.3 \text{ mg}$$

Similarly,

$$\bar{x} = 20 - 1.64(.8)$$
$$= 18.7 \text{ mg}$$

90% of the sample means ($\bar{x}$) will fall between the values 18.7 mg and 21.3 mg.

PROBLEM 17-14

An investigator measured the systolic blood pressures of 12 children in an age range of 5 to 16. The results are as follows where:

x = Age in years
y = Systolic blood pressure (in mm Hg)

Child	x	y
JR	5	94
AB	6	100
CL	7	101
MR	8	105
BS	9	107
JP	10	108
DW	11	110
ES	12	110
SP	13	115
NJ	14	114
HB	15	118
AD	16	119

Is there a relationship between age and systolic blood pressure? What type of relationship does it appear to be and what formula represents such a relationship?

Answer

Type of data: Quantitative; presents data on two variables, one dependent and one independent.

Method: Graph and visually inspect the plot for a relationship between the two variables.

Solution

See Fig. 17-1.

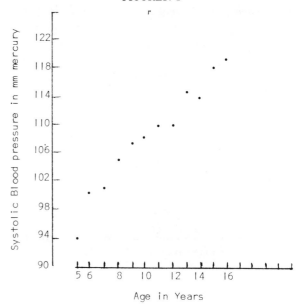

FIGURE 17-1

Conclusion: A relationship does seem to exist between the two variables. As the age increases, the systolic blood pressure also increases; therefore the relationship is positive.

The relationship appears to be that of a straight line and can be represented by the formula $y_c = a + bx$, where a is the y intercept and b is the slope or sample regression coefficient (i.e., average change in y per unit change in x).

PROBLEM 17-15

In a certain large area, 10% of the dwelling units are defective. If a random sample of 200 units is examined, what is the probability of finding 30 or more defective?

Answer

Type of data: Qualitative; shows an expected proportion and a sample outcome.

Method: Use the normal approximation to the binomial distribution of sample proportions around an expected proportion, and obtain areas of the standardized normal curve where

$$z = \frac{\left(\begin{array}{c}\text{Obs. sample} \\ \text{proportion}\end{array}\right) - \left(\begin{array}{c}\text{True} \\ \text{proportion}\end{array}\right)}{\text{Standard Error of proportion}}$$

Solution

$$z = \frac{\hat{p} - p}{\sqrt{\dfrac{pq}{n}}}$$

where

$$p = .10 \qquad q = .90$$
$$\hat{p} = \frac{30}{200} = .15$$
$$n = 200$$

$$z = \frac{.15 - .10}{\sqrt{\dfrac{(.10)(.90)}{200}}} = \frac{.05}{.0212} = 2.36$$

For $z \sim 2.4$, $P = .0164$ for both tails. However, we are interested in the upper tail only: $\frac{1}{2}P = .0082$, which is the probability of finding 30 or more defective dwelling units.

PROBLEM 17-16

Cyclamate salts fed to rats produced extensive hyperplasia and polyps in the bladders of 10 out of 20 animals. No such changes were found in any of the 20 control animals. Is the proportion of rats that developed hyperplasia and polyps significantly different in the experimental and control groups?

Answer

Type of data: Qualitative; shows outcomes of two independent samples.

Method: Since all expected values ≥ 5, use large sample methods, either (a) the Chi Square test for a 2×2 contingency table or (b) the test based on the normal distribution of chance differences between two sample proportions centered at a true difference of 0.

Solution

(a) Chi Square contingency test (Table 17-3):

TABLE 17-3

	Control	Cyclamate Treated	Total
Hyperplasia and polyps	0 (5)	10 (5)	10
No hyperplasia and polyps	20 (15)	10 (15)	30
Total	20	20	40

Overall $p' = \dfrac{10}{40} = .25$, overall $q' = \dfrac{30}{40} = .75$; expected numbers obtained from p' and $q' \times$ total in each group are shown in parentheses.

$$\chi^2 = \sum \frac{(O - E)^2}{E}$$
$$= \frac{(0 - 5)^2}{5} + \frac{(20 - 15)^2}{15} + \frac{(10 - 5)^2}{5}$$
$$+ \frac{(10 - 15)^2}{15}$$
$$= 5^2 \left(\frac{8}{15}\right) = 13.3$$

Critical $\chi^2_{.01,1df} = 6.63*$
Obs. χ^2 of $13.3 > 6.63$ $\therefore P < .01$

Since the numbers are small, we use Yates' correction

$$\chi^2_c = \sum \frac{\left(|O - E| - \frac{1}{2}\right)^2}{E}$$

although we are well beyond a borderline significance; $\chi^2_c = 10.8$ and the conclusion is the same.

---

* Since we suggested that cyclamate might increase the frequency of hyperplasia and polyps, it would have been reasonable here to make a one-tailed test for which the critical χ^2 value is 5.41 and the critical z value is 2.33.

TABLE 17-4

$$P\ (r = 0) = \frac{4!}{0!4!}\ (.2)^0 (.8)^4 = \ .4096 = \text{Probability that 0 will have an allergic reaction}$$

$$P\ (r = 1) = \frac{4!}{1!3!}\ (.2)^1 (.8)^3 = \ .4096 = \text{Probability that 1 will have an allergic reaction}$$

$$P\ (r = 2) = \frac{4!}{2!2!}\ (.2)^2 (.8)^2 = \ .1536 = \text{Probability that 2 will have an allergic reaction}$$

$$P\ (r = 3) = \frac{4!}{3!1!}\ (.2)^3 (.8)^1 = \ .0256 = \text{Probability that 3 will have an allergic reaction}$$

$$P\ (r = 4) = \frac{4!}{4!0!}\ (.2)^4 (.8)^0 = \ \underline{.0016} = \text{Probability that 4 will have an allergic reaction}$$

$$\text{Total} = 1.0000$$

Conclusion: Reject H_0 and conclude that the proportions of rats that developed hyperplasia and polyps in the experimental and control groups do differ significantly.

(b) Normal difference test:

$$n_1 = 20 \qquad n_2 = 20$$
$$\hat{p}_1 = 0 \qquad \hat{p}_2 = .50$$
$$p' = .25 \qquad q' = .75$$

$$z = \frac{(\hat{p}_1 - \hat{p}_2) - 0}{\sqrt{\dfrac{p'q'}{n_1} + \dfrac{p'q'}{n_2}}}$$

$$= \frac{(0 - .5) - 0}{\sqrt{\dfrac{(.25)(.75)}{20} + \dfrac{(.25)(.75)}{20}}} = -3.65$$

Critical $z_{.01} = 2.58$
Obs. z of $|3.65| > 2.58$ $\therefore P < .01$

Conclusion: Reject H_0.

Note: Same conclusion as with method (a) since $\chi^2_{1df} = z^2$. If the continuity correction for z is used, the results would be the same as χ^2 with Yates' correction.

PROBLEM 17-17

Suppose that the proportion of people who have an allergic reaction to a certain drug is known to be 0.2. A physician uses the drug in treating 4 patients. Find the theoretical distribution of the number of patients who have an allergic reaction in samples of size 4. What is the probability that there will be one or more reactors?

Answer

Type of data: Qualitative; shows an expected proportion and size of a sample.

Method: Use binomial distribution of sample proportions around an expected proportion (small sample method) since $n \times p$ (or $n \times q$) is < 5.

Solution

Expand the binomial formula

$$\frac{n!}{r!(n-r)!}\ p^r q^{n-r}$$

where p = .2, q = .8, n = 4, r = 0 to 4, n − r = 4 to 0. (See Table 17-4.)

Conclusion: There is a 60 percent chance that there will be one or more reactors as obtained from the sum of the last 4 terms, or from 1 − probability that there will be no reactors (.4096).

PROBLEM 17-18

The data in Table 17-5 give the hemoglobin concentration, in grams per 100 milliliters of blood, of two groups of infants who were 1

TABLE 17-5

Data in gm/100 ml	
Group A	Group B
18.6	22.5
17.3	25.3
15.7	22.0
22.0	22.3
18.7	25.1
18.1	22.8
18.3	23.5
21.6	24.0
19.7	20.8
21.0	21.1
19.3	22.2
21.0	24.7
18.0	20.5
21.0	
20.9	

week old. In Group A, the umbilical cord had been clamped immediately after the birth of the infant, and in Group B the cord was not clamped until the placenta began to descend the vagina.

(a) Test the hypothesis that the means of the populations from which the samples were drawn are the same. State the significance level you propose to use, accept or reject the Null Hypothesis, and give a statement in which you interpret your findings.

(b) State the assumptions made in carrying out the test.

(c) Find the 99% confidence limits on the true difference between the population means.

Answer

Type of data: Quantitative; shows the distributions of two independent samples.

Method: Use the t-test between two independent sample means where the population variance is not known and $n_1 \neq n_2$ (based on the distribution of chance differences between two independent sample means around a true difference of 0).

Solution

(a) Assume the Null Hypothesis, which states that the two samples were drawn from populations with the same means. Use a 5% significance level.

Data in gm/100 ml

	Group A	Group B
n	15	13
$\bar{x}$	19.413	22.831
$s^2 = \dfrac{\Sigma(x-\bar{x})^2}{n-1}$	3.2655	2.549

$$t = \frac{(\bar{x}_1 - \bar{x}_2) - 0}{\text{Est. SE}_{\bar{x}_1 - \bar{x}_2}}$$

Since $n_1 \neq n_2$, we use

$$s_p^2 = \frac{(n_1 - 1)s_1^2 + (n_2 - 1)s_2^2}{(n_1 - 1) + (n_2 - 1)}$$
$$= \frac{(14)(3.2655) + 12(2.549)}{26} = 2.9348$$

$$\text{Est. SE}_{\bar{x}_1 - \bar{x}_2} = \sqrt{\frac{s_p^2}{n_1} + \frac{s_p^2}{n_2}}$$
$$= \sqrt{\frac{2.9348}{15} + \frac{2.9348}{13}} = .649$$

$$t = \frac{(19.413 - 22.831) - 0}{.649} = \frac{-3.418}{.649} = -5.27$$

Degrees of freedom $= (n_1 - 1) + (n_2 - 1)$
$$= 26$$
Critical $t_{.05, 26df} = 2.06$
Obs. $t = |5.27| > 2.06$ ∴ $P < .05$
Reject H_0

Conclusion: From the above test statistic, one would conclude that the means of the populations from which these samples were drawn are significantly different. It would seem that the difference in treatment between the two groups had some effect on the hemoglobin concentration.

(b) The assumptions are that all sample means are drawn independently and from normal populations with equal variances. The Null Hypothesis of equality of means is then essentially that of identity of the two distributions.

(c) 99% confidence limits on the true difference between the two population means:

$$99\% \text{ C.L.} = (\bar{x}_1 - \bar{x}_2) \pm t_{.01, 26df} (\text{Est. SE}_{\bar{x}_1 - \bar{x}_2})$$
$$= -3.418 \pm 2.78 (.649)$$
$$= -3.418 \pm 1.804$$
$$= -5.22 \text{ gm/100 ml}$$
lower limit
$$= -1.61 \text{ gm/100 ml}$$
upper limit

Conclusion: These limits do not include zero; therefore the difference is significant. (If the 99% C.L. did include zero, the difference would not be significant at the .01 level).

PROBLEM 17-19

An entomologist carried out the following experiment as a test of a proposed mosquito repellent. Thirty-five volunteers had one forearm treated with a small amount of repellent and the other with a control solution. The subjects did not know on which forearm the repellent had been used. At dusk the volunteers exposed themselves to mosquitoes and reported which forearm was bitten first.

In 12 of the 35 subjects the forearm that had been treated with the test substance was bitten first. Make a statistical report on the findings.

Answer

Type of data: Qualitative; presents a sample outcome (expected proportion to be deduced).

Method: If the Null Hypothesis were true, we would expect half of the subjects to have their repellent-treated arm bitten first and half to have their control arm bitten first, i.e., the expected proportion $p = \frac{1}{2}$. Since $(n \times p)$ and $(n \times q) \geq 5$ use large sample method, (a) a test based on the normal curve of sample proportions centered around an expected proportion, or (b) a Chi Square Goodness of Fit test comparing an observed distribution with an expected distribution.

Solution

(a) Comparison of an observed with an expected proportion using the normal curve:

Expected proportion $p = \dfrac{1}{2}$, $q = \dfrac{1}{2}$

Obs. proportion $\hat{p} = \dfrac{12}{35} = .3429$

$$SE_{\hat{p}} = \sqrt{\frac{pq}{n}}$$

$$= \sqrt{\frac{\left(\frac{1}{2}\right)\left(\frac{1}{2}\right)}{35}} = .084$$

$$z = \frac{\hat{p} - p}{SE_{\hat{p}}} = \frac{.3429 - .50}{.084}$$

$$= -1.87$$

Critical $z_{.05} = 1.96$

Obs. $z = |1.87| < 1.96$

$\therefore P > .05$

Conclusion: Accept H_0.

(b) Chi Square Goodness of Fit test: see Table 17-6.

TABLE 17-6

	Observed Distribution	Expected Distribution
Repellent arm bitten first	12	$\frac{1}{2}$ or 17.5
Nonrepellent arm bitten first	23	$\frac{1}{2}$ or 17.5
Total	35	35

$$\chi^2 = \sum \frac{(\text{Observed} - \text{Expected})^2}{\text{Expected}}$$

$$\chi^2 = \frac{(12 - 17.5)^2}{17.5} + \frac{(23 - 17.5)^2}{17.5}$$

$$= 3.46$$

$$df = (r - 1) = 1$$

Critical $\chi^2_{.05,1df} = 3.84$

Obs. $\chi^{2*} = 3.46 < 3.84 \therefore P > .05$

---

* If Yates' correction is used,

$$\chi^2_c = \sum \frac{\left(|O - E| - \frac{1}{2}\right)^2}{E} = 2.86$$

Conclusion: We can accept the Null Hypothesis and conclude that there is no significant difference between the control solution and the proposed mosquito repellent. Note that this is in agreement with the results of method (a) since $\chi^2_{1df} = z^2$. If the continuity correction for z is used, the results would be the same as χ^2 with Yates' correction.

In both procedures just illustrated, however, significance at the .05 level would have obtained had we made a one-tailed test. The deviation from expectation was in the same direction as would have been anticipated had the repellent been effective. For a one-tailed test the critical z value would have been 1.64 and the critical χ^2 2.71.

Addendum

This is really an example of paired observations since the two arms on the same individual are not independent. A person may have a natural body odor which repels mosquitoes and therefore no arm is bitten, or both arms may be bitten at the same time. In these situations we ignore the tied pairs and proceed with McNemar's test. McNemar's test is:

$$\chi^2_{1df} = \frac{\left(\begin{array}{c}\text{No. of}\\\text{positive}\\\text{pairs}\end{array} - \begin{array}{c}\text{No. of}\\\text{negative}\\\text{pairs}\end{array}\right)^2}{\left(\begin{array}{c}\text{No. of}\\\text{positive}\\\text{pairs}\end{array}\right) + \left(\begin{array}{c}\text{No. of}\\\text{negative}\\\text{pairs}\end{array}\right)}$$

$$= \frac{(23 - 12)^2}{23 + 12} = 3.46$$

χ^2 corrected for continuity (χ^2_c) is

$$= \frac{(|23 - 12| - 1)^2}{23 + 12} = 2.86$$

Note: This is the same as the sign test as previously discussed in Problem 13-8. Also, since all pairs here are "contradictory," McNemar's test yields the same result as methods (a) and (b).

PROBLEM 17-20

In a particular "short-term" hospital, the average (mean) length of stay is 10 days and the standard deviation is 8 days. It is proposed to study a sample of 100 patients.

(a) What kind of distribution will the patients in the sample follow?

(b) If you took many such samples what

kind of distribution would the sample means follow?

(c) What would be the mean and standard deviation of the distribution of sample means?

(d) What proportion of sample means would be expected to exceed 11.6 days?

Answer

Type of data: Quantitative; gives the parameters (mean and standard deviation) of a population of individuals and the size of samples to be drawn from the population.

Method and Solution

(a) The distribution of a single random sample from a population will tend to resemble the parent population. (The shape of the parent population is not known but is most likely skewed to the right.[1])

(b) Generally a normal distribution even though the parent population may not be normal (see Central Limit theorem).

(c) The distribution of sample means would have as its center the population mean (μ): average $\bar{x} = \mu = 10$ days.

The standard deviation of the distribution of sample means ($SE_{\bar{x}}$) will depend on the sample size (n) and the population variability expressed by σ.

$$SE_{\bar{x}} = \frac{\sigma}{\sqrt{n}} = \frac{8}{\sqrt{100}} = .8 \text{ days}$$

(d) Determine the z value of the normal distribution of sample means as described above where $\bar{x} = 11.6$ and $\mu = 10$.

$$z = \frac{\bar{x} - \mu}{SE_{\bar{x}}} = \frac{11.6 - 10}{.8} = 2.0$$

The phrasing of this question requires use of only the upper tail of the distribution. For a z value of 2.0, P for both tails is .0455 and $\frac{1}{2}$ P for one tail is .0228. 2.28% of the sample means would be expected to exceed 11.6 days.

PROBLEM 17-21

The erythrocyte sedimentation rates for 10 subjects were measured both before and after treatment for a certain disease. The results are shown in Table 17-7.

---

[1] For this reason, the median should be calculated as well as the mean.

TABLE 17-7

| Subject | Erythrocyte Sedimentation Rate (mm/hr) | |
	Before Treatment	After Treatment
1	10	6
2	13	9
3	6	3
4	11	10
5	10	10
6	7	4
7	8	2
8	8	5
9	5	3
10	9	5

(a) Test the hypothesis that the true mean of the pair differences is zero. State the significance level you propose to use; accept or reject the Null Hypothesis; interpret your findings.

(b) Find the 95% confidence limits on the true mean of the pair differences.

Answer

Type of data: Quantitative; presents a series of paired values (before and after) on 10 subjects.

Method: (1) Use the modified *t*-test for paired data, based on the distribution of mean pair differences around a true difference of 0 (i.e., where the two samples are not independent of each other), or (2) use the non-parametric sign test.

Solution

(a) (1) For the paired *t*-test, assume H_0, that the true mean paired difference is zero. Set P = .05.

| Subject | d | (d − d̄) | (d − d̄)² |
	(mm/hr)		
1	+4	+1	1
2	+4	+1	1
3	+3	0	0
4	+1	−2	4
5	0	−3	9
6	+3	0	0
7	+6	+3	9
8	+3	0	0
9	+2	−1	1
10	+4	+1	1
	30	0	26
		(*check*)	

$$\bar{d} = \frac{30}{10} = 3.0$$

$$s_{\bar{d}}^2 = \frac{\Sigma(d - \bar{d})^2}{\text{No. of pairs} - 1} = \frac{26}{9} = 2.89$$

$$t = \frac{\bar{d} - 0}{\text{Est. SE}_{\bar{d}}} = \frac{\bar{d} - 0}{\sqrt{\dfrac{s_{\bar{d}}^2}{\text{No. of pairs}}}} = \frac{3.0 - 0}{\sqrt{\dfrac{2.89}{10}}}$$

$$= \frac{3.0}{.537} = 5.59$$

df = No. of pairs − 1 = 9
Critical $t_{.05, 9df} = 2.26$
Obs. $t = 5.59 > 2.26$ ∴ P < .05

Conclusion: Reject H_0 and conclude that there is a significant difference between the Before and After mean values, i.e., their difference is significantly different from the expected value of 0.

(2) For the sign test, nine of the Before treatment measurements are higher than the After treatment measurements (the tied pair is excluded); therefore 9 + signs are recorded and 0 − signs. By use of the binomial formula where n = 9, p = 0.5, and q = 0.5, we calculate the probability of 9 + signs or 0 + signs since this is a two-tailed test.

$$\text{Prob. (9)} = \frac{9!}{9!0!}(.5)^9(.5)^0 = \frac{1}{512} = .00195$$

$$\text{Prob. (0)} = \frac{9!}{0!9!}(.5)^0(.5)^9 = \frac{1}{512} = \frac{.00195}{.0039 = P}$$

Conclusion: Since P < .05, the difference is significant by the sign test.

(b) 95 C.L. on true mean difference = $\bar{d} \pm t_{.05}$ (Est. SE$_{\bar{d}}$):

df = No. of pairs − 1 = 9
$t_{.05, 9df} = 2.26$
SE$_{\bar{d}} = .537$
∴ 95% C.L. = 3.0 ± 2.26 (.537)
= 3.0 ± 1.21
= 1.79   4.21 (mm/hr)
lower   *upper*
limit   *limit*

Note that these limits do not include zero. Therefore, the result agrees with the significance test.

PROBLEM 17-22

It was reported from a village in India that in a certain week 350 out of a total of 976 deaths were due to cholera. If cholera had previously accounted for $\frac{1}{3}$ of the deaths, do the current figures indicate that the proportion of deaths from cholera has changed? Record the approximate P value and state your conclusion.

Answer

Type of data: Qualitative; shows an expected proportion and a sample outcome.

Method: Since (n × p) and (n × q) ≥ 5 for the sample use <u>large sample method</u>, either (a) the Chi Square Goodness of Fit test comparing an observed distribution with an expected distribution, or (b) a test based on the normal curve of sample proportions centered around an expected proportion.

Solution

(a) Chi Square Goodness of Fit test: see Table 17-8.

TABLE 17-8

	Observed Distribution	Expected (Theoretical) Distribution
Dead from cholera	350	1/3 or 325
Dead from other causes	626	2/3 or 651
Total	976	976

$$\chi^2 = \Sigma \frac{(\text{Obs. no.} - \text{Expected no.})^2}{\text{Expected no.}}$$

$$\chi^2 = \frac{(350 - 325)^2}{325} + \frac{(626 - 651)^2}{651}$$

$$= 625\left(\frac{1}{325} + \frac{1}{651}\right) = 2.88$$

df = (r − 1) = 1
Critical $\chi^2_{.05, 1df} = 3.84$
Obs. $\chi^{2*} = 2.88 < 3.84$ ∴ P > .05

Conclusion: H_0 is accepted. The current figures do not indicate that the proportion of deaths from cholera has significantly changed.

(b) Comparison of a sample proportion with an expected proportion using the normal curve:

$$p = .3333$$
$$\hat{p} = \frac{350}{976} = .3586$$

---

* If Yates' correction is used,

$$\chi_c^2 = \Sigma \frac{\left(|O - E| - \frac{1}{2}\right)^2}{E} = 2.80$$

$$SE_{\hat{p}} = \sqrt{\frac{pq}{n}} = \sqrt{\frac{(.33)(.67)}{976}} = .0148$$

$$z = \frac{\hat{p} - p}{SE_{\hat{p}}} = \frac{.3586 - .3333}{.0148} = 1.71$$

Obs. $z = 1.71 < 1.96$ ∴ P > .05

Note: Same conclusion as with method (a) since $\chi^2_{1df} = z^2$. If the continuity correction for z is used, the results would be the same as χ^2·with Yates' correction.

PROBLEM 17-23

(a) An epidemiologist proposes to study the diastolic blood pressure of a certain population. Suppose that he wishes to obtain with 95% confidence an estimate of the population mean that is within 2 mm Hg of the correct value. His best estimate of the standard deviation is that it lies in the range from 7 mm to 10 mm. What advice would you give him regarding the size of the sample he should use?

(b) In another study he wishes to estimate with the same degree of confidence the proportion of children that have been immunized against poliomyelitis. Based upon experience, he believes this proportion to be at least .30. He wishes his sample estimate to be within .05 of the true proportion. What should be the sample size?

Answer

Type of data: (a) Quantitative; gives estimates of the standard deviation σ of a population of individuals, an allowable error δ, and a confidence level.

(b) Qualitative; gives a minimum estimate of the true proportion, an allowable error δ, and a confidence level.

Method: Use the formula for calculating n given the above specifications.

Solution: (a)

$$n = \frac{z^2\sigma^2}{\delta^2}$$

where $z_{.05} \sim 2$, $\sigma = 10$ mm (we use 10 mm rather than 7 mm as an estimate of σ in order to be conservative in our determination of sample size), and δ is 2 mm. Then

$$n = \frac{(2)^2(10)^2}{(2)^2} = 100$$

Conclusion: A sample size of 100 should be used to obtain, with 95% confidence, an esti-

mate of the population mean that is within 2 mm of the correct value.

(b) His knowledge of p is that it is at least .30. It is prudent therefore to use .50 as an estimate of p in our calculations in order to allow for the maximum possible S.E. As noted in Chapter 15, at the 95% confidence level, the formula for the sample size with $p = .5$ reduces simply to

$$n = \frac{1}{\delta^2}$$

Since $\delta = .05$,

$$n = \frac{1}{(.05)^2} = 400$$

Conclusion: A sample size of 400 should be used to obtain with 95% confidence an estimate of the population proportion that is within .05 of the true proportion. (Note that if he sets the permissible error δ at .10 then the sample size need be only 100.)

PROBLEM 17-24

According to current information based on a large series of experiments, $\frac{2}{3}$ of the patients with a certain painful disease are relieved of the pain when they take drug X. A physician uses the drug on 6 subjects.

(a) Find the theoretical distribution of the number of patients who are relieved of the pain.

(b) What is the probability that the number relieved will be smaller than 3?

(c) Since the values of $p = \frac{2}{3}$ and $q = \frac{1}{3}$ are based on a "large series of data" they can be taken as population values and can provide valid answers to the types of questions raised in (a) and (b). Comment on the design of an experiment to determine whether a <u>new</u> drug Y is effective in relieving pain where information is gathered on only 6 subjects.

Answer

Type of data: Qualitative; shows an expected proportion and the size of a sample.

Method: Use the binomial distribution of sample proportions around an expected proportion (applicable to <u>small numbers</u>) since $(n \times p)$ or $(n \times q) < 5$.

Solution

(a) Expand the binomial formula

$$\frac{n!}{r!(n-r)!}\, p^r q^{n-r}$$

where $n = 6$, p (proportion relieved) $= \frac{2}{3}$, q (proportion not relieved) $= \frac{1}{3}$, as r varies from 0 to 6 and $n - r$ varies from 6 to 0.

Let $r = 0$; then

$$P\,(r = 0) = \frac{6!}{0!6!}\left(\frac{2}{3}\right)^0\left(\frac{1}{3}\right)^6 = \frac{1}{729}$$

Similarly

$$P\,(r = 1) = \frac{12}{729}$$

$$P\,(r = 2) = \frac{60}{729}$$

$$P\,(r = 3) = \frac{160}{729}$$

$$P\,(r = 4) = \frac{240}{729}$$

$$P\,(r = 5) = \frac{192}{729}$$

$$P\,(r = 6) = \frac{64}{729}$$

Total $\quad \frac{729}{729} = 1$

(b) The probability that the number who obtain pain relief will be less than 3 is

$$P = P\,(0) + P\,(1) + P\,(2) = \frac{73}{729} = \sim 10\%$$

(c) *Critique.* (1) No provision has been made for placebo controls, which could be important to include if spontaneous relief occurs. If it is known that spontaneous relief ordinarily does not occur, it may still be desirable to include placebo controls just in case we have encountered an unusual situation. However, ethically placebos may not be allowed since we do have available the relatively effective drug X. Drug X controls could help alert us to unusual situations where pain relief rates are unusually high or unusually low, but drug Y results could be compared with historical spontaneous rates of pain relief. If spontaneous relief occurs with some degree of frequency, then a study size involving only 6 patients may be too small.

(2) The purpose of the study must be considered. Are we trying to determine whether drug Y provides any pain relief, or are we trying to establish that it may be superior to drug X? The study size with only 6 patients cannot establish such superiority: Even if relief occurred for <u>all 6 patients</u> on drug Y, such an event would still have a probability of $64/729 = 9\%$, assuming Y were only as good as X (where $p = \frac{2}{3}$).

(3) Other considerations which should be taken into account are: (a) Proper definition of patients to be entered into the study. (b) Proper randomization into treatment groups if more than one group is employed. (c) Study should be double blind so that neither the patient nor the physician (nor the hospital staff) knows to which group the patient has been assigned. (d) Carefully defined end points of pain relief should be established.

PROBLEM 17-25

Red-green color blindness was found in 14 out of a sample of 100 adult males. Test the hypothesis that 10% of males are color-blind. State the significance level you propose to use, and give a non-technical summary of your findings.

Answer

Type of data: Qualitative; presents an expected proportion and a sample outcome.

Method: Since ($n \times p$) and ($n \times q$) > 5 for the sample, use large sample methods, either (a) the Chi Square Goodness of Fit test comparing an observed distribution with an expected distribution, or (b) a test based on the normal curve of sample proportions centered around an expected proportion.

Solution

Choose 5% significance level. Assume the hypothesis that 10% of males are color-blind.

(a) Chi Square Goodness of Fit test: see Table 17-9.

TABLE 17-9

	Observed No.	Expected No.
Color-blind	14	10
Not color-blind	86	90
	100	100

$$\chi^2 = \sum \frac{(\text{Observed} - \text{Expected})^2}{\text{Expected}}$$

$$= \frac{(14-10)^2}{10} + \frac{(86-90)^2}{90} = 1.78$$

df $= (r-1) = 1$

Critical $\chi^2_{.05,1df} = 3.84$

Obs. $\chi^{2*} = 1.78 < 3.84 \quad \therefore P > .05$

Conclusion: Accept H_0. From the information available, one would conclude that the sample proportion does not differ significantly from 10% and therefore that the percent of males in the population who are color-blind may well be 10%.

(b) Normal curve test:

$$p = .10 \qquad q = .90$$
$$\hat{p} = .14 \qquad n = 100$$

$$z = \frac{\hat{p} - p}{\sqrt{\dfrac{pq}{n}}} = \frac{.14 - .10}{\sqrt{\dfrac{(.10)(.90)}{100}}} = \frac{.04}{.03} = 1.33$$

Critical $z_{.05} = 1.96$

Obs. $z = 1.33 < 1.96 \quad \therefore P > .05$

Note: Accept H_0. Same conclusion as with method (a) since $\chi^2_{1df} = z^2$. If the continuity correction for z is used, the results would be the same as χ^2 with Yates' correction.

PROBLEM 17-26

The graph in Fig. 17-2 shows the simultaneous measurement of central venous pressure (CVP) and pulmonary capillary wedge pressure (PCW) on 50 subjects with acute myocardial infarction. The coefficient of correlation (r) is (+0.45). Does knowledge of the CVP aid you in predicting PCW?

Answer

Type of data: Quantitative; presents plots on simultaneous measurements on two variables.

Method: Visually inspect the plots for relation between the two variables. Obtain the coefficient of determination (r^2).

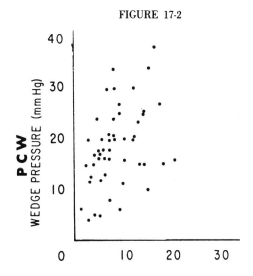

FIGURE 17-2

FIG. 17-2. Adapted from Forrester, J. S., et al., Filling Pressures in the Right and Left Sides of the Heart in Acute Myocardial Infarction: A Reappraisal of Central-Venous-Pressure Monitoring, New Eng. J. Med. 285:191–193, 1971.

Conclusion: The r of (+0.45) is significantly different from zero ($t \sim 3.5$).[1] Therefore we can say that on the average there is a relationship between CVP and PCW. The PCW tends to be low for low CVP's and high for high CVP's. However, the coefficient of determination (r^2) is $(.45)^2 = .2025$; i.e., only 20% of the variance in PCW is explained by the variance in CVP. The prediction of PCW from CVP is only a small improvement over that yielded by assigning each person the overall average PCW value. (Another way of stating this is that the standard deviation of the estimate for PCW values around the regression line ($s_{y \cdot x}$) is 89% of the standard deviation of PCW values around the mean value: $\sqrt{1 - r^2} = 0.89$.)

PROBLEM 17-27

Whiting, R. B., et al., in an article titled "Idiopathic Hypertrophic Subaortic Stenosis in the Elderly," (New Eng. J. Med. 285:196–200, 1971) compare certain parameters of 30 patients 60 years of age and under and 14 pa-

---

* If Yates' correction is used,

$$\chi^2_c = \sum \frac{\left(|O - E| - \dfrac{1}{2}\right)^2}{E} = 1.36$$

---

[1] From the formula

$$t_r = \frac{r}{SE_r} = \frac{r}{\sqrt{\dfrac{1-r^2}{n-2}}} \qquad \text{with } n - 2 \text{ df}$$

tients over 60 years of age with this disorder. The following data are excerpted from their abstract: Older patients had a mean resting left ventricular outflow tract gradient of 53.3 ± 8.8 mm (mean $\pm$ S.E.M.[1]) of mercury, and younger patients a mean resting gradient of 32.2 ± 5.2 mm (mean $\pm$ S.E.M.) of mercury (P less than 0.05).

From the information presented, how would you verify the P value?

Answer

Type of data: Quantitative; gives the parameters (mean and Standard Error of the Mean) of each of two independent samples.

Method: Compute the 95% Confidence Limits on each true mean. If these limits do not overlap, one can be certain that a *t*-test on the difference between means would be significant. If they do overlap, then it is necessary to carry out a *t*-test.

Solution

(1) 95% C.L. on true mean

$$= \bar{x} \pm t_{.05, n-1df} \ (\text{Est. SE}_{\bar{x}})$$

For Sample 1 (patients 60 years of age and under):

$\bar{x}_1 = 32.2$ mm, Est. $SE_{\bar{x}_1} = 5.2$ mm, $n_1 = 30$, $df_1 = 29$

$\therefore$ 95% C.L. $= 32.2 \pm 2.04 \ (5.2)$
$= 21.6$ mm   42.8 mm Hg
   lower   *upper*
   limit   *limit*

For Sample 2 (patients over 60 years of age):

$\bar{x}_2 = 53.3$ mm, Est. $SE\bar{x}_2 = 8.8$ mm, $n_2 = 14$, $df_2 = 13$

$\therefore$ 95% C.L. $= 53.3 \pm 2.16 \ (8.8)$
$= 34.3$ mm   72.3 mm Hg
     lower   *upper*
     limit   *limit*

The confidence intervals on the true mean do overlap (see Fig. 17-3). Therefore we must determine the S.E. of the Difference ($SE_{\bar{x}_1 - \bar{x}_2}$) and do a *t*-test. We could also determine the 95% confidence limits on the true difference.

(2) *t*-test: Since $n_1 \neq n_2$ it is necessary to work backwards to derive the individual sample variances. We then compute a pooled or weighted sample variance to obtain the $SE_{\bar{x}_1 - \bar{x}_2}$.

(a)   <u>Patients 60 yrs and under</u>

$$\bar{x}_1 = 32.2 \text{ mm Hg}$$

$$\text{Est. SE}_{\bar{x}_1} = \frac{s_1}{\sqrt{n_1}}$$

$$5.2 = \frac{s_1}{\sqrt{30}}$$

$$5.2\sqrt{30} = s_1 \sim 28.5$$
$$811 = s_1^2$$

<u>Patients over 60 yrs</u>

$$\bar{x}_2 = 53.3 \text{ mm Hg}$$

$$\text{Est. SE}_{\bar{x}_2} = \frac{s_2}{\sqrt{n_2}}$$

$$8.8 = \frac{s_2}{\sqrt{14}}$$

$$8.8\sqrt{14} = s_2 \sim 33$$
$$1084 = s_2^2$$

(b) Next, we compute a pooled or weighted average variance where $(n_1 - 1)$ and $(n_2 - 1)$ or (df_1 and df_2) are the weights:

$$s_p^2 = \frac{(n_1 - 1)s_1^2 + (n_2 - 1)s_2^2}{(n_1 - 1) + (n_2 - 1)}$$
$$= \frac{(29)(811) + (13)(1084)}{(29) + (13)} = 895.5$$

Note that this value is intermediate between s_1^2 and s_2^2 since it is a weighted average.

(c) Using s_p^2 we compute the S.E. of the difference between the two means:

$$\text{Est. SE}_{\bar{x}_1 - \bar{x}_2} = \sqrt{\frac{s_p^2}{n_1} + \frac{s_p^2}{n_2}}$$

$$= \sqrt{\frac{895.5}{30} + \frac{895.5}{14}} = 9.6 \text{ mm Hg}$$

FIGURE 17-3

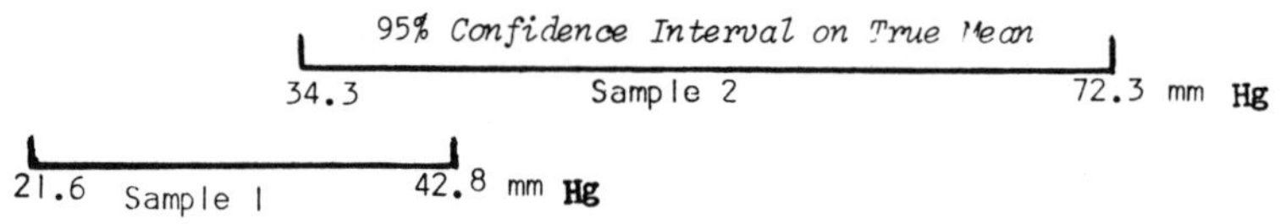

95% Confidence Interval on True Mean

34.3   Sample 2   72.3 mm Hg

21.6   Sample 1   42.8 mm Hg

---

[1] Standard Error of the Mean, same as $SE_{\bar{x}}$.

FIGURE 17-4

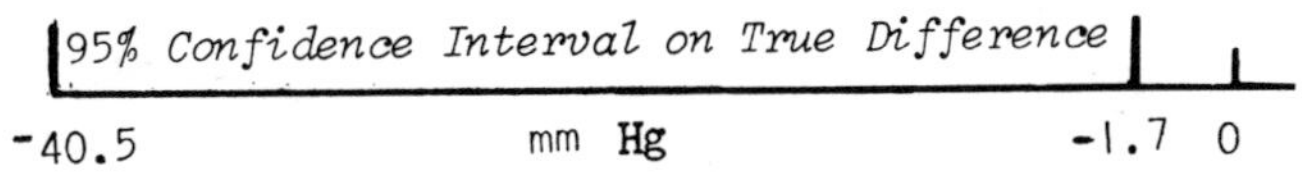

| 95% Confidence Interval on True Difference |

-40.5   mm Hg   -1.7 0

Note that the S.E. of the <u>difference</u> is <u>greater</u> than either S.E. of the <u>mean</u> since sampling errors of <u>two</u> independent means are involved.

(d) We can now compute the t ratio:

$$\text{Obs. } t = \frac{(x_1 - x_2) - 0}{\text{Est. SE}_{\bar{x}_1 - \bar{x}_2}} = \frac{32.2 - 53.3}{9.6}$$
$$= |2.2| > 2.02 \text{ (critical } t_{.05} \text{ for 42 df)}$$
$$\therefore P < .05$$

Conclusion: Reject H_0. Difference is significant.

(3) We can also compute the 95% C.I. on the true difference to see if it includes 0.

$$95\% \text{ C.L.} = (\bar{x}_1 - \bar{x}_2) \pm t_{.05} \text{ (Est. SE}_{\bar{x}_1 - \bar{x}_2})$$
$$= -21.1 \pm 2.02 \text{ (9.6)}$$
$$= -40.5 \text{ mm}, -1.7 \text{ mm Hg}$$

The 95% C.I. does not include 0 (see Fig. 17-4). The difference is significant.

Note that, while the observed difference of −21.1 mm Hg is significant at the 5% level, the limits on the true difference vary from −40.5 mm (which would be an extremely important difference) to only −1.7 mm (which would suggest the age effect to only a minor degree).

The high variability[1] between patients in their measurements might suggest that the study was too small. That is, to compensate for such "inherent" variability, larger samples are needed in order to reduce the S.E. Alternatively, it is noted in the article that the group 60 years of age and under covered individuals as young as 16 with equal numbers of males and females. Therefore, the high variability for this age group may reflect only gross heterogeneity; for a fixed age and sex, variability may be only moderate. (The patients over 60 ranged in age from 61–76, with females predominating.) A different analysis might have been sought based on a more refined age categorization and taking sex into account.

---

[1] Coefficients of Variation for the two groups are:

	60 yrs and under	Over 60 yrs
C.V. in % $= \frac{s}{\bar{x}} \times 100$	$\frac{28.5}{32.2} = 89\%$	$\frac{33}{53.3} = 62\%$

PROBLEM 17-28

In a certain experiment, serum chloride levels were recorded to the <u>nearest</u> milliequivalent of chloride per liter (meq/liter) of serum for 100 mice. The data were grouped as follows:

Serum chloride levels, in meq/liter of serum	No.
120–121	4
122–123	8
124–125	23
126–127	35
128–129	18
130–131	7
132–133	5
	100

(a) Draw a cumulative percentage distribution.
(b) Calculate Q_1, Q_2, Q_3.
(c) Estimate the standard deviation from the plot.

Answer

Type of data: Quantitative; presents a frequency distribution of grouped data.

Solution

(a)

Serum chloride levels, in meq/liter of serum (end points of class intervals)	Cumulative (% less than given value)
121.5	4
123.5	12
125.5	35
127.5	70
129.5	88
131.5	95
133.5	100

(b) $Q_1 = 123.5 + \dfrac{25\% - 12\%}{35\% - 12\%} (2) = 124.630$

$Q_2 = 125.5 + \dfrac{50\% - 35\%}{70\% - 35\%} (2) = 126.357$

$Q_3 = 127.5 + \dfrac{75\% - 70\%}{88\% - 70\%} (2) = 128.056$

FIGURE 17-5

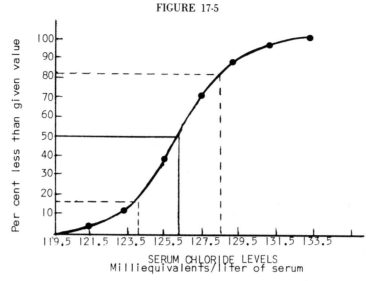

(c) From Fig. 17-5:
At 16%, serum level = 123.9.
At 50%, serum level = 126.2.
At 84%, serum level = 128.4.

$$126.2 - 123.9 = 2.3$$
$$128.4 - 126.2 = 2.2$$
$$\text{Est. } s = \frac{2.3 + 2.2}{2} = 2.25 \text{ meq/liter of serum}$$

PROBLEM 17-29

Rats in which anemia had been produced by restriction to a milk diet were subsequently treated by the administration of iron. Hemoglobin levels before and after treatment are shown in Table 17-10.

TABLE 17-10

| Rat No. | Hemoglobin (gm/100 ml blood) | |
	Before Treatment	After Treatment
1	3.4	4.9
2	3.0	2.3
3	3.0	3.1
4	3.4	2.1
5	3.7	2.6
6	4.0	3.8
7	2.9	5.8
8	2.9	7.9
9	3.1	3.6
10	2.8	4.1
11	2.8	3.8
12	2.4	3.3

(a) Test the hypothesis that the mean of the pair differences is zero. State the significance level you propose to use, accept or reject the Null Hypothesis, and interpret your findings.

(b) Find the 95% confidence limits on the true mean pair difference.

Answer

Type of data: Quantitative; presents a series of two readings (before and after) on 12 individuals.

Method: (1) Use the modified t-test for paired data, based on the distribution of mean pair differences around a true difference of 0 (i.e., where the two samples are not independent of each other), or (2) use the non-parametric sign test.

Solution

(a) (1) For the paired t-test, assume H_0, that the mean of the pair differences is zero. Set $P = .05$. (See Table 17-11.)

TABLE 17-11

| Rat No. | (gm/100 ml) | | |
	$d = (\text{After} - \text{Before})$	$(d - \bar{d})$	$(d - \bar{d})^2$
1	+1.5	+0.675	.4556
2	−0.7	−1.525	2.3256
3	+0.1	−0.725	.5256
4	−1.3	−2.125	4.5156
5	−1.1	−1.925	3.7056
6	−0.2	−1.025	1.0506
7	+2.9	+2.075	4.3056
8	+5.0	+4.175	17.4306
9	+0.5	−0.325	.1056
10	+1.3	+0.475	.2256
11	+1.0	+0.175	.0306
12	+0.9	+0.075	.0056
	+9.9	0	34.6822

$$\bar{d} = \frac{\Sigma d}{\text{No. of pairs}} = \frac{9.9}{12} = .825$$

$$s_{\bar{d}}^2 = \frac{\Sigma(d - \bar{d})^2}{\text{No. of pairs} - 1} = \frac{34.68}{11} = 3.15$$

$$t = \frac{\bar{d} - 0}{\text{Est. SE}_{\bar{d}}} = \frac{\bar{d} - 0}{\sqrt{\dfrac{s_{\bar{d}}^2}{\text{No. of pairs}}}}$$

$$= \frac{.825 - 0}{\sqrt{\dfrac{3.15}{12}}} = \frac{.825}{.513} = 1.61$$

Degrees of freedom = No. of pairs $- 1 = 11$
Critical $t_{.05,11df} = 2.20$
Obs. $t = 1.61 < 2.20$ $\therefore$ P $> .05$

Conclusion: Accept H_0 and conclude that the mean of the pair differences could well be zero, i.e., that there is no significant difference between the Before and After treatment groups based on the available data.

(2) For the sign test, 8 of the After Treatment measurements are higher than the Before Treatment; therefore we record $8 +$ signs and $4 -$ signs. By use of the binomial formula, where $n = 12$, $p = 0.5$, and $q = 0.5$, we can calculate the probability of 8 or more $+$ signs. This is a symmetrical distribution; therefore, we can double this value to obtain the area for both tails, since this is a two-tailed test.

However, since there are a large number of pairs, and

$$(n \times p) = (12 \times .5) = 6 > 5$$

we can use the normal approximation to the binomial:

$$z = \frac{\hat{p} - p}{\sqrt{\dfrac{pq}{n}}}$$

$$= \frac{\dfrac{8}{12} \text{ (or .67)} - .5}{\sqrt{\dfrac{(.5)(.5)}{12}}} = 1.17, \text{ P} > .05$$

Conclusion: Since P $> .05$, the difference is not significant by the sign test (or its equivalent). Where the data are normally distributed, for a test on the difference between means the sign test is less powerful than the paired *t*-test because it does not take into account the magnitude of the differences but only their direction. Therefore, a difference may be found insignificant with the sign test but significant with the *t*-test. Therefore, if the sign test had been done initially, it would be desirable to now do a paired *t*-test. As is

indicated by (1) above, however, the paired *t*-test also is not significant.

(b) 95% C.L. on true mean difference:

$$95\% \text{ C.L.} = .825 \pm t_{.05,11df} \text{ (Est. SE}_{\bar{d}})$$
$$= .825 \pm 2.20 \, (.513)$$
$$= .825 \pm 1.130$$
$$= \underset{\substack{\text{lower} \\ \text{limit}}}{-.305} \qquad \underset{\substack{\text{upper} \\ \text{limit}}}{1.955} \text{ (gm/100 ml)}$$

Note that the Confidence Limits include 0, which agrees with the significance test.

PROBLEM 17-30

FAILURE TO TRANSFORM SKEWED DATA[1]

Following are the daily fecal blood losses from 27 patients treated with a drug:

Ml.	No. of patients
0.1	1
0.2	4
0.3	2
0.4	2
0.5	4
0.6	4
0.7	2
0.8	1
0.9	1
1.0	1
1.3	1
1.7	1
2.0	1
2.4	1
4.1	1

$$\bar{x} = 0.83$$
$$\text{S.D.} = 0.86$$
$$95\% \text{ spread} = 0.83 \pm 2(0.86)$$
$$= -0.9, \, 2.6 \text{ ml}$$

The lower limit is estimated as a negative quantity, which is not possible. The data are markedly skewed to the right and a logarithmic transformation would seem to be indicated. Let

$$x^* = \log x$$

This gives

$$\bar{x}^* = -0.242 \text{ (in logs)}$$
$$\text{S.D.} = 0.3735$$
$$95\% \text{ spread} = -0.242 \pm 2(0.3735)$$
$$= -0.989, \, 0.505$$

---

[1] Problem provided by J. Ciminera.

Taking antilogarithms, we have

Geometric mean x = 0.57
95% spread = 0.1, 3.2 ml

Thus, transformation has yielded more "reasonable" summary measures.

PROBLEM 17-31

FAILURE TO TAKE PAIRING INTO ACCOUNT[1]

Following are the results from skin testing 282 patients with two types of penicillin placed on the 2 arms of each patient by random allocation (see Table 17-12).

TABLE 17-12

Type of Penicillin	Positive Skin Reaction	Negative Skin Reaction	Totals
G	28	254	282
BT	21	261	282
Totals	49	515	564

When tested by the chi square test corrected for continuity but not taking into account the fact that the same patients were used with both types of penicillin, we obtain for 1 df:

$$\chi_c^2 = 0.80 < \chi_{.05}^2 = 3.84$$

Since χ_c^2 is less than the critical value, no statistically significant difference is observed.

However, the table does not give the complete classification reflecting the pairing in the subjects. A more complete classification (still incomplete since right and left arms are not differentiated) and analysis is shown in Table 17-13 and Table 17-14.

TABLE 17-13

Type of Response	Type G	Type BT	No. of Patients
A	Reaction	Reaction	20
B	Reaction	No Reaction	8
C	No Reaction	Reaction	1
D	No Reaction	No Reaction	253

TABLE 17-14

		Type BT		
		Reaction	No Reaction	Totals
Type G	Reaction	A = 20	B = 8	28
	No reaction	C = 1	D = 253	254
	Totals	21	261	282

McNemar's test:

$$\chi_c^2 = \frac{(|B - C| - 1)^2}{B + C} = \frac{(|8 - 1| - 1)^2}{8 + 1} = \frac{36}{9}$$
$$= 4.0 > \chi_{.05}^2 = 3.84$$

Since χ_c^2 is larger than the critical value, a statistically significant difference is observed.

[1] Problem provided by J. Ciminera.

Appendix

TABLE A. *Random Numbers*

22 17 68 05 84	68 95 23 92 35	87 02 22 57 51	61 09 43 95 06	58 24 82 03 47	10 27 53 96 23
19 36 27 59 46	13 79 93 37 55	39 77 32 77 09	85 52 05 30 62	47 83 51 62 74	28 41 50 61 88
16 77 23 02 77	09 61 87 25 21	28 06 24 25 93	16 71 13 59 78	23 05 47 47 25	34 21 42 57 02
78 43 76 71 61	20 44 90 32 64	97 67 63 99 61	46 38 03 93 22	69 81 21 99 21	61 81 77 23 23
03 28 28 26 08	73 37 32 04 05	69 30 16 09 05	88 69 58 28 99	35 07 44 75 47	61 15 18 13 54
93 22 53 64 39	07 10 63 76 35	87 03 04 79 88	08 13 13 85 51	55 34 57 72 69	91 76 21 64 64
78 76 58 54 74	92 38 70 96 92	52 06 79 79 45	82 63 18 27 44	69 66 92 19 09	00 97 79 08 06
23 68 35 26 00	99 53 93 61 28	52 70 05 48 34	56 65 05 61 86	90 92 10 70 80	36 46 18 34 94
15 39 25 70 99	93 86 52 77 65	15 33 59 05 28	22 87 26 07 47	86 96 98 29 06	88 98 99 60 50
58 71 96 30 24	18 46 23 34 27	85 13 99 24 44	49 18 09 79 49	74 16 32 23 02	04 37 59 87 21
57 35 27 33 72	24 53 63 94 09	41 10 76 47 91	44 04 95 49 66	39 60 04 59 81	63 62 06 34 41
48 50 86 54 48	22 06 34 72 52	82 21 15 65 20	33 29 94 71 11	15 91 29 12 03	78 47 23 53 90
61 96 48 95 03	07 16 39 33 66	98 56 10 56 79	77 21 30 27 12	90 49 22 23 62	87 68 62 15 43
36 93 89 41 26	29 70 83 63 51	99 74 20 52 36	87 09 41 15 09	98 60 16 03 03	47 60 92 10 77
18 87 00 42 31	57 90 12 02 07	23 47 37 17 31	54 08 01 88 63	39 41 88 92 10	56 88 87 59 41
88 56 53 27 59	33 35 72 67 47	77 34 55 45 70	08 18 27 38 90	16 95 86 70 75	02 57 45 86 67
09 72 95 84 29	49 41 31 06 70	42 38 06 45 18	64 84 73 31 65	52 53 37 97 15	31 54 14 13 17
12 96 88 17 31	65 19 69 02 83	60 75 86 90 68	24 64 19 35 51	56 61 87 39 12	28 50 16 43 36
85 94 57 24 16	92 09 84 38 76	22 00 27 69 85	29 81 94 78 70	21 94 47 90 12	63 29 62 66 50
38 64 43 59 98	98 77 87 68 07	91 51 67 62 44	40 98 05 93 78	23 32 65 41 18	45 65 58 26 51
53 44 09 42 72	00 41 86 79 79	68 47 22 00 20	35 55 31 51 51	00 83 63 22 55	39 65 36 63 70
40 76 66 26 84	57 99 99 90 37	36 63 32 08 58	37 40 13 68 97	87 64 81 07 83	73 71 98 16 04
02 17 79 18 05	12 59 52 57 02	22 07 90 47 03	28 14 11 30 79	20 69 22 40 98	72 20 56 20 11
95 17 82 06 53	31 51 10 96 46	92 06 88 07 77	56 11 50 81 69	40 23 72 51 39	75 17 26 99 76
35 76 22 42 92	96 11 83 44 80	34 68 35 48 77	33 42 40 90 60	73 96 53 97 86	37 48 60 82 29
26 29 13 56 41	85 47 04 66 08	34 72 57 59 13	82 43 80 46 15	38 26 61 70 04	68 08 02 80 72
77 80 20 75 82	72 82 32 99 90	63 95 73 76 63	89 73 44 99 05	48 67 26 43 18	14 23 98 61 67
46 40 66 44 52	91 36 74 43 53	30 82 13 54 00	78 45 63 98 35	55 03 36 67 68	49 08 96 21 44
37 56 08 18 09	77 53 84 46 47	31 91 18 95 58	24 16 74 11 53	44 10 13 85 57	78 37 06 08 43
61 65 61 68 66	37 27 47 39 19	84 83 70 07 48	53 21 40 06 71	95 06 79 88 54	37 21 34 17 68

Source: Abridged from Table XXXIII, Fisher, R. A., and Yates, F., *Statistical Tables for Biological, Agricultural and Medical Research*, ed. 6, Edinburgh and London, Oliver and Boyd Ltd., 1963, by permission of the authors and publisher.

TABLE B. *Areas of the Standard Normal Curve* (z)

z	I — P	P	z	I — P	P	z	I — P	P	z	I -- P	P
0.0	0.0000	1.0000	1.0	0.6827	.3173	2.0	0.9545	.0455	3.0	0.9973	.0027
0.1	.0797	.9203	1.1	.7287	.2713	2.1	.9643	.0357	3.1	.9981	.0019
0.2	.1585	.8415	1.2	.7699	.2301	2.2	.9722	.0278	3.2	.9986	.0014
0.3	.2358	.7642	1.3	.8064	.1936	2.3	.9786	.0214	3.3	.9990	.0010
0.4	.3108	.6892	1.4	.8385	.1615	2.4	.9836	.0164	3.4	.9993	.0007
0.5	0.3829	.6771	1.5	0.8664	.1336	2.5	0.9876	.0124	3.5	0.9995	.0005
0.6	.4515	.5485	1.6	.8904	.1096	2.58	.9901	.0099	3.6	.9997	.0003
0.7	.5161	.4839	1.64	.9000	.1000	2.6	.9907	.0093	3.7	.9998	.0002
0.8	.5763	.4237	1.7	.9109	.0891	2.7	.9931	.0069	3.8	.9999	.0001
0.9	.6319	.3681	1.8	.9281	.0719	2.8	.9949	.0051	3.9	.9999	.0001
			1.9	.9426	.0594	2.9	.9963	.0037			
			1.96	.9500	.0500						

P = two-tailed area of the Normal Cuve or area beyond ± z.

P/2 = one-tailed area of the Normal Curve.

See Table 4-1 for more complete explanation.

TABLE C. *Distribution of Chi-Square (χ^2)*

Degrees of Freedom df	Probability of a Greater Value (P)				
	0.100	0.050	0.025	0.010	0.005
1	2.71	3.84	5.02	6.63	7.88
2	4.61	5.99	7.38	9.21	10.60
3	6.25	7.81	9.35	11.34	12.84
4	7.78	9.49	11.14	13.28	14.86
5	9.24	11.07	12.83	15.09	16.75
6	10.64	12.59	‖14.45	16.81	18.55
7	12.02	14.07	16.01	18.48	20.28
8	13.36	15.51	17.53	20.09	21.96
9	14.68	16.92	19.02	21.67	23.59
10	15.99	18.31	20.48	23.21	25.19
11	17.28	19.68	21.92	24.72	26.76
12	18.55	21.03	23.34	26.22	28.30
13	19.81	22.36	24.74	27.69	29.82
14	21.06	23.68	26.12	29.14	31.32
15	22.31	25.00	27.49	30.58	32.80
16	23.54	26.30	28.85	32.00	34.27
17	24.77	27.59	30.19	33.41	35.72
18	25.99	28.87	31.53	34.81	37.16
19	27.20	30.14	32.85	36.19	38.58
20	28.41	31.41	34.17	37.57	40.00
21	29.62	32.67	35.48	38.93	41.40
22	30.81	33.92	36.78	40.29	42.80
23	32.01	35.17	38.08	41.64	44.18
24	33.20	36.42	39.36	42.98	45.56
25	34.38	37.65	40.65	44.31	46.93
26	35.56	38.89	41.92	45.64	48.29
27	36.74	40.11	43.19	46.96	49.64
28	37.92	41.34	44.46	48.28	50.99
29	39.09	42.56	45.72	49.59	52.34
30	40.26	43.77	46.98	50.89	53.67
40	51.80	55.76	59.34	63.69	66.77
50	63.17	67.50	71.42	76.15	79.49
60	74.40	79.08	83.30	88.38	91.95
70	85.53	90.53	95.02	00.42	104.22
80	96.58	101.88	106.63	12.33	116.32
90	107.56	113.14	118.14	24.12	128.30
100	118.50	124.34	129.56	35.81	140.17

Source: Condensed from table with six significant figures by Catherine M. Thompson, by permission of the Editor of *Biometrika;* from *Tables for Statisticians*, Vol. 1, ed. 3, 1966.

TABLE D. *Distribution of t*

Level of significance for one-tailed test

Degrees of Freedom df	0.10	0.05	0.025	0.01	0.005	0.0005
	Level of significance for two-tailed test					
	0.20	0.10	0.05	0.02	0.01	0.001
1	3.078	6.314	12.706	31.821	63.657	636.619
2	1.886	2.920	4.303	6.965	9.925	31.598
3	1.638	2.353	3.182	4.541	5.841	12.941
4	1.533	2.132	2.776	3.747	4.604	8.610
5	1.476	2.015	2.571	3.365	4.032	6.859
6	1.440	1.943	2.447	3.143	3.707	5.959
7	1.415	1.895	2.365	2.998	3.499	5.405
8	1.397	1.860	2.306	2.896	3.355	5.041
9	1.383	1.833	2.262	2.821	3.250	4.781
10	1.372	1.812	2.228	2.764	3.169	4.587
11	1.363	1.796	2.201	2.718	3.106	4.437
12	1.356	1.782	2.179	2.681	3.055	4.318
13	1.350	1.771	2.160	2.650	3.012	4.221
14	1.345	1.761	2.145	2.624	2.977	4.140
15	1.341	1.753	2.131	2.602	2.947	4.073
16	1.337	1.746	2.120	2.583	2.921	4.015
17	1.333	1.740	2.110	2.567	2.898	3.965
18	1.330	1.734	2.101	2.552	2.878	3.922
19	1.328	1.729	2.093	2.539	2.861	3.883
20	1.325	1.725	2.086	2.528	2.845	3.850
21	1.323	1.721	2.080	2.518	2.831	3.819
22	1.321	1.717	2.074	2.508	2.819	3.792
23	1.319	1.714	2.069	2.500	2.807	3.767
24	1.318	1.711	2.064	2.492	2.797	3.745
25	1.316	1.708	2.060	2.485	2.787	3.725
26	1.315	1.706	2.056	2.479	2.779	3.707
27	1.314	1.703	2.052	2.473	2.771	3.690
28	1.313	1.701	2.048	2.467	2.763	3.674
29	1.311	1.699	2.045	2.462	2.756	3.659
30	1.310	1.697	2.042	2.457	2.750	3.646
40	1.303	1.684	2.021	2.423	2.704	3.551
60	1.296	1.671	2.000	2.390	2.660	3.460
120	1.289	1.658	1.980	2.358	2.617	3.373
∞	1.282	1.645	1.960	2.326	2.576	3.291

Source: Abridged from Table III of Fisher, R. A., and Yates, F., *Statistical Tables for Biological. Agricultural and Medical Research*, ed. 6, Edinburgh and London, Oliver and Boyd Ltd., 1963, by permission of the authors and publisher.

Originally called "Student's" t.

TABLE E. *Table of Squares, Square Roots, and Reciprocals*

n	n²	√n	√10n	1/n	n	n²	√n	√10n	1/n
1	1	1.000	3.162	1.00000	51	2601	7.141	22.583	.01961
2	4	1.414	4.472	.50000	52	2704	7.211	22.804	.01923
3	9	1.732	5.477	.33333	53	2809	7.280	23.022	.01887
4	16	2.000	6.325	.25000	54	2916	7.348	23.238	.01852
5	25	2.236	7.071	.20000	55	3025	7.416	23.452	.01818
6	36	2.449	7.746	.16667	56	3136	7.483	23.664	.01786
7	49	2.646	8.367	.14286	57	3249	7.550	23.875	.01754
8	64	2.828	8.944	.12500	58	3364	7.616	24.083	.01724
9	81	3.000	9.487	.11111	59	3481	7.681	24.290	.01695
10	100	3.162	10.000	.10000	60	3600	7.746	24.495	.01667
11	121	3.317	10.488	.09091	61	3721	7.810	24.698	.01639
12	144	3.464	10.954	.08333	62	3844	7.874	24.900	.01613
13	169	3.606	11.402	.07692	63	3969	7.937	25.100	.01587
14	196	3.742	11.832	.07143	64	4096	8.000	25.298	.01562
15	225	3.873	12.247	.06667	65	4225	8.062	25.495	.01538
16	256	4.000	12.649	.06250	66	4356	8.124	25.690	.01515
17	289	4.123	13.038	.05882	67	4489	8.185	25.884	.01493
18	324	4.243	13.416	.05556	68	4624	8.246	26.077	.01471
19	361	4.359	13.784	.05263	69	4761	8.307	26.268	.01449
20	400	4.472	14.142	.05000	70	4900	8.367	26.458	.01429
21	441	4.583	14.491	.04762	71	5041	8.426	26.646	.01408
22	484	4.690	14.832	.04545	72	5184	8.485	26.833	.01389
23	529	4.796	15.166	.04348	73	5329	8.544	27.019	.01370
24	576	4.899	15.492	.04167	74	5476	8.602	27.203	.01351
25	625	5.000	15.811	.04000	75	5625	8.660	27.386	.01333
26	676	5.099	16.125	.03846	76	5776	8.718	27.568	.01316
27	729	5.196	16.432	.03704	77	5929	8.775	27.749	.01299
28	784	5.292	16.733	.03571	78	6084	8.832	27.928	.01282
29	841	5.385	17.029	.03448	79	6241	8.888	28.107	.01266
30	900	5.477	17.321	.03333	80	6400	8.944	28.284	.01250
31	961	5.568	17.607	.03226	81	6561	9.000	28.460	.01235
32	1024	5.657	17.889	.03125	82	6724	9.055	28.636	.01220
33	1089	5.745	18.166	.03030	83	6889	9.110	28.810	.01205
34	1156	5.831	18.439	.02941	84	7056	9.165	28.983	.01190
35	1225	5.916	18.708	.02857	85	7225	9.220	29.155	.01176
36	1296	6.000	18.974	.02778	86	7396	9.274	29.326	.01163
37	1369	6.083	19.235	.02703	87	7569	9.327	29.496	.01149
38	1444	6.164	19.494	.02632	88	7744	9.381	29.665	.01136
39	1521	6.245	19.748	.02564	89	7921	9.434	29.833	.01124
40	1600	6.325	20.000	.02500	90	8100	9.487	30.000	.01111
41	1681	6.403	20.248	.02439	91	8281	9.539	30.166	.01099
42	1764	6.481	20.494	.02381	92	8464	9.592	30.332	.01087
43	1849	6.557	20.736	.02326	93	8649	9.644	30.496	.01075
44	1936	6.633	20.976	.02273	94	8836	9.695	30.659	.01064
45	2025	6.708	21.213	.02222	95	9025	9.747	30.822	.01053
46	2116	6.782	21.448	.02174	96	9216	9.798	30.984	.01042
47	2209	6.856	21.679	.02128	97	9409	9.849	31.145	.01031
48	2304	6.928	21.909	.02083	98	9604	9.899	31.305	.01020
49	2401	7.000	22.136	.02041	99	9801	9.950	31.464	.01010
50	2500	7.071	22.361	.02000	100	10000	10.000	31.623	.01000

Indexes

Index to Definitions
of Symbols* and Abbreviations

---

*For algebraic symbols, see pages 25 and 73.

Subject Index*

---

*Includes references to selected examples and graphs. Page references to glossaries or definitions are in italics.